ADVANCED PRAISE FOR

BEYOND PTSD

"This is a first-class compilation of accessible, compassionate, and expert guidance on understanding and supporting traumatized young people and their families. *Beyond PTSD* provides a superb foundational understanding of the impact of trauma on adolescent development, with detailed chapters addressing common specific challenging behaviors in traumatized youth and explicit strategies for the systems and settings these youth occupy to better help them. The rolling case-based approach in each chapter skillfully lays out the practical approaches to helping these young people overcome their challenges, making this work useful to a broad range of stakeholders, including clinicians, educational, child welfare and juvenile justice workers, and families."

> **Jennifer F. Havens, M.D.,** Professor and Vice Chair, Department of Child and Adolescent Psychiatry, NYU Langone Medical Center

"Using case studies to illustrate key concepts and valuable takeaways, Gerson, Heppell, and colleagues have provided us with an invaluable resource that greatly enhances our understanding of adolescent trauma and its impact and treatment. This highly accessible volume by some of America's most experienced trauma treatment providers will undoubtedly become a go-to referral for clinicians, parents, and teachers alike for years to come."

> **Jess P. Shatkin, M.D., M.P.H.,** Professor of Child and Adolescent Psychiatry and Pediatrics, NYU School of Medicine, and author of *Born to Be Wild: Why Teens Take Risks, and How We Can Help Keep Them Safe*

"Over the past 20 years there has been a rapidly growing body of research and increasing public and professional awareness of the critical role that traumatic life experiences, especially those during childhood, play in subsequent illness and behavioral problems. This book edited by Gerson and Heppell provides a comprehensive overview of this accumulating knowledge and how to integrate this new knowledge into care for children and adolescents presenting with serious mental health crises. By listening and addressing the stressors and life circumstances driving these psychological crises, health care professionals can begin to treat sources of pain rather than just focusing on symptoms. This trauma-informed approach leads more often to healing than to the revolving door of psychiatric crises and symptom-focused short-term interventions."

David L. Corwin, M.D., Professor and Director of Forensic Services, Pediatrics Department, University of Utah School of Medicine; President, American Professional Society on the Abuse of Children; Immediate Past Board Chair of the Academy on Violence and Abuse

BEYOND PTSD

Helping and Healing
Teens Exposed to Trauma

BEYOND PTSD

Helping and Healing Teens Exposed to Trauma

Edited by

Ruth Gerson, M.D.

Patrick Heppell, Psy.D.

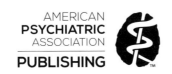

AMERICAN
PSYCHIATRIC
ASSOCIATION
PUBLISHING

If you wish to buy 50 or more copies of the same title, please go to www.appi.org/specialdiscounts for more information.

Copyright © 2019 American Psychiatric Association Publishing

ALL RIGHTS RESERVED

First Edition

Manufactured in the United States of America on acid-free paper
22 21 20 19 18   5 4 3 2 1

American Psychiatric Association Publishing
800 Maine Avenue SW
Suite 900
Washington, DC 20024-2812
www.appi.org

Library of Congress Cataloging-in-Publication Data
Names: Gerson, Ruth, editor. | Heppell, Patrick, editor. | American Psychiatric Association Publishing, publisher.
Title: Beyond PTSD : helping and healing teens exposed to trauma / edited by Ruth Gerson, Patrick Heppell.
Description: First edition. | Washington, DC : American Psychiatric Association Publishing, [2019] | Includes bibliographical references and index.
Identifiers: LCCN 2018034928 (print) | LCCN 2018036187 (ebook) | ISBN 9781615372171 (ebook) | ISBN 9781615371105 (pbk. : alk. paper)
Subjects: | MESH: Stress Disorders, Traumatic | Psychological Trauma— therapy | Psychology, Adolescent | Dangerous Behavior | Psychosocial Support Systems | Child Welfare
Classification: LCC RJ506.P55 (ebook) | LCC RJ506.P55 (print) | NLM WM 172.5 | DDC 616.85/2100835—dc23
LC record available at https://lccn.loc.gov/2018034928

British Library Cataloguing in Publication Data
A CIP record is available from the British Library.

With this book we honor those who have taught us so much, especially Myer, Alexandre, Maggie, Ellie, Ayla, Callen, Vikram, Sanjay, Rohan, Will, Meg, Aviva, Luis, Leila, Tiffani, Jeff, Tania, Itzel, Lorenzo, Eleni, Mia, Jane, Mary, Brad, Blakely, Neko, Sunhi, Max, Louise, Chloe, Audrey, and all of the children and families we've had the privilege to work with.

Dedicated to the beloved memory of Dr. Fadi Haddad, who taught many of us, and countless others, how to listen and how to love.

Traumatic events of the earliest years of infancy and childhood are not lost but, like a child's footprints in wet cement, are often preserved life-long. Time does not heal the wounds that occur in those earliest years; time conceals them. They are not lost; they are embodied.

Vincent J. Felitti (2010)

Contents

PART 2

Working With Systems and Traumatic Stress

Contributors

Komal Bhasin
Building Principal, Leonard School, Lawrence Public Schools, Lawrence, Massachusetts

Jennifer Cabrera, M.D.
Clinical Assistant Professor, Department of Child and Adolescent Psychiatry, New York University School of Medicine, New York, New York

Gabrielle Carson, Ph.D.
Clinical Psychologist and Clinical Instructor, Department of Child and Adolescent Psychiatry, New York University School of Medicine, New York, New York

Sin Chu, M.D.
Resident (PGY-3), Department of Psychiatry, Michigan State University, East Lansing, Michigan

Sophie de Figueiredo, Psy.D.
Licensed Clinical Psychologist, Division of Adolescent and Young Adult Medicine, Children's Hospital Los Angeles, Los Angeles, California

Ruth Gerson, M.D.
Assistant Professor, Department of Child and Adolescent Psychiatry, New York University School of Medicine, New York, New York

Fadi Haddad, M.D.
Clinical Assistant Professor, Department of Child and Adolescent Psychiatry, New York University School of Medicine, New York, New York

Schuyler W. Henderson, M.D., M.P.H.
Associate Professor, Department of Child and Adolescent Psychiatry, New York University School of Medicine, New York, New York

Patrick Heppell, Psy.D.
Clinical Assistant Professor, Department of Child and Adolescent Psychiatry, Hassenfeld Children's Hospital at NYU Langone School of Medicine, New York, New York; Clinical Director, ACS/Bellevue Mental Health Team at the New York City Administration for Children's Services Nicholas Scoppetta Children Center

Aron Janssen, M.D.
Clinical Associate Professor, Department of Child and Adolescent Psychiatry, Hassenfeld Children's Hospital at NYU Langone, New York, New York

xii Beyond PTSD

Jessica Linick, Ph.D.
Clinical Assistant Professor, Department of Child and Adolescent Psychiatry, New York University School of Medicine, New York, New York

Rachel Mandel, M.D.
Clinical Assistant Professor, Department of Child and Adolescent Psychiatry, New York University School of Medicine, New York, New York

Bruce D. Perry, M.D., Ph.D.
Senior Fellow, The Child Trauma Academy, Houston, Texas; Adjunct Professor, Department of Psychiatry and Behavioral Sciences, Feinberg School of Medicine, Northwestern University, Chicago, Illinois

Blake Phillips, M.D.
Medical Director, Bellevue Home-Based Crisis Intervention Program; Attending Psychiatrist, Bellevue Child and Adolescent Partial Hospitalization Program, New York University School of Medicine Medical Center/Bellevue Hospital Center, New York, New York

Moises Rodriguez, Ph.D.
Clinical Director, Homeless Adolescent Wellness Center, Division of Adolescent and Young Adult Medicine, Children's Hospital Los Angeles, Los Angeles, California

Karen C. Rogers, Ph.D.
Associate Professor of Clinical Pediatrics (Clinician Educator) and Program Area Leader, Project Heal, USC University Center for Excellence in Developmental Disabilities, Children's Hospital Los Angeles, Los Angeles, California

Jeanette M. Scheid, M.D., Ph.D.
Associate Professor, Department of Psychiatry, Michigan State University, East Lansing, Michigan

J. Rebecca Weis, M.D.
Clinical Assistant Professor, Department of Child and Adolescent Psychiatry, New York University School of Medicine, New York, New York

Jeremy A. Wernick, L.M.S.W.
Clinical Assistant Professor, Department of Child and Adolescent Psychiatry, Hassenfeld Children's Hospital at NYU Langone, New York, New York

Alexis K. Yetwin, Ph.D.
Pediatric Psychologist, USC University Center for Excellence in Developmental Disabilities, Department of Pediatrics, and Division of Pain Management, Department of Anesthesiology and Critical Care Medicine, Children's Hospital Los Angeles, Los Angeles, California

About the Editors

Dr. Gerson is an assistant professor of child and adolescent psychiatry at the NYU School of Medicine. She is the director of the Children's Comprehensive Psychiatric Emergency Program (CCPEP), a specialized emergency room for children and adolescents in psychiatric crisis. The CCPEP serves youth suffering from acute or complex mental health symptoms, referred from schools, therapists, pediatricians, child welfare, juvenile justice, and family members. Dr. Gerson has lectured nationally on assessment and treatment of youth with acute, complex psychiatric symptoms such as suicidality or aggression, and on the impact of trauma on such symptoms in youth. She has won two teaching awards for her work training child and adolescent psychiatry and psychology students in how to connect with and evaluate youth in crisis and how to work effectively within complex systems of care. She is co-editor of *Helping Kids in Crisis: Managing Psychiatric Emergencies in Children and Adolescents*, which won the Medical Book of the Year award in psychiatry from the British Medical Association in 2015. She has worked in psychiatric emergency, inpatient, outpatient, state hospital, and day-treatment programs for children, adolescents, and adults.

Dr. Heppell is a clinical assistant professor of child and adolescent psychiatry at the NYU School of Medicine. He currently serves as the clinical director for the Bellevue Hospital–ACS Mental Health Team (MHT) at the Administration for Children Services' Children's Center. Dr. Heppell and MHT provide clinical evaluation, support, and treatment to youth entering New York City's child welfare system and for youth in the system who have complex psychiatric and/or medical needs. Dr. Heppell and his team have also trained more than 120 child welfare staff in understanding and working with traumatized youth, specifically through the Think Trauma model. Dr. Heppell supervises child psychology trainees at NYU and Bellevue Hospital and has taught child psychiatry residents, social work staff, and others on working effectively and sensitively with youth in the child welfare system. Dr. Heppell has advanced-level training in Trauma-Focused Cognitive Behavior Therapy (TF-CBT) for child and adolescent maltreatment issues, grief, and bereavement. Previously, he was a child psychologist at Bellevue Hospital's Children's Comprehensive Psychiatric Emergency Program and has also worked at the Children's Hospital Los Angeles, in the University of Southern California Center for Excellence in Developmental Disabilities, and in family therapy and day-treatment programs.

Foreword

Fifty thousand years ago, human beings genetically equivalent to us walked this earth. In some ways, these ancestors had dramatically different lives—absent all of the technological, demographic, and sociocultural elements of our modern world. Yet in many important ways, these humans were very similar to us. The basic processes of neurodevelopment, the use-dependent organization and modification of neural networks (a key aspect of neuroplasticity), the neurophysiology of the stress responses, the basics of neurosociology, and the importance of early bonding experiences in shaping the neurobiology of reward, regulation, and relational capacities—among other things—were just the same in the past as they are for babies born today in Chicago, New York, or Bismarck, North Dakota. Also, in each "community" there was food and housing insecurity, material poverty, natural disasters, intra- and intertribal violence, postpartum depression, psychosis, domestic violence, tribalism, war, and a host of other unpredictable, overwhelming, and traumatic experiences. It would not be unreasonable to suggest that adversity has been common to the majority of individual humans during the entire history of humankind. In truth, it seems we in the United States are spared much of the more pervasive and traumatic elements of life of past generations—and of life in many of the communities and cultures of our current world. We are a lucky people. Yet even with this luck, the rate of adversity in our population is remarkably high—as you will read in many of the chapters in this book.

Trauma has always shaped us. Sometimes it breaks us, and mostly we will heal, stronger but different, at the broken places. In the past, when humans lived together in small multifamily, transgenerational groups, they were well aware of this. Each culture developed beliefs about death, warfare, injury, and many other potentially traumatizing experiences. Song, dance, ritual, and ceremony emerged to provide a cognitive framework to "make sense" of the insensible, to restore connectedness to community and nature, and to provide regulating rhythms. These are the three essential elements of all successful "trauma-informed" practices: providing meaning, supplying relational supports, and regulating somatosensory dosing. The development of these practices was, in part, an effort to become aware of, sensitive to, and informed about trauma. To the degree that these practices helped human living groups to survive and thrive, they were successful.

A remarkable property of our species is our brain's capacity to store and manipulate experience. The capacity of the cortex (predominantly) to change in response to experience has allowed a remarkable process of sociocultural evolution. We have invented ourselves into this modern world, each generation adding new tools, practices, beliefs, and technologies. As time passes, each generation needs to problem-solve about the unintended consequences of the choices and "inventions" of the previous generations. An example is seen with the child welfare system. Mobility, urbanization, agricultural advances, single-family dwellings, tenements, and other factors contributed to greater isolation for young parents and increased risk for our youngest children. Poverty, despair, social isolation, and other issues resulted in more abuse and neglect. As a result, our society was forced to invent the child welfare system to protect children. We care for the maltreated children of a despairing depressed mother in a very different way now than humans would have in a hunter-gatherer clan 10,000 years ago.

Our societies have become much more complex and fragmented. We have had to invent law, to create systems to deliver education, to provide health and mental health care, and to monitor and intervene with those who "violate" our society's rules. In the recent past, the rate of sociocultural evolution—the rate of inventing—has accelerated beyond the capacity of our systems to adjust. Our systems lost track of the tools and frameworks that they had previously utilized to combat the effects of adversity. Education forgot that movement, song, dance, sport (all regulating and rhythmic), and "connectedness" are the best ways to make the cortex capable of processing and internalizing cognitive content. Mental health forgot that exposure to chaos, threat, relationally mediated abuse, and traumatic experiences create emotional, behavioral, and cognitive symptoms that can mimic essentially all of the neuropsychiatric disorders. The juvenile justice system did not take into consideration the impact of trauma on judgment, impulsivity, and aggressive behavior; instead, youth in the system were merely deemed "bad kids." The relationship between exposure to trauma and physical health—something well known to our ancestors—was never mentioned in medical school. Yet, as this book illustrates, trauma-related problems permeate all of our systems.

From this distant perspective, the true power of this book becomes evident. The authors in this book come from many different systems, yet they all appreciate the complex and diverse effects of trauma on youth. A primary value of this book resides in the "defragmenting" impact it has; the unifying thread is developmental adversity. Each chapter has its own voice, putting forth the challenges (and importance) of working with and understanding youth exposed to developmental adversity or trauma; the essential role of mental health and medical personnel as leaders in the "trauma-informed" systems movement; the benefits of understanding the emotional, social, cognitive, and physiological effects that may arise following childhood trauma; the various manifestations of developmental trauma in educational and juvenile justice systems; and the need to create developmentally sensitive practice, programs, and policy. When put together, like a choir, the collective creates a deeper and more vibrant effect. The awareness and integration of a more developmental and trauma-aware perspective shared by the authors in this book represent a refreshing and positive shift in how we can understand and better help the youth we serve.

So, dear reader, this book should be viewed as a snapshot of an important inflection point—a change in direction—in the implementation of more "inventions" in the never-ending problem-solving process that must accompany human sociocultural evolution. As it is the nature of our species to adapt, and it is the nature of the world to change, we will always be in the exploring, examining, experimenting, inventing, implementing, revising, and reinventing business. The cycles and rhythms of systemic change keep us moving—mostly forward. In each chapter of this book, the authors share their insights for those doing the difficult and painstaking work of caring for traumatized adolescents and improving our systems. This book reflects a broader, yet just emerging, awareness of the need to understand, quantify, qualify, and respond to trauma-related problems in every segment of our culture and across all of our systems.

Bruce D. Perry, M.D., Ph.D.
Senior Fellow, The Child Trauma Academy, Houston, Texas;
Adjunct Professor, Department of Psychiatry and Behavioral Sciences,
Feinberg School of Medicine, Northwestern University, Chicago, Illinois

CHAPTER 1

Teens and Traumatic Stress

A Toxic Combination

Ruth Gerson, M.D.

Erika, age 14, started cutting herself after her mom's new boyfriend, Joe, moved in. Even though Erika always got along well with Joe before, she has been withdrawn and testy with him since he moved in. Her mom sees the cuts on her daughter's arms, but when her mom tries to ask about them, Erika just gets irritated and insists she's fine. She's doing well at school and is always smiling and laughing with her friends. It feels to her mom that Erika is jealous and trying to get her mother's attention by being dramatic.

Javhon, age 16, took on a "fuck it" attitude after his dad left. First his grades and attendance started dropping, and now he stays up all night, smoking pot in his room and playing video games. When his mom tries to wake him in the morning for school, he snaps at her and refuses to go. Sometimes, if she begs and shares how worried she is for him, he'll relent and say that he'll go to school tomorrow, but then he never does. He knows he's failing this year but doesn't seem to care.

Is this typical adolescence? The beginning of delinquency? Or what if there is more to these stories? What if we knew the things that these youth wish we knew about them but can't tell us?

Erika was molested 2 years ago, by her mom's last boyfriend. It happened intermittently for close to a year after the guy moved in with them. She didn't tell anyone because she was ashamed and felt that it must be her fault. And she didn't want to upset her mother, who finally seemed happy. When her mom and the guy broke up, Erika was relieved and thought about telling

1

her mom but could never get the words out. Erika likes her mom's new boy-friend, Joe, who has always been kind and never made her feel uncomfort-able. But having a man in the house again reminds her of what happened, and she's scared that there's something bad about her that will make Joe try to touch her too. Cutting helps distract her from the shame and the intru-sive memories, and in some ways it feels right to hurt and mark this body of hers that has been the cause of so much pain.

Javhon feels overwhelmed with sadness and anger since his dad left. The years before his dad left, as far back as Javhon can remember, were peppered with screaming fights between Javhon's parents. Sometimes Javhon would hear his dad threaten his mom or hear the thud of him hitting her. A few times Javhon had crept out of his room to see what was happening, but his father would roar at him to go back to his room. Seeing his mom with a black eye or a bruise on her neck, Javhon would be filled with rage at his father and shame that he himself hadn't stepped in to protect her. But at other times Javhon's dad was affectionate, fun, and kind, and Javhon loved him. He misses his dad every day, and is torn between sadness that he left and relief that his mom is safe. Overwhelmed by conflicting feelings, Javhon can't focus in school and finds himself snapping at his friends and his mom. Smoking mari-juana gives him relief from his internal conflict, and video games give him something to focus on. He smokes and plays online through the night and sleeps most of the day. He feels awful, but this pattern lets him avoid seeing his mom and experiencing the flood of guilt and anger he feels around her.

Hearing Erika and Javhon's full stories, no one would write them off as just "bad" kids. Traumatic experiences are behind their behaviors, but Erika and Javhon aren't able to tell us that right away. We rarely get the full story up front with teens in such circumstances, so with limited information, we may write off their behavior as either "normal teenage drama" or the begin-ning of delinquency.

Youth who have been abused or traumatized tend to keep their secrets to themselves. They often feel eaten up by shame and guilt, afraid to trust anyone, and alone in a world that has no idea what they've been through. To help teens like Erika and Javhon, we have to be able to see their behaviors as warning signs, as smoke signals from fires hidden deep inside. If we can see through the behavior to what's underneath, we can understand what's really going on. Once we start to understand, we can approach, connect with, and support traumatized adolescents who desperately need our help.

Understanding Adolescents

Adolescents—moody, unpredictable, and stubbornly illogical beings who ping-pong between brilliantly insightful and incredibly stupid—are mysteries to the adults around them. Teens can show impressive wisdom, selfless-ness, and dedication to others or to important ideals. In such moments, an adolescent can be endearing and even inspiring to parents, teachers, and other adults. But at other times, impulsivity, poor judgment, and short-sighted stubbornness can make the same teen seem like a completely different per-son. Parents often joke that some alien creature took possession of their child's body when he or she turned 13.

Adolescents themselves sometimes don't know why they seem to change from moment to moment. Even if they do know, they are certainly not go-ing to explain to an adult who could "never" understand. As teens shift from parents to peers as their main source of social support, the teenage mind be-comes increasingly opaque to parents, teachers, and other adults. At best, this leads to misunderstandings and drama that families look back on with amusement. But when teens start to struggle, it doesn't feel as funny to the parents, teachers, therapists, and others striving to understand the enigmatic young person before them. Instead adults can feel that raising, teaching, or just connecting with teenagers is impossible.

Emotional or behavioral problems in adolescents like Erika and Javhon can be especially hard for parents and other adults to understand. Adults wonder where to draw the line between the normal storms of teenage drama and behaviors that are more concerning. Often adults try to use adult rea-soning with teens. For example, they might remind youth of the conse-quences they will face if they keep skipping school or using drugs. They try to push teens to weigh pros and cons and take responsibility for their actions. If reasoning doesn't work, they try to force the teens to make better choices by taking away privileges or giving punishments. But these interventions might not help if an adult doesn't understand why a teen is engaging in the negative behavior. Because major parts of teens' lives (school, social inter-actions, online life) are unseen by adults, it can be hard for adults to know why teens are doing what they do. As a result, adults fall easily into a think-ing trap that psychologists call the *fundamental attribution bias*.[1]

What is the fundamental attribution bias? We've all had moments in which we do something we wouldn't usually do—cut someone off on the highway, lie to a loved one, jump the line at the store—because of unusual or problematic circumstances. Maybe we cut someone off at the highway or jumped the line because we were racing to pick up a sick child from school. Or maybe we lied to a loved one to protect them or because we couldn't get into the complicated truth at the time. When we think about our own be-havior in these moments, we think about context: we are doing out-of-character things because of the unusual circumstances. When we look at others doing these same things—when someone lies to us or cuts in line—we are generally blind to context, because of course we don't know the other person's circumstances. But because we can't see the context, we assume that there is none and that the behavior is due to some fundamental characteristic of that person. The person who lied to us did so because he's a liar, and the person who cut us off in line did so because she thinks her time is more important and doesn't care about anyone else. This is the fundamental attribution bias. Rather than trying to consider what kinds of circumstances would cause the person to lie to us or otherwise behave in a certain way, we attribute the behavior to some fundamental characteristic of that person. Unfortunately, adults do fall into the thinking trap of the fundamental attribution bias with kids (even young children, and even our own children) all the time: "My toddler's constant tantrums are because he's spoiled, and my teenager lies to me because she doesn't want to take responsibility for her screw-ups. In contrast, when I lose my temper, I know it's because I'm overtired and overstressed from work, and when I lie to my teenager it's because certain things are too adult or too complicated to explain to her." The truth may be somewhere in the middle: "My toddler is a little spoiled but also sometimes tantrums because she's overtired. I need to get enough sleep myself and learn to deal with stress from work so I'm not always losing my temper with my kids." Looking at the context increases our understanding and helps us find solutions. But adults often don't fully know the context in which teens are working. This means we are vulnerable to the fundamental attribution bias and generally fail to consider the context for a teen's behaviors and the reasons a teen might have for acting the way he or she does. This leads to simplistic, out-of-context explanations and misunderstandings that frustrate everyone involved.

Usually, the context that drives any of us to act in uncharacteristic ways is some sort of stress. Stress can make us distracted, emotional, or depleted. This is especially true when we are first learning to deal with stress, cope with new challenges, or solve new problems, such as during adolescence. That said, stress is a normal and even desirable part of adolescence. Adolescents need to be challenged. They are learning and growing academically and socially, developing independence and responsibility, and discovering how to cope with conflicts and consequences. These challenges are necessary for adolescents to grow, but they create stress. In the moment the stress may make teens (like adults) irritable, stubborn, or prone to overreacting, and teens may try to avoid their stress through distraction (video games, social media, etc.). This can be a normal part of learning how to cope with stress, but it can also be upsetting and frustrating for the adults around the teens. Not knowing the context, adults often fall into the fundamental attribution bias and assume the teen is just being a typical obnoxious adolescent.

What if, instead, adults try to understand what might be behind an adolescent's behavior? Imagine that my teenager is extra irritable this week and keeps bingeing on Facebook rather than doing her homework. I can yell at her or punish her, but this will put anger and distance between us at a time when she clearly needs help. If I can identify that this change is related to a big fight with her best friend last weekend, I can help her talk about the fight, reflect on how it has affected her mood and behavior, and help her learn to cope with it. Understanding the context for her behavior does not excuse her behavior. She is still responsible for her reactions to stress, and by helping her see how stress makes her behave in negative ways, I can help her take responsibility and learn to respond better in the future.

> Taking an empathic, curious stance will help you ask about what's happening in a way the teen might actually answer. Saying, "I can't believe you're on Facebook again when your homework's not done! What's going on with you?" puts the teen on the defensive. You might try saying instead, "You haven't seemed like yourself recently—like you're distracted or something's bothering you. Is everything okay?" If the teen says, "No, I'm fine," you might say, "Hmm, I've noticed that you've been looking kind of down, and things seem to be frustrating you more than normal, and you haven't been able to focus on your homework. Is there something bothering you?" Being genuinely curious and empathic is key; ask yourself, "If I was acting this way, what might be underneath it for me?"

Even a small stress can lead to problematic or out-of-character behaviors. A fight with a friend, worries about upcoming state tests or sports tryouts, adjusting to a new sibling or a new school, and many other things can make a teen irritable, edgy, or distracted. If a small stress has such impact, imagine the effects of traumatic experiences such as the ones experienced by Javhon and Erika.

Trauma is the kind of stress that overwhelms the ability of our minds and bodies to cope. Just as normal stress can push youth to act in occasionally problematic ways, trauma can completely derail them with psychiatric symptoms and severe behavioral problems. These problems might show up right away, or can manifest years later because trauma can create a stress that never goes away. Unfortunately, many youth experience trauma in childhood. Up to 68% of youth experience domestic violence, community violence, traumatic loss of a loved one (due to an accident, illness, or violent act), terrorism, physical abuse, sexual assault or abuse, severe bullying, neglect, violence in dating relationships, or other types of trauma before they turn age 16.[2,3] This book will help adults better understand how trauma can be behind symptoms and behaviors such as self-harm, aggression, substance use, and school problems, among others. By trying to piece together the context for a traumatized teen's behavior, we can better understand and empathize with why the teen is acting this way. Then we can help him or her learn to cope and get back on track.

What Is Trauma?

Certain kinds of trauma are obvious: facing combat as a soldier, being attacked or sexually assaulted on the street, and living through a terrorist attack or natural disaster. But adults often forget the experiences that can be traumatizing to children. Many of us who have experienced serious problems in our childhood have managed to come to terms with and grow from those experiences, so we may no longer see them as being a "trauma" on par with combat or assault. Many common experiences of childhood—for example, severe bullying, domestic or community violence, or coping with a parent abusing drugs or alcohol—can be traumatic for youth. *Trauma* is, by definition, when an experience feels so threatening to one's safety and well-being that it overwhelms one's ability to cope. Human beings, especially children, are amazingly resilient. Not only can we humans survive terrible things, but often we commit incredible acts of strength and heroism in the face of adversity, such as the soldier who carries a wounded friend out of battle despite her own wounds, or a father who rescues his children from a raging fire. But just because we survive something does not mean we are not marked by the experience.

Trauma is the Greek word for "wound." Just as there are many physical wounds, large and small, visible and invisible, there are also many psychological wounds caused by traumatic experiences. Even when we seem fine immediately after a traumatic experience, trauma leaves traces on our brains and in our minds in ways that may not manifest until much later. This is especially true for children, who may seem to recover quickly in the moment but who are deeply vulnerable to the effects of trauma because their brains and selves are developing.

We tend to idealize childhood as a typically happy time filled with loving family, play, learning, and few responsibilities. However, trauma in childhood is extremely common. The following gives a sense of the extent: Trauma is most associated in many people's minds with war and combat. Approximately 1.5 million American men and women served in the Iraq War between 2003 and 2011. By comparison, every single year about 3 million children and adolescents in the United States are reported to authorities as victims of child abuse or neglect—and these are only the instances of abuse that get reported.[4] Surveys of youth suggest that trauma is even more common, especially if we ask about a broader range of traumatic experiences. In a nationally representative survey of adolescents aged 12–17 years, 8% reported having experienced sexual assault, 17% reported physical assault, and 39% reported having witnessed violence.[5] As reported on the National Child Traumatic Stress Network (NCTSN) "Facts and Figures" page,[6] a survey of elementary and middle school students found that 30% had witnessed a stabbing and 26% had witnessed a shooting, while in another study as many as 41% of youth had witnessed such violence. In national surveys of high school students, 17% report that they have experienced a serious physical assault, 8% have experienced sexual assault, and 39% have witnessed serious interpersonal violence.[7] As stated on NCTSN's "Facts and Figures" page, up to 33% of adolescent boys reported they themselves had been shot or shot at.[6]

Even these reports may underestimate the prevalence of trauma in children and adolescents. A large national survey found that 71% of youth had experienced child abuse, domestic violence, a serious car accident or major medical trauma, traumatic loss of a significant other, sexual assault, dating violence, or hate crimes in the past year. Nearly 70% of children and adolescents had experienced more than one type of trauma, with an average of three different types of traumatic experiences reported.[8]

Repeated or multiple traumatic experiences can be particularly damaging for children and teens. A child who experiences a single trauma—for example, witnessing a shooting while walking to school—will feel shaken and afraid for some time. A child who lives in a community where shootings, stabbings, and other violent incidents occur daily or weekly will never stop feeling afraid (although a teenager will never admit it). Repeated abuse, especially physical or sexual abuse, can be especially harmful to children and teens. Youth who are abused repeatedly over a period of time feel trapped and unable to predict or escape the horror. The abuser often threatens to kill or harm the child or someone the child loves if the child speaks up, and may tell the child it's the child's fault or that the child deserves or enjoys what is happening. If the abuser is the child's own parent or caregiver, the child feels even more trapped because he or she is dependent on the abuser.

The child may also love the parent or caregiver despite the abuse, especially if the abuse is intermittent and the abuser is kind or loving at other times (or if the abuser is the only parent or caregiver the child has). This type of repeated abuse or trauma, termed *developmental trauma* or *complex trauma*, is some of the most damaging to children. Developmental trauma happens at a time when children are physically and emotionally vulnerable. They are too weak to fight and too dependent and vulnerable to escape. Children are neuro-biologically vulnerable as well, because their growing brains are affected by everything they experience. Because of these vulnerabilities, developmental trauma leaves a legacy of shame, confusion, self-blame, and physical and psychological problems that creates one of the most pervasive and least understood syndromes in medicine. The impact of developmental trauma lasts through adolescence and into adulthood, affecting every aspect of a person's health and behavior.

The Marks of Trauma

Trauma affects everyone slightly differently. The effects depend on what happened and how often, how old the child is, what his or her personality is, and whether he or she has close family and other supports to turn to (or if those family members were the ones perpetrating the abuse). The largest study ever done to understand the long-term effects of trauma was the Adverse Childhood Experiences (ACE) study.[9] The ACE study asked more than 17,000 adults about traumatic experiences in their childhood. Of the respondents, 30% reported having been physically abused, 20% reported having been sexually abused, 11% were emotionally abused, 25% were physically or emotionally neglected, 24% had a parent struggling with alcoholism, 5% had a parent struggling with drug addiction, 19% had a parent struggling with mental illness, 5% had a parent go to jail, and 13% witnessed domestic violence in their home. Two-thirds of the people in the study had experienced at least one of these traumas, and more than one in five had experienced three or more different traumas.[9]

The ACE study found that for each trauma an individual had experienced, he or she had an increased rate of medical illnesses, such as heart disease, emphysema, liver disease, autoimmune diseases, cancers, and sexually transmitted diseases. Individuals with multiple traumas also had increased rates of psychiatric illness, such as depression, suicide attempts, or drug or alcohol abuse, and were more likely to have social or life problems such as difficulty at work or school, teen pregnancy or unintended pregnancy, and financial stress. Individuals who had experienced traumas were also at increased risk of later trauma, including being the victim of sexual assault or domestic violence. The relationship between these outcomes and trauma was linear, clearly showing that with each additional trauma, an individual experienced more medical, psychological, or social problems (as the number of traumatic experiences went up, so did all the person's other problems). Although the adults in the ACE study had experienced trauma in childhood, even decades later the trauma was still affecting them physically and psychologically.

Trauma and Adolescence: A Toxic Combination

The ACE study clearly showed that the effects of trauma are widespread. But the ACE study looked at adults, years or decades after the trauma happened. What are the effects of trauma on adolescents?

We typically think of posttraumatic stress disorder (PTSD) as the most common effect of trauma. PTSD was first described in adults after a single severe trauma, such as military combat or a sexual assault. Trauma in childhood, however, can have effects that go far beyond PTSD, as we see in the ACE study. This is particularly true in adolescents. Adolescents who have experienced trauma (either recently or earlier in their childhood) can have a wide range of social and psychological problems. They show changes in their mood and behavior, problems with attention and impulse control, and problems in relationships. Their grades and academic performance often start to slip, and they are more likely to drop out of school. They engage in more risky behaviors, including substance abuse, risky or promiscuous sexual behavior, gang involvement, and criminal behavior. They are more at risk for sexual assault, dating violence, and teen pregnancy. They also are more likely to develop depression, anxiety, sleep problems, or thoughts of suicide.[10]

How do we understand the pervasive effects of trauma on children and adolescents? The damaging effects of traumatic stress in youth start with two pathways: The first is related to the immediate impact of trauma, the body's natural fight-or-flight response. The second is related to the ways growing up in a dangerous and unpredictable world affects how individuals think, learn, and relate to others, on both a neurobiological and a psychological level. Each of these topics is discussed in turn to explain how these effects can be particularly harmful to children and adolescents.

Fight-or-Flight and Freeze Responses

Erika doesn't like to think about the man who abused her. When he first came into her room and tried to touch her, he was so much bigger and stronger than she was. She tried to fight back and even bit him, but he said that if she did that again or told anyone, he would hurt her mom. When he came to her room the second time, she felt frozen in place. The third time, he started telling her that she liked it, and even though she didn't, she couldn't shake the feeling that she had made this happen somehow.

Once, when he was age 11, Javhon tried to intervene when his dad was beating on his mom. But his dad shoved him away, and Javhon was so afraid he ran back to his room in tears. He spent days fantasizing about punching his dad. A few weeks later a kid at school shoved him, and Javhon punched the kid in the stomach over and over until the teacher pulled him away. It felt amazing and powerful. Then the principal called Javhon's mom in, and seeing the look of disgust and fear on his mom's face when she looked at him made Javhon feel ashamed and angrier than ever.

The *fight-or-flight response* is the body's natural and automatic response to a life-threatening event. Epinephrine (more commonly called *adrenaline*), its sister hormone norepinephrine, and the stress hormone cortisol are released from the brain, triggering a series of steps to prepare the body to fight back or run. Blood pressure and blood sugar rise to boost the flow of energy to the muscles. The senses intensify and focus. Blood flow in the brain changes, increasing in brain areas that focus attention to threats and negative or hostile things in the environment. Youth (and adults) having a fight-or-flight response describe feeling hyperfocused, with tunnel vision and with every muscle tense and every hair on end. Teens might describe it as getting "hyped" or feeling like "turning it up." The fight-or-flight response also cuts off blood flow to areas of the brain that won't help with fighting or running. For example, blood flow drops to the brain's language areas and auditory processing, making it hard for youth to put what they're feeling into words or to respond to the reassuring words of others.

Although most people have heard of the fight-or-flight response, there is another natural trauma response that is actually more common in many children: the *freeze response*. Children are too small to fight and too weak to flee, so like a deer in the headlights of an oncoming car, they freeze. Like children having a fight-or-flight response, they are less able to speak or process what others are saying, or to form conscious memories, because of changes in the blood flow in their brains. These youth feel numb, dissociated, sometimes as if they were separated from their bodies or as if the terrible thing were happening to someone else. They might describe it as feeling like they're losing it or blacking out.

The fight-or-flight and freeze responses happen automatically when a child (or adult) is faced with a life-threatening event, but they can also happen when the child or teen experiences a reminder of, or trigger for, the trauma. Triggers can happen at any moment, and may be external (something in the environment that reminds the youth of the trauma) or internal (a physical sensation, memory, or thought related to what happened). Triggers can bring back the fight-or-flight or the freeze response in full force. Some youth are self-aware enough to describe feeling as though the trauma is happening again, but most don't know why they are suddenly freaking out. Some teens alternate between these stress responses. This is especially true for those who have experienced multiple traumas. They can become extremely anxious, agitated, or aggressive (the fight-or-flight response) in some circumstances, or numb and shut down (the freeze response) in others.

Further complicating the situation, most teens are not conscious or aware of the trauma triggers or don't connect what is happening now with trauma from the past. Imagine how excruciating it is to know that out of nowhere, for no reason you can understand, you might suddenly feel terrified, rageful, or numb; there is nothing you can do to predict or prevent the feeling and no end in sight. Many youth start to feel anxious or depressed or to fear they are "going crazy." Others turn to drugs and alcohol to try to mellow or escape the feelings. If adults are not aware that the youth has been through a traumatic event, these unpredictable and bizarre swings of behavior can look like psychiatric illness, ranging from oppositional behavior or anger problems to bipolar disorder or psychosis. Or worse, the youth can look like a "bad" teen going off the rails.

Brain Development in a Traumatizing World

> That first fight wasn't the end of Javhon getting into trouble at school. Even though he tried to "stay calm" like his mom advised him, he couldn't seem to control his reactions. Every time a kid bumped into him in the hall or a teacher yelled at him for some little thing, he felt like punching something (and often did). But he also felt violent at times that didn't make sense, such as when his grandma died or when his dog ran away. He broke up with his first girlfriend even though he really liked her, because sometimes when she couldn't hang out (because her parents were strict), he'd have an urge to shake her or choke her. He didn't want to hurt her or be like his dad, so he dumped her. Smoking pot became the only way he could keep his anger in check. After his dad left, Javhon felt so on edge, even with the pot to calm him down, that it was better not to be around people because he could never be sure he wouldn't lash out and hurt someone.

The second way in which trauma can be damaging to children and adolescents is by changing the ways their brains and minds develop. Our brains are designed to adapt to the world around us, to learn from what we experience so that we can successfully navigate the environment we live in. Our brains are most sensitive in childhood and adolescence. When children grow up in a world that is safe and predictable, their brains grow and develop to fit that world. But trauma makes a child's world dangerous or unpredictable. Brains develop differently in children who grow up in a dangerous or unpredictable world than in children who grow up feeling safe. Importantly, the effects of trauma on brain development can be lasting and make it difficult for a child to adjust to environments that are safe or secure.

The brain develops in stages, starting with the basics. Babies learn to eat, sleep, and deal with physical sensations from a mother's loving touch to hunger to a sudden need to poop. Babies learn what each of these sensations means (*hunger means I need to eat, being tired means I need to sleep, feeling scared means I need a hug*) from experiencing the sensation and its resolution (*when my caregiver feeds me and I feel better, I learn that uncomfortable thing I was feeling before is hunger*). The brain areas (located in the brain stem) that help us manage hunger, fatigue, arousal, touch, and other key sensations develop through these experiences. When a child is abused or neglected, when a mother's touch is a slap, or when crying in hunger is met with no response, these brain areas develop differently than they do in children who are well cared for. Teens who have been neglected as children often find it difficult to distinguish these basic sensations and may confuse hunger or fatigue for sadness or loneliness. They may binge on food or alcohol without knowing why they are doing it, because their brain signals for hunger and loneliness or anxiety or other sensations have gotten mixed up by the early neglect. Others have long-standing problems with sleep or are hyperreactive to even a gentle or caring touch.

The next part of the brain to develop is the emotional brain. Think of toddlers: They need to learn to recognize and articulate what they are feeling (anger, sadness, frustration, fear, excitement) and learn to manage those feelings without devolving into a tantrum. Parents and caregivers help toddlers learn how to recognize and manage their emotions and how to get help from others to feel better. The adults do this by responding to the toddlers' outsized emotions with calm and caring, by putting words to the experience ("You don't want to go to bed, I know! It's so hard!"), and providing a safe environment for the toddlers to express themselves. But children who are abused, neglected, or exposed to violence during infancy and early childhood never get a chance to learn how to recognize or manage their feelings. This is why Javhon feels angry and violent when he experiences sad things, such as when his grandma died, his dog ran away, or his girlfriend had to go home. Being exposed to domestic violence from an early age disrupted the areas of his brain that allow emotion recognition and self-control. These brain areas are called the *limbic system*. They include the amygdala, which judges what is scary or exciting; the hippocampus, which controls learning and memory; the thalamus, which integrates what we hear, see, and feel; and other regions that network between these and other areas (e.g., to manage the fight, flight, or freeze response). According to developmental trauma expert Bessel van der Kolk,[11] children who grow up frightened and abused are wired to respond to fear and hurt. When the limbic system is disrupted by trauma, children and adolescents may perceive threat where there is none and may experience a small frustration or rejection as soul destroying. They can have difficulty articulating their emotions (e.g., differentiating anger from sadness). When upset, they can have adolescent-size tantrums (losing control, breaking things around them, or hurting themselves), because like a toddler, they don't know how to articulate what they're feeling and to work with others to resolve it. Children who consistently receive comfort from others when they are upset learn to feel safe and know to ask for help. Those who don't often come away with the lesson that no one can help them or that violence is the only way to get what they need.

The most sophisticated part of the brain (and the part that develops the latest, from childhood through early adulthood) is the prefrontal cortex. This is the area of the brain in which conscious thought happens. The prefrontal cortex lets us consciously process what we see and hear and keeps the limbic system from freaking out. If we're startled by someone grabbing us from behind, it's the prefrontal cortex that processes the friendly face and familiar voice to realize it's just a friend surprising us with a hug. Or if a fierce-looking dog rushes toward us, the prefrontal cortex balances between the amygdala's automatic fear response and our visual observation that the dog is on a leash, so we step back a bit but don't flee in panic. The prefrontal cortex serves what is called *executive functions*: the ability to observe our own thoughts, feelings, and impulses and calmly choose between them.

The prefrontal cortex is still developing in the average adolescent, which is why teens can be impulsive, illogical, and overly driven by emotion at times. In youth who have been traumatized, these functions can completely break down. The prefrontal cortex is less able to regulate other brain areas including the amygdala and the fight-or-flight or the freeze response. The brains of traumatized teens are more controlled by the amygdala and the automatic fear reactions than by the conscious thinking of the prefrontal cortex. This makes sense in a way; because the amygdala processes much faster than conscious thinking can, a kid can identify and escape a dangerous situation more quickly. But even if automatic responses and impulses are necessary for survival, being driven by them is disconcerting. Javhon feels unable to control his anger because his prefrontal cortex (his conscious mind) is not in control of his impulses.

It is not really a fair question when we ask teens like Javhon, "What were you thinking?" Their automatic fear and stress responses had them acting (running, fighting, etc.) before their conscious mind (the prefrontal cortex) even had a chance to respond. When we try to reason with them in the moment of acute stress—for example by reminding them of consequences or questioning why they're making a bad "choice"—we're trying to reason with the prefrontal cortex, when that isn't what's running the show. The automatic and emotional brain is in charge at this point in their lives.

The last way in which trauma during childhood and adolescence, particularly developmental trauma, can change the brain is through the cortisol system. Cortisol, known as the "stress hormone," is made in the adrenal glands, not in the brain. But it has huge impact on the function of all the brain areas described above. We all know how small amounts of stress, such as arise when we're facing an upcoming test or deadline, help us to focus, give us self-discipline, sharpen our memory, and let us learn faster. This occurs because in these moments of minor stress, cortisol triggers the brain areas for attention, self-regulation, learning, and memory. But traumatic stress, being stress that overwhelms the body's systems, derails the cortisol response. Cortisol response in traumatized youth is either persistently too high, so the teen is constantly on edge and overreacts to tiny slights or even benign interactions, or completely shut down, so the teen is not reacting to even real threats. Either of these is dangerous. Youth with a too-high cortisol response feel constantly anxious or irritable, and may turn to alcohol or drugs to get some relief. Those whose cortisol response is too low feel numb much of the time. They don't get that "hair on the back of the neck" feeling most people get during threatening situations, such as while being followed by a creepy guy or attending a party with a weird vibe. As a result, teens with too-low cortisol have difficulty recognizing unsafe situations and are more at risk for being hurt or victimized by others. They may also turn to thrill-seeking, dangerous behavior, or self-harm to escape the numbness and to "feel something."

Trauma in childhood and adolescence can affect some or all of these different brain areas and systems. The impact depends on the type of trauma, how often it happened, and how old (in what developmental stage) the child was when hurt. If trauma happened repeatedly, there can be disruptions to all of these brain systems. These effects can be lasting, so even if the teen is now in a safe environment, the brain and body still react in the only way they know how. Unlike a reaction to simple stress (which occurs only when that stress is present), the reaction to childhood trauma persists, ingrained in a person's body and mind. Over time, connections in the brain and ways of responding to stress get reinforced over and over, especially if the trauma is repeated or goes untreated and unresolved. The right treatment can reverse these effects, but they are unlikely to go away on their own.

Understanding all of the ways in which trauma can affect the brain of a child helps us understand why the effects of trauma can go way beyond PTSD. Thinking about trauma's effects on the brain also helps us understand why traumatized teens might need more than a "think about the consequences of your actions" talk to get back on track.

Beyond PTSD

Youth who have experienced trauma or abuse rarely walk into our offices and announce, "Hi, I've been abused and I'm acting up as a result. Can you help?" Their inability to state this need isn't just the usual adolescent obfuscation. Instead, the trauma has changed their brains in important ways. Trauma and trauma triggers cut off blood flow to the speech and language processing areas of the brain, making it impossible for youth to express verbally in the moment what it is that they are experiencing. As a result of these areas being cut off, and trauma's effects on memory formation, youth are unable to form integrated, narrative memories of the trauma and to understand and articulate their experiences in a linear way. Trauma disrupts the connections between the emotional, intuitive right side of the brain and the logical, analytical, language-generating, story-telling left side of the brain. When youth talk about their experience of the trauma or about why they lose control in the face of a trauma reminder, they can rarely tell us the whole story. Their stories are often fragmented, confusing, and devoid of emotion or self-awareness. They may be able to tell the facts of the story (using their left brain) but without any emotional content; this can make their reports feel insincere or untrustworthy. Alternatively, they may be able to express the emotional experience (using their right brain), but these versions of the story tend to lack any sense of time or order (which requires the left brain). This can make their reports confusing, inconsistent, or even hard to believe.

Trauma makes it harder for youth to talk to us on a psychological level as well as a neurobiological one. Many traumatized youth carry around intense feelings of guilt and blame themselves for the trauma they experienced. This is especially true if someone else (a parent, friend, or sibling) was also hurt. Many who have experienced physical abuse or assault feel that they deserved it in some way, or that if they had really wanted to they could have fought back or gotten away. Those who survived accidents or experienced traumatic loss of a loved one often feel that they could and should have prevented the event and carry terrible guilt that they did not. And of course, if someone has hurt a youth terribly, that youth will be wary and distrusting of others as well. Trauma makes it harder for teens to trust and get close to others, so they are even more likely to keep their experiences to themselves.

As adults, then, we can't simply wait for teens to come to us. Youth who have experienced trauma and abuse are in our offices, classrooms, clinics, hospitals, foster homes, and jails every day. Because trauma can affect the developing brain in so many ways, the symptoms and difficulties experienced by traumatized youth are broad-ranging and confusing. Thus, in the search for youth who might have been traumatized, it is not enough merely to screen for PTSD, because although PTSD is one consequence of traumatic stress, it is not the only one or even the most common.

About one-third of youth who have experienced trauma develop PTSD. Sleep problems should be a red flag for PTSD in teens who have experienced trauma. PTSD in youth usually presents with nightmares, although the nightmares will not be specifically related to the trauma and the teen may not remember them. Teens might instead just describe insomnia or trouble falling asleep. Similarly, PTSD usually brings flashbacks, but teens may not be fully aware of or able to describe the flashbacks as such. They might only be aware that their mood shifts quickly, that they get angry easily, or that it's hard to concentrate at school or on homework. Many youth with PTSD feel either constantly on edge or chronically numb and disconnected. Adults get frustrated at teens with PTSD for being irritable, checked out, or withdrawn. Teens with PTSD often struggle to feel connected with others, even with peers, and may start using drugs or alcohol to feel more "normal" in social situations. Some experience chronic numbness and dissociation and may cut themselves or engage in risky behaviors in an attempt to "feel something." Adults often struggle to understand why traumatized teens put themselves in harm's way through substance use and risky behaviors, and may start to wonder if a teen somehow wants to be hurt.

After trauma, teens more commonly experience depression and other mood changes than they experience PTSD. Traumatic experiences often leave long-lasting feelings of shame and guilt, low self-esteem, and a pessimistic view of the future. These changes can mimic depression, and youth who have experienced trauma are also at high risk for full-fledged major depression. They have more suicidal ideation, more suicide attempts, and more

TABLE 1–1. **The different impacts of trauma**

	Keyed-up type (hyperarousal)	Numb or depressed type (dissociation)
Symptoms	Hypervigilance, anxiety, exaggerated responses	Numbing, anhedonia, detachment
Behavioral effects	Distractibility, frequent fights or aggression, self-injury, substance use, learning problems, impulsive actions	Self-injury, withdrawal, substance use, inattention, "spacing out"
Misidentified as and/ or comorbid with	Oppositional defiant disorder, conduct disorder, bipolar disorder, psychosis	Depression, attention-deficit/hyperactivity disorder–inattentive type, psychosis

Source. Adapted from American Academy of Pediatrics: *Helping Foster and Adoptive Families Cope With Trauma.* Itasca, IL, American Academy of Pediatrics, 2016. Available at: https://www.aap.org/en-us/Documents/hfca_foster_trauma_guide.pdf. Accessed February 21, 2018.

frequent self-injurious behavior than depressed teens who haven't experienced trauma. Their depression can be harder to treat (particularly if the trauma is not addressed), which can worsen their sense of being hopeless and alone. The fight-or-flight and freeze responses to trauma reminders or triggers can also make teens moody and irritable, which might look like psychiatric disorders such as bipolar disorder, especially when combined with risky behaviors. Other youth have such severe flashbacks, hallucinations, and dissociation that they look psychotic (Table 1–1). Still others have such difficulties with relationships, oppositional behavior, distrust of others, self-regulation, and self-harm that adults are tempted to label them with personality disorders such as borderline or antisocial personality. As a result, traumatized adolescents are disproportionally represented in special education, child welfare, and juvenile justice systems.

But these labels and systems unfairly write off traumatized youth—an additional unfairness for teens who have already been through so much. Understanding the role of trauma in their symptoms and behaviors doesn't mean that we let the youth off the hook for their behavior or that we don't take their symptoms seriously. Understanding the role of trauma helps us to understand the context for the teens' behaviors, to help them make better choices, and to design treatments that will work to reduce their symptoms. The rest of this book will explain how to do just that, in our work with youth who have different types of symptoms or behaviors, and in different settings (such as school or juvenile justice systems) that serve teens. We can break the bonds of the fundamental attribution bias to really understand our teens—what they have been through and what they are going through. And we can help ensure that eventually trauma becomes just a thing that happened to them, not the thing that defines them for the rest of their lives.

Resources and Additional Reading

Online Resources

ACESTooHigh (ACEs=Adverse Childhood Experiences) collaborative: https://acestoohigh.com

American Academy of Pediatrics Early Brain and Child Development: https://www.aap.org/ebcd

American Academy of Pediatrics Healthy Foster Care America: https://www.aap.org/fostercare

American Academy of Pediatrics Medical Home for Children and Adolescents Exposed to Violence. https://www.aap.org/en-us/Documents/resilience_webinars_medical_home.pdf

Center on the Developing Child, Harvard University: https://www.developingchild.harvard.edu

Child Trauma Academy: http://www.childtrauma.org

Matanick N, Kisiel C, Fehrenbac T; Center for Child Trauma Assessment, Services and Interventions: Remembering Trauma: Connecting the Dots Between Complex Trauma and Misdiagnosis in Youth (educational film), 2017. Available at: http://www.rememberingtrauma.org

National Child Traumatic Stress Network, Learning Center: https://learn.nctsn.org

National Child Traumatic Stress Network, Resources for Parents and Caregivers: http://www.nctsn.org/resources/audiences/parents-caregivers

National Child Traumatic Stress Network: What Is Complex Trauma? A Resource Guide for Youth and Those Who Care About Them. http://www.nctsn.org/sites/default/files/assets/pdfs/ct_guide_final.pdf

Substance Abuse and Mental Health Services Administration (SAMHSA) National Center for Trauma-Informed Care and Alternatives to Seclusion and Restraint: https://www.samhsa.gov/nctic

Additional Reading

Neufeld G, Mate G: Hold on to Your Kids: Why Parents Need to Matter More Than Peers. New York, Ballantine Books, 2008

Perry BD, Szalavitz M: The Boy Who Was Raised as a Dog: And Other Stories from a Child Psychiatrist's Notebook—What Traumatized Children Can Teach Us About Loss, Love, and Healing. New York, Basic Books, 2006

Shatkin J: Born to Be Wild: Why Teens Take Risks and How We Can Help Keep Them Safe. New York, TarcherPerigree, 2017

van der Kolk B: The Body Keeps the Score: Brain, Mind, and Body in the Healing of Trauma. New York, Penguin, 2014

References

1. Ross L: The intuitive psychologist and his shortcomings: distortions in the attribution process, in Advances in Experimental Social Psychology. Edited by Berkowitz L. New York, Academic Press, 1997, pp 173–220

2. Copeland WE, Keeler G, Angold A, et al: Traumatic events and posttraumatic stress in childhood. Arch Gen Psychiatry 64(5):577–584, 2007 17485609

3. Costello EJ, Erkanli A, Fairbank JA, et al: The prevalence of potentially traumatic events in childhood and adolescence. J Trauma Stress 15(2):99–112, 2002 12013070

4. Baiocchi D: Measuring army deployments to Iraq and Afghanistan. Rand Corporation, 2013. Available at: https://www.rand.org/content/dam/rand/pubs/research_reports/RR100/RR145/RAND_RR145.pdf. Accessed June 2018.

5. Hamblen J, Barnett E: PTSD in children and adolescents. National Center for PTSD, February 23, 2016. Available at: https://www.ptsd.va.gov/professional/treatment/children/ptsd_in_children_and_adolescents_overview_for_professionals.asp. Accessed June 2018.

6. National Child Traumatic Stress Network (NCTSN): Facts and Figures. Available at: http://www.nctsn.org/resources/topics/facts-and-figures. Accessed June 2018.

7. Kilpatrick DG, Saunders BE: The Prevalence and Consequences of Child Victimization. National Institute of Justice Research Preview. Washington, DC, U.S. Department of Justice, 1997

8. Finkelhor D, Ormrod R, Turner H, et al: The victimization of children and youth: a comprehensive, national survey. Child Maltreat 10(1):5–25, 2005 15611323

9. Centers for Disease Control and Prevention: Violence Prevention: About the CDC-Kaiser ACE Study—data and statistics. Available at: https://www.cdc.gov/violenceprevention/acestudy/about.html. Accessed June 2018.

10. Gerson R, Rappaport N: Traumatic stress and post-traumatic stress disorder in youth: recent research findings on clinical impact: assessment, and treatment. J Adolesc Health 52(2):137–143, 2013 23332476

11. van der Kolk BA: Developmental trauma disorder: toward a rational diagnosis for children with complex trauma histories. Psychiatric Annals 35(5):401–408, 2005

CHAPTER 2

Recognition and Treatment

Patrick Heppell, Psy.D.
Ruth Gerson, M.D.

Jason, age 17, walks confidently into the clinic. Short and muscular, with blingy earrings and new Jordan sneakers, he draws attention naturally. But the clinic staff know him as a "frequent flyer" who has been seen there by different therapists, intermittently, for years. Jason's last therapist (his fourth in 3 years) is out on maternity leave, so Jason is seeing a new clinician, Mark. As Mark goes through the usual intake interview questions, Jason is respectful and engaged but generally vague. He says he is chronically depressed and doesn't "feel safe," but denies wanting to hurt himself or experiencing any danger. He describes long-standing bouts of rage and violent thoughts toward strangers, but he has never hurt anyone. When Mark asks Jason why he's here today, Jason replies, "I got these urges to hurt someone, anyone. It's mad strong, like I can't fight it anymore." Mark asks what has helped him in the past, and Jason shakes his head: "Nothin' can help me." Later Mark attempts to ask Jason about past or current traumatic experiences: "Ever experienced anything traumatic in your life?" he asks. "Not really," Jason replies. Mark asks, "You've never been abused by anyone, like, physically or sexually, right?" "Nah, man," says Jason, rolling his eyes. Mark is confused by Jason's incongruous presentation and wonders if there is something more to Jason's case. Flipping through Jason's chart, Mark sees an extensive list of psychiatric disorders: cannabis abuse, substance-induced psychotic disorder, oppositional defiant disorder, bipolar disorder, attention-deficit/hyperactivity disorder (ADHD), and schizophrenia. There is no diagnosis of posttraumatic stress disorder (PTSD) or any mention of trauma history. However, Mark notices in the social history that Jason was adopted out of foster care when he was age 10, and recognizes Jason's address as being in a dangerous, gang-infested part of town. Mark asks Jason what he's looking for in therapy. Jason shrugs and says, "Therapy don't work."

Teens who have experienced trauma show up to mental health treatment every day, although we do not always recognize them. They are sent by parents, teachers, social workers, judges, probation officers, and pediatricians. They are referred for "problem" behaviors: defiance, oppositionality, violence, self-harm, drug use, truancy, social withdrawal, seeming depression, bizarre behavior, running away from home, nonadherence to medical treatment, promiscuity, criminal behavior, or "failing out" of the child welfare system. Occasionally, they are referred for treatment by someone who knows about their trauma history, but usually, as with Jason, nobody knows. Even if their trauma history is known, typically no one connects the individual's trauma to the current symptoms or problems. Trauma is not even part of the equation.

When traumatized adolescents present for treatment, we often find that they have been struggling for a long time but have not previously sought or received help. Teens face many barriers to getting care. Often families can't find or afford treatment, or they have had negative experiences of mental health care themselves. Pediatricians, teachers, counselors, and caseworkers might not have the time or training to notice the early red flags for trauma and refer a teen for treatment early. Sometimes youth themselves avoid treatment, because of stigma, fear of being forced to talk about traumatic experiences, or just being a teenager. Often it is not until the teen is completely off the rails that adults (or rarely, a very self-aware teen) are forced to act and get professional help. The help the teen receives, however, is often the wrong help. If no one asks about or knows about the teen's trauma history, or if no one connects the history of trauma to the current problems or symptoms, treatment will not address the core issues and will not be very effective. If the therapist tries to address behaviors without understanding their source or context, the youth may feel judged or "crazy." Getting the wrong treatment and having treatment "fail" makes teens like Jason skeptical or blatantly avoidant of mental health treatment.

Over the years, Jason has seen a dozen well-intentioned therapists for play therapy, unstructured talk therapy, and substance use treatment. Not one has asked about, understood, or addressed the abuse he experienced before and during foster care, or the community violence he has witnessed. All this treatment has left a bitter taste in Jason's mouth about therapy. "It doesn't work," he tells Mark, and he's not wrong. Research has repeatedly shown that trauma-focused therapy is the most effective treatment for youth like Jason, but like Jason, many traumatized teens never get it.

What's Wrong With the Wrong Treatment?

As in Jason's case, when adolescents enter treatment but the treatment providers fail to ask about trauma, understand the history, or connect the past to current behaviors, treatment will likely be ineffective or downright counterproductive. In each of the case examples below, adults see the teen's problem behavior but, not thinking about trauma, reach only a superficial understanding of the issue. Because they don't understand the deeper issue, the adults choose simplistic solutions that are well intentioned but ineffective.

- Becca's falling grades are easily explained by her poor attendance and bad attitude. Her counselor tells her dad to implement tougher consequences. This response leads to even more parent-teen conflict and to Becca's being more distracted and anxious at school.
- Jon's being withdrawn and irritable recently is attributed to a bad attitude and substance use. His caseworker and parents tell him that he should make better decisions and stop hanging out with his "bad-influence" friends. Jon then either hangs out with those friends in secret, or obeys his parents but feels isolated and depressed.
- Aimee runs away from home, an action that her therapist and mother understand as a lack of respect for authority. They call in "help" from the child welfare or juvenile justice system, which leads to Aimee being even more mistrustful of adults, escalating her running away and eventually landing her in a detention center.

The adults in these examples care deeply about their kids and want what is best for them. But a lot gets in the way of adults really understanding when a teen is struggling. Adults have expectations for their teen (that he or she be respectful, want to learn, make good choices, and so forth), feel pressure to raise the teen correctly, and are busy with work and other children and other responsibilities. The adults are left with little time and patience to consider the teen's perspective and the context for the teen's behavior. Even if the adults do try to ask their teenage child about the behavior, odds are they get a "whatever" or "nothing" in reply, especially if they asked in the midst of an argument or in a moment when the teen was feeling criticized or judged. And without knowing the context, adults fall into the *fundamental attribution bias* (as described in Chapter 1, "Teens and Traumatic Stress") and never consider alternative explanations for the concerning problem or behavior. Imagine how differently we would approach the teens in the examples if we knew that Becca was being bullied, or that smoking marijuana with friends is the only thing that gives Jon relief from the flash-backs about the car accident that killed his brother, or that Aimee's step-brother has been molesting her and she no longer feels safe at home.

Therapists may also be quick to jump to simple explanations and solutions for behaviors and psychiatric symptoms. The hypervigilant, hyperaroused, hyperreactive teen is seen as hyperactive and impulsive and is started on a stimulant medication and told to work on his "executive functioning skills." The quiet, avoidant teen is diagnosed with depression and put on an anti-depressant medication. Meanwhile, the angry teen is labeled as oppositional or "conducty" and is subjected to anger management treatment and a behavioral program of rewards and consequences.

As discussed in Chapter 1, trauma in childhood can lead to a wide range of emotional and behavioral problems, including depression, anger, self-harm, substance use, impulsivity, dissociation, social problems, and insomnia.[1,2] If clinicians and parents don't see how these symptoms relate to trauma, they might see the symptoms as being part of major depression, ADHD, bipolar disorder, conduct disorder, or psychosis and design a treatment for those disorders. Such treatments can be helpful as part of a more comprehensive treatment that also addresses trauma; however, without any recognition or discussion of how the current symptoms and the earlier trauma are connected, these treatments alone aren't effective and can leave teens feeling blamed and misunderstood. Therapies that don't consider trauma also miss the ways in which there might be ongoing exposure to trauma reminders or triggers in their environment that unleash a new wave of symptoms or problematic behaviors.

The Challenge of Recognizing Traumatic Stress in Adolescents

Most of us shy away from asking about or openly sharing personal traumatic experiences in everyday conversations. We pretend that trauma is not a part of our lives, even though traumatic experiences are actually very common. As a result, adolescents who have experienced trauma feel alone with these experiences in schools, hospitals, child welfare systems, juvenile justice systems, and even mental health clinics. Our own discomfort keeps us from asking and keeps them from telling, so the trauma remains unspoken. When we can't even speak or know about trauma, we can't fully understand the teens in front of us or address what has happened to them in treatment.

Multiple factors make conversations about trauma uncomfortable for both the adult—even a caring, trained clinician—and the youth. Let's be honest:

Engaging adolescents in serious conversation is complicated in the best of circumstances. Asking about sensitive topics such as trauma is harder, especially for those who aren't used to asking and talking about such matters.

> Asking about trauma can be hard if you're not used to doing it. Try practicing with a friend until the questions and phrases feel more natural to you. Teens will pick up on your discomfort, but rather than thinking "she's nervous and self-conscious about her own interviewing skills," they think, "she's uncomfortable with what I might tell her; she doesn't want to hear this from me," so they clam up.

We often worry about upsetting or triggering the teen, angering the parents, or opening a conversation that we won't know how to handle. These are normal concerns, and the reality is that traumatic experiences can be uncomfortable to hear about, both in content and in affect. Sometimes we don't really want to know about the heartbreaking realities of teens' lives, which can burden us personally (triggering our own traumatic memories or worries about keeping our own children safe) or professionally (leading to vicarious trauma or feelings of being inadequate to help the teen). So we don't ask, or we ask just once, quickly or in passing, and the teen senses that we don't really want to know.

Even if adults ask and ask well, there are many reasons that teens don't talk about trauma. Adolescents are wired not to trust adults, especially adults whom they feel don't look like them, don't share a background, or with whom they "can't relate." Traumatized teens are often even more mistrusting of adults. Some have been hurt (physically or emotionally) by adults who were supposed to care for them. Others feel damaged or ashamed about what happened and assume that others see them the same way. Still others are angry at adults for not protecting them, not realizing what happened, or not believing them. PTSD makes teens avoid talking about traumatic experiences (avoidance is a key symptom of PTSD), and so does depression, which makes youth feel that no one cares and problems are their fault alone. Finally, many youth have heard well-meaning adults state a variety of messages aimed at helping the teens to move on: "You'll get over it," "Everything happens for a reason," "Just forget about it," "Others have it worse than you do." These statements, while generally well intentioned, feel very invalidating to teens, who are probably trying their best to forget and move on but can't, because their brains and their bodies won't let them. Other teens have heard more nefarious messages, stated explicitly or implied, suggesting, for example, that the abuse never happened, the violence they experienced is normal or okay, or the whole thing was their own fault. Sometimes adults deny the trauma or blame the teen without really meaning to: "Are you sure that was what happened?"; "I can't imagine he would do that"; "If you hadn't gone out with those people…"; "If you hadn't been drinking…"; "Why didn't you just call me?" These statements make the youth feel ashamed, think that the trauma should not be talked about, and feel that no one will be able to help them because the experience was all their fault.

This can be particularly problematic for teenagers, for whom shame and helplessness are especially terrifying emotions. The teenage brain has a biological need to feel independent, competent, and in control; gaining such independence and competence is the key task as children move through adolescence into adulthood. Feeling shame or helplessness is painful at any age, but teens are much less able to tolerate that vulnerability and often react with anger, aggression, or even self-harm behaviors such as cutting. These behaviors help them feel more in control. Teens rarely have insight into these reactions, because they don't recognize triggers and are unaware of their own responses. Even when they are aware of their behavior, they rarely connect it to the past traumatic events or reminders and triggers in the environment. Therefore, when a teacher, counselor, social worker, or mental health professional genuinely and sensitively asks a question (e.g., "Why the decline in school performance?" "Why the substance use?" "Why are you running away from home?" "What's going on lately?"), the answer from the teen is rarely "Oh see, it's because of this trauma I went through." Unless the adult can ask in a way that is sensitive, direct, normalizing, and validating, most teens are quick to deny, avoid, and move on to the next question.

Screening and Recognition: How to Ask About Trauma

Screening tools and assessments can be very helpful in asking about trauma, and below we'll talk about some good and accessible tools to use. Trauma screening tools shouldn't be used in isolation, however. They should be an adjunct to a caring, sensitive adult asking appropriately and directly about traumatic experiences. Even if you are using a screening tool to help you ask about trauma, knowing how to engage, relate to, and interview a teen about trauma is a critical first step. The New Haven Trauma Competency Guidelines include evidence-based consensus recommendations on the essential components and approaches for any assessment of trauma.[3] They recommend, as we do, asking directly about trauma exposure and reactions with all patients, whether or not you suspect that they have experienced trauma. Unfortunately, experiencing frightening events, hardship, and abuse crosses all lines of gender, race, socioeconomic status, and geography. Building rapport and therapeutic alliance with the individual in front of you requires thinking about the youth's strengths, culture, and beliefs, which is another of the guidelines' recommendations. Experiencing an adult "seeing" them in this light lessens their feelings of helplessness and gives them a sense of agency. The guidelines also highlight that to reduce avoidance and minimization, it is important that we show youth that we can tolerate both the content of their trauma history and the affect they show. Although these guidelines are helpful in outlining evidence-based key principles, they fall short in providing concrete examples of the "how to" and "what to" ask for clinicians. When you ask about trauma, the following techniques can help put the teen at ease and demonstrate that you want to hear and to help.

Generalize

- "I'm going to ask you a bunch of questions that I ask all the teenagers I see, because a lot of us experience these things."

Normalize

- "Lots of teens who are dealing with depression [or cutting themselves, or smoking weed a lot, or getting into fights] tell me that part of it is about dealing with [or escaping from] bad memories or painful feelings from things that have happened in the past. A lot of times those memories and feelings are really hard to talk about or even think about."

Validate

- "That must have been so hard [sad, confusing, frustrating]."
- "I bet it hurts to talk or think about this."

Explain

- "I ask these questions because I want to make sure you are safe."
- "I also ask because it happens to a lot of people."
- "I'm trying to understand what is behind the behavior. You're a smart, reasonable guy, so I'm sure you're not skipping school [or cutting, or getting into fights] for no reason. Most of the time, there is a good reason for a smart kid to miss school [or run away, or cut, or use drugs]."

Ask specifically, but start generally

- "Have you ever been through anything very scary? Something you have been through and that you have kept thinking about? Like being part of

or witnessing an accident? Violence in the neighborhood? Bullying at school?"
- "Has there been a time when you had to live apart from one of your parents?"
- "Have you ever lost someone close to you?"
- "Has anyone ever hit you? Smacked you? Pushed you? Punched you? Threatened you? Harmed you in any way?"
- "Who yells the most in your house? Who fights in your house? Do the fights ever get physical?"
- "If you get in trouble at home, what happens as punishment?"
- "Has someone ever touched you inappropriately? Touched your private areas without permission? Made you touch them in a way that made you uncomfortable? Made you feel uncomfortable in any sexual way?"
- "You mentioned you're dating someone. Does he treat you well? Has he ever threatened you? Hit you? Made you do anything sexually that you didn't want to do?"
- "Have you ever done sexual things in exchange for money? A place to stay? Drugs? Or anything else?"

Ask often

- The teen may not tell you the first time, or the second time. Keep asking.

Show respect

- "It's up to you how much you want to share with me right now…."
- "We don't have to talk about this anymore right now if you don't want to. If you need a break or want to come back to this at another time, that's cool, but I really want to make sure we talk about it because it's important to me to understand what you've been through."

Show empathy

- "I'm sorry you had to go through that."
- "I'm sorry they couldn't take care of you the way you deserved to be taken care of."
- "It's so unfair that you had to go through that."

Respect avoidance

- "I get it why you haven't talked about this…."
- "It makes sense you've been trying not to think about this—it sounds like it's just too hard to think about this sometimes."

Respect resiliency

- "You've been through so much. How have you been able to handle all of this?"
- "Even with all of this, you've still been keeping up with school [or taking care of your siblings, or staying focused on your music or basketball]. How do you do that? Is there anyone who helps you, or do you just do this on your own?"

Expect ambivalence and look for intrinsic motivation for change

- "I can see how smoking weed [or cutting, or running away, or avoiding thinking about what happened] has helped you to deal with all of this. How has it impacted you in other ways? Has it always been helpful? Do you wish there were other ways to manage those painful memories [or thoughts, or emotions]?"

> For more on *motivational interviewing* techniques to bring out motivation for change, check out the tips and tools at: http://www.motivationalinterviewing.org.

Get familiar with cultural differences

- Don't make assumptions that you know the teen's cultural background or beliefs, even if you have seen other kids from the same background or if you come from the same culture yourself. Every kid and family are different, so ask about how this individual adolescent's culture, beliefs, and background might have made it easier or harder for him to cope with this trauma.

Know your limits/acknowledge

- "I can't imagine how it feels to go through all of this…"
- "I wish I could change what happened, or fix this situation for you now. I feel angry and frustrated that you've had to go through this, so I can only begin to imagine how it feels for you being in it."

Praise

- "I know it's hard to talk about this. You are very strong for doing so, and I'm really grateful that you're sharing it with me."
- "I'm really impressed at how articulate and insightful you are about this. This is hard stuff to talk about."

Screening and Recognition: Using Trauma Screening Tools

Trauma screening tools can be used in two ways. One option is to give the screening tool to the youth to complete on his or her own, as a way to give the teen another opportunity to share about his or her experiences. Make sure to introduce and describe the purpose of the screening tool, generalizing ("This is something I ask all the teens I see to fill out"), normalizing ("because lots of kids have had these kinds of experiences"), explaining ("and knowing about these experiences helps me understand where you're coming from and what you've been through"), and showing respect ("You can answer as much or as little as you want today, and we can talk about it together or go over it next time if you prefer"). Alternatively, go through the screening tool with the adolescent, using the screening tool as a guide in how to ask. Trauma screening tools should ask both about traumatic experiences and about symptoms of and reactions to traumatic stress. The National Child Traumatic Stress Network (NCTSN) lists trauma screening and assessment tools, provides links to how to get them (including those that are available and free online), and even gives case examples of how they can be best used (http://www.nctsn.org/resources/topics/trauma-informed-screening-assessment/trauma-screening). If parents or others who know the teen well are involved, you can also ask them to complete the same screening tools, in case they might share something the teen forgets or doesn't feel comfortable mentioning.

Screening tools can also be used to assess for other types of symptoms, such as suicidal thoughts (Columbia Suicide Severity Rating Scale [CSSRS] or the Ask Suicide-Screening Questions [ASQ]), depression (Patient Health Questionnaire–9 [PHQ-9]), or substance abuse (CRAFFT). (The section "Resources and Additional Reading" at the end of this chapter lists Web sites for these specific scales.)

You should always go over the results of any screening tools with individual teens, making sure that you understand what they wrote, asking follow-up questions, highlighting their strengths and resilience, praising their willingness to share the information, and clarifying any confusing or inconsistent areas. Remind them that you'll be asking these questions again in the future, not to be annoying, but because it's important and you want them to know they can talk about these things with you anytime.

Most importantly, any assessment of trauma should be with the goal of understanding the teen so as to develop an effective, individualized treatment that makes sense for the youth and his family.

Trauma-Informed Treatment: What Does It Look Like?

Susan is 58 years old and has always been terrified of flying. Her first and only time flying, when she was newly married, was harrowing. Since then, she has relied on long car drives, buses, and trains, or skipping certain destinations altogether. It even makes her nervous when her husband or children fly, or when a character in a movie gets on a plane. But then her pregnant daughter announces that she is moving to Hawaii and says, "Mom, I know your thing about flying. We'll just travel to you a few months after the birth."

Susan can't imagine missing the birth of her first grandchild. But when she imagines herself on a plane, she starts hyperventilating. She asks her doctor about taking medication for the flight, but he says it's not safe because of her blood pressure problem. One friend tells her, "Just don't think about it until you have to go, and then just face your fear!" Susan knows trying this in the past has ended with her standing in the doorway with her suitcase, watching the cab drive away, unable to will herself to actually go to the airport. Another friend who used to have a similar fear says, "Your daughter isn't due for 4 months? Then you've got plenty of time to practice and get ready," and then shows her pictures from his own recent trip to the Caribbean.

The "practice" Susan's friend is referring to is the basis for cognitive behavioral therapy (CBT). CBT starts with psychoeducation, teaching the connections between thoughts, feelings, behavior, and symptoms like anxiety, then moves to teaching and practicing coping skills. Next CBT uses gradual exposure, meaning that people expose themselves slowly and incrementally to the emotionally triggering or anxiety-provoking thing, so that they learn to manage the anxiety and find the scary thing less frightening over time. Rather than trying to force herself onto a plane, Susan would start by reflecting on what is behind her fear of flying, learning (and believing) facts about airplane safety, learning relaxation techniques, and learning reassuring and accurate statements that she can think about when facing anxious thoughts or situations. Once she is more comfortable, she would incrementally start to imagine herself in a plane (feeling the anxiety that comes with it, and practicing relaxing and reassuring herself), take a few trips to the airport with a close friend, watch airplanes take off and land safely over and over, and maybe even get on a plane or take a short flight (and practicing tolerating and managing her anxiety). All the while she would be starting to make specific plans for her trip (who is going to travel with her, when they will go, and how she can help herself feel better if she gets scared).

Trauma treatment is similar in some ways. The reason that childhood trauma comes out as so many emotional and behavioral problems is that the trauma is never addressed or processed. Unfortunately, when it comes to trauma, time heals no wounds, contrary to popular belief. We need to process and understand trauma to heal it. However, most teens (and adults) do anything they can to avoid thinking or talking about their trauma, just as Susan shies away from anything that has to do with airplanes. Their fears are just too scary. But for the emotional and behavioral problems to go away, the trauma needs to be understood and processed. Trying to change all at once would be like Susan's first friend telling her to "just face your fear"—such a rapid change generally doesn't work and can make the teen feel overwhelmed, shut down, or "freak out." Trauma treatment works in phases to help the traumatized teen get ready to gradually think about and process the trauma. The teen initially spends time preparing, understanding why this will be useful and how the trauma is connected to current problems, before learning relaxation and coping skills to manage the symptoms associated with the avoidance, reactivity, and maladaptive coping skills that are so common as responses to traumas.

Trauma treatment may be a bit more complicated than addressing Susan's fear of flying, but the concepts are the same. The phase-based approach ensures that the teen is not forced to confront the trauma until she is ready. The phases of trauma treatment typically address four goals: ensuring safety, developing skills, finding meaning in past traumatic events, and enhancing resiliency and integration into a social network.[4]

Safety is the goal of the first phase because addressing trauma is only possible once the teen's safety can be ensured. Just as an FBI agent wouldn't remove her protective vest until the crime scene is deemed safe, a teen shouldn't be expected to (and will not) remove his defenses and make himself vulnerable if his living situation is or feels unsafe. Thus, safety is required before having the teen gradually expose himself to his or her trauma history. If the environment is unsafe, involving the court system, child protective services, family members, and the school may be necessary to create a safer environment for the teen. If safety cannot be achieved, treatment should focus on psychoeducation (understanding normal responses to ongoing traumatic stress) and "surviving" with skill building, refraining from any exposure or meaning until safety has been attained.

After ensuring the teen's safety and before moving on to the next goal, the therapist needs to get the adolescent to "buy in" to the treatment. The techniques described above (show respect, explain, normalize, etc.) can be helpful in this regard, as can engaging the teen in identifying his or her own goals or targets for treatment. Maybe a teen doesn't particularly want to stop smoking marijuana but also doesn't want to feel so jumpy; or maybe a teen is not so worried about her cutting but doesn't want to dissociate or go numb every time someone touches her. After treatment goals are identified, the therapist should provide trauma-informed treatment to educate the teen (and family or other adults who are involved) about the effects of trauma and to explain how triggers or trauma reminders can lead to flashbacks, anger, dissociation, or other distressing reactions. This psychoeducation is the beginning of the gradual exposure process, as it assists the teen and family with connecting the behaviors to the trauma.

The next goal is to learn coping skills such as relaxation skills, distraction, grounding, cognitive techniques such as reframing or positive self-talk, and getting help effectively from others. These skills will help the teen to deal with triggers and reduce the symptoms or behaviors that the therapist and teen have identified as the targets of treatment. In addition to teaching coping skills, the therapist should work to get the teen engaged with positive activities and supportive peers or adults. The therapist should work with the teen's family or any available supports (e.g., school, social worker, court) to better understand the teen. Through this process, the adolescent is building a good foundation of skills and supports and establishing trust with the therapist.

Once the teen and therapist feel ready (usually after there has been a reduction in symptoms or problem behaviors), the therapy shifts to directly addressing the past trauma. This will require gradually developing a narrative or story of what happened, filling in details, reflecting on thoughts and feelings in the moment and after, and slowly processing or coming to terms with what happened and even sharing the story with trusted others. Lastly, building on strengths and resiliency moves the teen away from further revictimization and integrates the teen into a more positive and engaged future.

This explanation might sound straightforward, but addressing trauma with wary and skeptical teens (which is most of them) can be harder than it sounds. We return to Jason as an example. Let's imagine that Mark, Jason's therapist, used the strategies described above to build a connection with Jason and to ask more effectively about what Jason has been through. Jason doesn't admit to ever being abused, but he does acknowledge that his years in foster care were "hard" and that he has seen some violence in his neighborhood. Mark recognizes that Jason's time in foster care may have been traumatic and may be related to the issues Jason says he wants help with (feeling depressed, rageful, unsafe). Mark tries to get Jason on board with the idea of trauma-focused treatment.

> "Jason, I have two scenarios for you," Mark begins. "There is a question at the end that I ask most teens I meet with here (*normalizing, generalizing*):

Two young guys join the Marine Corps. They're both 19 and both love their country and want to serve, but their backgrounds are different. The first guy never knew his dad and was adopted at a young age after losing his mom to drugs. He and his siblings were in foster care for a bit before being adopted, and they lived in a rough neighborhood. The guy never joined a gang growing up, but he lost a few friends to shootings and worked hard to keep his siblings safe at home. (*The therapist makes the story similar to Jason's, normalizing and beginning the process of gradually and sensitively exposing Jason to his story.*) The other soldier grew up in a different part of town with a stable family and a pretty safe, easy childhood. The two soldiers trained together, were deployed together, and became close friends. They share the same war stories. They feared for their lives a few times together and buried a few of their troop members together. They both came back to the United States on the same plane with the same plan: to go to college and meet a nice girl. But one of them really struggled with coming back from deployment. He always felt on edge—feeling weird, having flashbacks, not being able to keep up at his classes, and getting upset at his girlfriend for no reason (*normalizing common responses to trauma*). The other one jumped right back into life and seemed to be okay. So my question for you, Jason, is which one do you think had a harder time coming back to the United States: the first guy who had gone through some hard stuff as a kid or the second one who'd had a pretty easy life?"

Jason thinks about it for a while as he seems to know this might be a trick question. He responds with confidence, "The second one for sure. He never saw anything like this before. It freaked him out when he was over there, you know, so he couldn't really hang when he came back. The first guy was used to all of this, so it don't affect him, it don't touch him, like you know, he's able to handle it." Mark smiles: "Your answer is the same as what most adolescents and adults respond to this question. But, surprisingly, it's the opposite. We know from talking to real guys like these, that soldiers who have had difficult experiences in their childhoods and adolescence are more affected by the hard stuff on deployment and have a harder time with school, work, relationships, and such when they get back." Jason cocks an eyebrow, incredulous, but Mark continues: "Everyone is a little different, but this is true for most people (*generalizing*). This is surprising to a lot of the soldiers themselves, even. Those who have been through hard things in the past expect to be able to get through it and not be affected. Why do you think that the first soldier might have a harder time with this (*asking for reflection rather than telling*)? Jason thinks for a bit before replying: "Yeah, I see, it's all catching up to him…it's just too much and you just can't get away from it all. You go to war and then you come back home to the same crap." Mark notes that Jason used "you" instead of "he" and wonders if Jason is starting to relate to or internalize the story, but then Jason's face darkens and he says, "I'm not talking about this anymore, man."

Mark stays calm: "I get it and I'll respect that. We'll talk more about this stuff another time (*explaining the plan for treatment*). It will be up to you when and how much (*showing respect*). It's hard for that first soldier and for most people to talk about this kind of stuff (*normalizing and respecting avoidance*). It's too hard to even think about. That soldier feels like he is still at war, surviving, even though he is back. Thinking about that stuff only gets his guard down, and he can't do that, not where he lives. It's easier for the second soldier to talk about it because he can separate himself from those war experiences and think, 'Man, war was ff-ed up,' when for the first guy, life has been and continues to be 'ff-ed up.' It's not fair (*generalizing, using a broad concept such as unfairness rather than a more personal emotion such as sadness or fear*)."

Jason responds with a simple "Yeah" while looking defeated. Mark empathizes with Jason's sad affect: "You may not have gone to war, but you have kind of been at war for a while now." Jason shrugs, "Yeah, I guess you can say that."

Mark continues, "The first soldier might never ask for help. He might be too proud, or not know how. But you, Jason, you are doing it differently. I'm proud of you for always finding us when things get real hard and for asking for help (*praising and showing respect*). I'm glad you came in today. What do you want to focus on today (*showing respect, eliciting the teen's goals*)?"

While exploring Jason's goals for treatment, Mark provides psychoeducation on how Jason's confusing feelings of rage and despair might relate to the "hard" experiences he faced in the past. Mark also empathizes with Jason's ambivalence about treatment while arguing that earlier treatment didn't work because it didn't address the trauma. Jason is wary, expressing hesitance to talk about "that stuff." Mark is gentle but persistent: "My goal is to help you get ready to talk about it. This treatment has been around for a while and has helped lots of teenagers who experience some of the stuff you have (*normalizing*). For example, it's clear to me that the thoughts you've been dealing with have been hard to manage, and I think that's related to some of the things you've been through that are hard to talk about (*explaining, providing psychoeducation*). I'm guessing that those thoughts make it hard to focus at school or on the basketball court." "And it's messing up my sleep, too," Jason jumps in. Mark uses this moment of buy-in from Jason to increase his motivation for treatment, explaining, "We'll work together in addressing those thoughts and the stress you've been experiencing. Those thoughts would keep anyone awake, and anyone who has gone through as much as you have would have these reactions (*normalizing*). Another thing that happens to a lot of teens is that they're up a lot at night because their body is used to being on edge, because when they were younger the night was when scary or bad things happened (*connecting past traumas to current behaviors or symptoms*). Or sometimes something has happened during the day that pulled up lots of bad memories, and our minds can't quiet down and sleep because we're processing all that (*psychoeducation about triggers*). Part of what I'd like to work on together is finding ways to manage this stuff, so you can sleep better and focus and everything. Then once you're feeling a little better, and when you feel up for it, we'll get to a place where you'll share your story, little by little. You'll start with the easier stuff to talk about and move toward harder things to talk about—the things you've never talked to anyone about. If we can talk about them in a safe way here together, they won't be as likely to pop into your head when you don't want them to, like when you're trying to sleep or hanging with friends. Teens tell me that after this process, when faced with a trauma reminder or unpleasant thoughts, rather than feeling panicky or overwhelmed, they're able to step back, choose whether or not they want to think about it or deal with it later, and know that they have the skills to stay in control of their thoughts and feelings."

Getting adolescents on board with treatment is difficult but critical. Explaining the point of treatment and the connections between symptoms/behaviors and memories/thoughts/flashbacks can help the teen see why talking about "the past" can be worthwhile. The techniques of showing respect, normalizing, and empathizing with the teen's avoidance (without giving in to that avoidance) help the teen feel safe rather than judged or "crazy." If Jason can learn adaptive coping skills to gradually expose himself to his own trauma narrative, he'll learn that he can tolerate thinking and talking about his trauma and being vulnerable without losing control. Doing this in therapy is the first step to doing it in the real world, to once again be open to relationships and new experiences and the idea of a future.

Parents and caregivers should be part of trauma treatment too. Parents need to understand the teen's behavior in the context of his past traumatic experiences and current stressors. Trauma therapists help parents learn parenting skills, improve the parent-child relationship, and address behaviors in an empathic and effective way. The clinician should be transparent with the adolescent about involving parents or caregivers. The teen may not be ready to share the trauma narrative with the caregivers. Generally, however, teens will be open to the idea of the therapist helping the caregivers to understand the teen's perspective or helping the teen and parents to find a middle ground in conflicts. This can be a starting point to get the adolescent on board with eventually sharing more, and even the trauma narrative, with family.

Finding the Frame: Finding the Trauma-Focused Treatment That Is Right for Your Teen

Although trauma-informed treatments may be difficult to find and access, there are numerous evidence-based trauma models that are appropriate for teenagers. These vary in format, but most follow the phase-based approach described in the previous section. Most treatments operate in a typical "therapy" model as found in mental health clinics and hospitals. Other treatments are delivered in the teenager's environmental context, such as in home-based or family services and in school mental health programs. Group therapy models are also available and effective. Most treatments rely on cognitive behavioral strategies (talking, processing), whereas others incorporate other means such as meditation, mindfulness, and music. No matter the format, there always should be a significant component focusing on working with the teen's caregiver(s).

In considering which treatment is the "right one" for a specific adolescent, consult with colleagues and other professionals (school employees, pediatrician, social worker) who know the youth and her particular symptoms and difficulties. Talk to her care coordinator, case worker, or insurance provider to find out which providers are trained in trauma-focused treatment. Most importantly, talk to the adolescent and have her consider the following: Where would she prefer to receive services? Is she likely to initially attend on her own? Would she prefer a group format? Does she like expressing herself verbally or through artistic, musical, or physical means?

The following are resources that can help in locating empirically based trauma treatments:

- National Child Traumatic Stress Network (NCTSN): http://www.nctsn.org/resources/topics/treatments-that-work/promising-practices

- Substance Abuse and Mental Health Services Administration (SAMHSA) Mental Health Services Locator: http://www.mentalhealth.samhsa.gov/databases/

See also American Academy of Child and Adolescent Psychiatry (AACAP) for general information for families and their Child and Adolescent Psychiatrist Finder.

In addition to inquiring about trauma-informed services or specific treatment modalities as mentioned above, if you suspect that trauma may have *anything* to do with the adolescent's current concerning behavioral or emotional distress, ask potential providers if they have experience working with teens who may have been traumatized. Also, inquire if the providers incorporate working with a caregiver and other sources of supports for the teenager, as this should be a part of any good trauma therapy.

Table 2–1 describes specific individual and family treatments, and Table 2–2 describes group and school-based treatments. These tables do not list all treatments available but provide a summary of widely available, well-respected, evidence-based, trauma-focused treatments for teenagers.

The Role of Psychiatric Medications

Trauma-focused therapy, even when done with empathic, experienced clinicians, is not exactly fun or easy for adolescents. Confronting trauma is hard work at best and can at times be painful and difficult. Asking adolescents who have experienced trauma to engage in a therapy in which they will confront and discuss the most upsetting things they have experienced is like asking someone to get up and walk after they've broken their leg in two places. While doctors do push people to try to walk after a broken leg—slowly, in physical therapy—the doctors also often give them medication, such as anti-inflammatories or pain medication, to make that "try" possible. For youth experiencing severe posttraumatic symptoms, psychiatric medications can serve a similar function, to ease the most debilitating symptoms in order to make trying therapy possible.

Unfortunately, there is no one medication that addresses or targets the core symptoms of PTSD or other posttraumatic stress symptoms. Similarly, at the time of this writing, there are no medications that reverse or cure the effects of trauma on the brain. Different psychiatric medications can, however, be helpful to address specific symptoms. Choosing the right medication requires a balance of potential benefits and side effects. Talking with parents or guardians about a range of issues—the target symptoms, the risks and benefits of the medication, how to know if the medication is working, and how to know when the patient might be ready to go off the medication—helps the parents or guardians make an informed decision about consent for medication. The teen should be a part of this decision, too. Reversing the negative effects of trauma includes empowering adolescents to make safe and healthy decisions for their own bodies and minds. Giving them opportunities to understand, ask questions about, and make informed choices about medication lets them practice this safely while you communicate that you trust and care about their experience. Even if youth refuse or announce they are stopping medication, doing so is safer if they are honest and open about this with their prescriber than if they cheek the medication or stop it in secret.

Many of the chapters that follow will discuss specific medication classes that can be useful for the psychological symptoms that typically follow traumatic experiences. Briefly, medications are typically used to address either

TABLE 2–1.	Individual and family treatments					
	Trauma-Focused Cognitive Behavioral Therapy (TF-CBT)	Trauma System Therapy (TST)	Prolonged Exposure (PE)	Child-Parent Psychotherapy (CPP)	Cognitive Processing Therapy (CPT)	Eye Movement Desensitization and Reprocessing Therapy (EMDR)
What kind of treatment is this?	Combines trauma-sensitive interventions with CBT strategies Addresses difficulties related to traumatic life events	Uses a multidisciplinary team of providers to address both the teen's emotional needs and the environment in which he or she lives	A form of CBT Focuses on processing the traumatic event through remembering it and engaging with it, rather than avoiding it	Attachment-based treatment for teen parents with young children who have experienced trauma Focuses on ways the trauma has affected the parent-child relationship	A form of CBT Teaches how to evaluate and change upsetting thoughts since the trauma	A form of CBT Uses saccadic eye movements to promote learning and processing

TABLE 2–1.	Individual and family treatments (continued)				
	Trauma-Focused Cognitive Behavioral Therapy (TF-CBT)	Trauma System Therapy (TST)	Prolonged Exposure (PE)	Child-Parent Psychotherapy (CPP)	Cognitive Processing Therapy (CPT)	Eye Movement Desensitization and Reprocessing Therapy (EMDR)
What will the teen do?	Learn skills to regulate affect, behavior, thoughts, and relationships Process the trauma Enhance safety, trust, and communication (Caregiver will also learn parenting skills)	Identify links between triggering stimuli and the teen's symptoms or behaviors Learn skills to self-regulate (Caregivers learn how to help the teen self-regulate)	Talk about the trauma Start doing safe things that he or she has been avoiding	Learn safety and affect regulation skills, all with the goal of improving the relationship between the teen parent and the child and returning the child to a normal developmental trajectory	Talk about his or her thoughts associated with the trauma	Recount traumatic memories while focusing on following the therapist's finger with his or her eyes (or another physical sensation, like hand tapping) to stay grounded in the moment
Where does it take place?	Mental health clinics, hospitals, and community (foster care, home, schools, RTF, group settings)	Home- and community-based services	Mental health clinics, hospitals	Mental health clinics, hospitals, foster care agencies, schools, home and community	Mental health clinics, hospitals	Mental health clinics

TABLE 2-1. Individual and family treatments (continued)

	Trauma-Focused Cognitive Behavioral Therapy (TF-CBT)	Trauma System Therapy (TST)	Prolonged Exposure (PE)	Child-Parent Psychotherapy (CPP)	Cognitive Processing Therapy (CPT)	Eye Movement Desensitization and Reprocessing Therapy (EMDR)
How long does treatment last?	12–25 sessions (60–90 minutes each), divided equally between youth and parent or caregiver	Weekly or more frequent sessions for 7–9 months	Weekly sessions for about 3 months	Average of 50 sessions	Weekly sessions for about 3 months	Weekly sessions for 1–3 months
Whom may this be best for?	Appropriate for everyone (including teens with developmental delays) Requires caregiver's participation	Most appropriate for teens with chronic traumas Requires involvement of caregivers, providers, and others	Most appropriate for teens who have experienced a single traumatic experience Requires that the teen be living in a "safe" environment	Teenage parents (with children ages 0–6 years who have experienced trauma) who are committed to parenting for the "long run"	Most appropriate for teens who have experienced a single traumatic experience Requires that the teen be living in a "safe" environment	Most appropriate for teens who have experienced a single traumatic experience Requires that the teen be living in a "safe" environment

Note. CBT = cognitive behavioral therapy; RTF = residential treatment facility.

TABLE 2–2.   Group and school-based treatments

	Structured Psychotherapy for Adolescents Responding to Chronic Stress (SPARCS)	Skills Training in Affective and Interpersonal Regulation/ Narrative Story-Telling (STAIR/NST)	Cognitive Behavioral Intervention for Trauma in Schools (CBITS)	Adapted Dialectical Behavior Therapy for Special Populations (DBT-SP)
What kind of treatment is this?	A group therapy designed to address the needs of chronically traumatized teens who may still be living with ongoing stress and are experiencing problems in several areas of functioning	Group and/or individual therapy that is aimed to reduce symptoms of PTSD and other trauma-related symptoms, and builds and enhances specific social and emotional competencies	A skills-based group therapy that is aimed at relieving symptoms of PTSD, depression, and general anxiety among children and teens exposed to trauma	Family, group, and individual therapy that addresses general symptoms of trauma rather than being a method of processing a specific trauma
What will the teen do?	Learn to cope more effectively in the moment Enhance self-efficacy Connect with others for supportive relationships Cultivate awareness Create meaning	Learn emotion regulation skills, social skills, positive self-definition exercises, and goal-setting skills Process the traumas in detail and develop a positive life narrative	Receive education about reactions to trauma Learn relaxation techniques and problem-solving skills Process the trauma	Learn skills for emotion regulation, distress tolerance, relationship effectiveness, and mindfulness Not discuss the specific trauma

TABLE 2–2. Group and school-based treatments (*continued*)

	Structured Psychotherapy for Adolescents Responding to Chronic Stress (SPARCS)	Skills Training in Affective and Interpersonal Regulation/Narrative Story-Telling (STAIR/NST)	Cognitive Behavioral Intervention for Trauma in Schools (CBITS)	Adapted Dialectical Behavior Therapy for Special Populations (DBT-SP)
Where does it take place?	Mental health clinics, schools, group homes, boarding schools, residential treatment centers and facilities, and foster care	Mental health clinics, hospitals	Schools, mental health clinics	Mental health clinics, hospitals
How long does treatment last?	16 sessions	10 sessions (there is also an adapted version that is shorter)	10 sessions	Multiple times per week, for about 18 weeks
Whom may this be best for?	Appropriate for most typically developing teens	Appropriate for most typically developing teens	Most appropriate for younger teens	Most appropriate for teens with acute behavioral concerns such as self-injurious or suicidal behaviors

Note.   PTSD=posttraumatic stress disorder.

fight-or-flight–related symptoms (e.g., anxiety, nightmares, mood swings, irritability, flashbacks) or freeze-related symptoms (e.g., depression). For anxiety, hyperarousal, and irritability, α-adrenergic agonists (e.g., clonidine, guanfacine) and β-blockers (e.g., propranolol) can be very effective,[5] without the abuse potential seen in other antianxiety medications (e.g., benzodiazepines). A related medication, prazosin, seems to specifically target nightmares.[6,7] When α-adrenergic and β-blocker medications have failed, atypical neuroleptic medications such as aripiprazole or risperidone may be used, although these can have a high side-effect burden and can worsen numbing.[8] Antidepressant selective serotonin reuptake inhibitors (SSRIs) can be useful when freeze-related symptoms become persistent and develop into a major depressive episode; keep in mind, however, that these medications do not have approval from the U.S. Food and Drug Administration for use in adolescent PTSD in the absence of a major depressive episode.

Remember that medication is an adjunct to therapy for PTSD and all psychiatric symptoms that follow trauma, something that can make therapy easier or more tolerable but that is not a cure in itself. Trauma-focused therapy, like physical therapy after a physical injury, is what helps teens get their strength back and feel safe getting back out into the world.

Getting Trained in Trauma-Informed Treatment

Clinicians, counselors, and caseworkers can receive specific training to improve their knowledge about trauma-informed treatment strategies and/or become certified in specific trauma therapies. There may be in-person trainings at a local school of counseling or social work, but there are also rich resources online and at the library.

The NCTSN Learning Center, a free online education program, provides everything from curricula, to webinars, conferences, and consultation on training and implementation initiatives. The Medical University of South Carolina offers free Web-based training in Trauma-Focused Cognitive Behavioral Therapy (TF-CBT) (see "Resources and Additional Reading").

Many evidence-based treatments have treatment manuals written by the developers of the treatments. Although reading such a treatment manual will not certify you in providing a particular treatment, most of the manuals are easily accessible and offer a comprehensive description of treatment delivery through activities and helpful vignettes.

Resources and Additional Reading

Screening Resources

Ask Suicide-Screening Questions (ASQ): https://www.nimh.nih.gov/news/science-news/ask-suicide-screening-questions-asq.shtml

Columbia-Suicide Severity Rating Scale (CSSRS): http://cssrs.columbia.edu

CRAFFT Screening Tool for substance abuse: http://www.ceasar-boston.org/CRAFFT

Guide to Trauma-Informed Screening and Assessment (screening tools): http://www.nctsn.org/resources/topics/trauma-informed-screening-assessment/trauma-screening

Patient Health Questionnaire–9 (PHQ-9) screen for depression: http://www.phqscreeners.com

Treatment Manuals

Briere JN, Lanktree CB: Treating Complex Trauma in Adolescents and Young Adults. Los Angeles, CA, Sage, 2012

Cohen JA, Mannarino AP, Deblinger E: Treating Trauma and Traumatic Grief in Children and Adolescents, 2nd Edition. New York, Guilford, 2006

Saxe GN, Ellis BH, Brown AD: Trauma Systems Therapy for Children and Teens, 2nd Edition. New York, Guilford, 2016

Online Resources

The National Child Traumatic Stress Network Learning Center: https://learn.nctsn.org; see also http://www.nctsn.org/resources/training-and-implementation

Medical University of South Carolina TF-CBT Web 2.0: https://tfcbt2.musc.edu/

Additional Reading

Ford JD, Courtois CA (eds): Treating Complex Traumatic Stress Disorders in Children and Adolescents: Scientific Foundations and Therapeutic Models. New York, Guilford, 2013

Greenwald R: Child Trauma Handbook: A Guide for Helping Trauma-Exposed Children and Adolescents. New York, Routledge, 2005

Perry BD, Szalavitz M: The Boy Who Was Raised as a Dog: And Other Stories From a Child Psychiatrist's Notebook—What Traumatized Children Can Teach Us About Loss, Love, and Healing. New York, Basic Books, 2006

Silva PR: Posttraumatic Stress Disorder in Children and Adolescents Handbook. New York, WW Norton, 2004

Steele W, Malchiodi CA: Trauma-Informed Practices With Children and Adolescents. New York, Routledge, Taylor & Francis 2012

References

1. D'Andrea W, Ford J, Stolbach B, et al: Understanding interpersonal trauma in children: why we need a developmentally appropriate trauma diagnosis. American Journal of Orthopsychiatry 82(2):187–200, 2012

2. Ford JD, Grasso D, Greene C, et al: Clinical significance of a proposed developmental trauma disorder diagnosis: results of an international survey of clinicians. J Clin Psychiatry 74(8):841–849, 2013 24021504

3. Cook JM, Newman E: A consensus statement on trauma mental health: the New Haven Competency Conference process and major findings. Psychological Trauma: Theory, Research, Practice, and Policy 6(4):300–307, 2014

4. Cook A, Blaustein M, Spinazzola J, et al: Complex trauma in children and adolescents. National Child Traumatic Stress Network Complex Trauma Task Force, 2003. Available at: https://nursebuddha.files.wordpress.com/2011/12/complex-trauma-in-children.pdf. Accessed February 27, 2018.

5. Lubit RH, Giardino ER: Posttraumatic stress disorder in children: treatment and management. Medscape 2016. Available at: http://emedicine.medscape.com/article/918844-treatment#d9. Accessed February 27, 2018.

6. Akinsanya A, Marwaha R, Tampi RR: Prazosin in children and adolescents with posttraumatic stress disorder who have nightmares: a systematic review. J Clin Psychopharmacol 37(1):84–88, 2017 27930498

7. Kung S, Espinel Z, Lapid MI: Treatment of nightmares with prazosin: a systematic review. Mayo Clin Proc 87(9):890–900, 2012 22883741

8. van der Kolk BA: The Body Keeps the Score: Brain, Mind, and Body in the Healing of Trauma. New York, Viking, 2014

PART 1

Working With Symptoms of Traumatic Stress

CHAPTER 3

Aggression

Jennifer Cabrera, M.D.
Jessica Linick, Ph.D.

Kevin, age 15, is admitted to juvenile detention for a felony. This is Kevin's first time in "juvie," though he has been in foster care and residential treatment programs since he was age 3 and had run away from a residential facility a few weeks before his arrest. His charge, robbery in the first degree, came after police arrested him for stealing at gunpoint an expensive winter coat off an elderly man on the street. When Kevin enters juvenile detention, he is guarded and emotionally shut down and doesn't speak to many people. The other kids find him "weird" and "too quiet." They watch as Kevin sits alone in the cafeteria, eyes darting to take in his surroundings, seeming on high alert at all times. He gets in trouble often for not following rules, and the staff roll their eyes at Kevin when he seems set on disobeying even simple instructions and basic routines. Though he projects a cold indifference, he sometimes becomes explosively angry and gets into a lot of fights with peers and the staff. A month into his stay, he has had so many fights that staff start to question what is really going on with him. But whenever they talk to him, Kevin acts like he doesn't care and shows little remorse for his behaviors. He says he "blacks out" and doesn't remember what sets him off or what he's done. His legal aid social worker warns Kevin that his poor behavior in detention will prevent him from getting released. She wants to believe there's more to Kevin than cold-hearted anger and aggression but isn't sure what lies beneath it all. When she tries to find out more about him and help him with his case, he won't talk to her, saying, "Nah, Miss, I don't talk about that."

Many of us, as therapists, teachers, psychiatrists, probation officers, judges, parents, and counselors, see kids with aggressive behaviors. These can range from overblown tantrums in which a teen screams obscenities and slams doors, to destruction of property, to threatening behavior and violence toward others. When we see teens with these aggressive behaviors, we fear that these youth might be on a path like Kevin's and wonder if it can be averted. When a teen shows a persistent pattern of aggression, especially with little remorse or response to consequences, we may fear that the teen is a psychopath—someone unable to feel empathy, someone who enjoys hurting others, someone beyond help.

Yet, most teens with aggressive behavior do not end up escalating to violent crime or juvenile detention, and most aggressive youth are aggressive for reasons that have nothing to do with psychopathy. Often, aggression is rooted in trauma. Understanding different types of aggression and where they come from can help us treat teens more effectively to stop violent behaviors in the future.

Take a moment to think about the aggressive youth that you've worked with. Answer these three questions:

- What have been their major challenges?

- What situations in their lives (e.g., family circumstances, community issues, mental health issues) might be impacting their behavior?

- How well do the interventions you have in place target all these issues?

Before his placement in juvenile detention, Kevin had run away from his residential treatment program for about 2 months. When he left, Kevin thought that he'd be able to go back to his old neighborhood and find somewhere to stay. But when he got there, things didn't go as planned. He spent most of those first few weeks on the street or sleeping on the subway. He kept running into Joey, a kid he used to know from the neighborhood, who always seemed to have money and helped Kevin out a few times with a meal or a drink. Kevin knew that Joey, now age 19, had been in trouble with the law, but it was nice to have the help. After a few weeks, Joey convinced Kevin to join his "crew" and told him he'd be able to "make some easy money" by selling drugs. Joey got Kevin his first gun, showed him the ins and outs of the drug game, and soon had Kevin stealing or beating up other kids at Joey's command. Kevin was scared initially, but what he was doing wasn't that much more frightening than some of what he'd seen in foster care, plus it gave him a path toward the money and freedom that he'd always wanted. He knew that what he was doing was wrong, but he initially told himself the risk was worth it to save up some money and get out of the foster care system. Eventually, however, the guilt got so bad that he left the gang—landing back on the street, homeless, cold, and with no family. One night, Kevin was so cold that he tried to steal a coat from someone on the street. He used the gun that Joey had given him and threatened to shoot the man if he screamed. He thought he would feel bad about robbing an old guy, but he'd gotten so used to pushing his feelings away that

---

TABLE 3–1. Categorizing aggression

Level	Type, severity, and frequency of aggression acts.
	Types of aggression include yelling/cursing, verbal threats, destruction of property, and aggression to others. Aggression can also be covert (hidden, such as stealing or fraud) or relational (targeting the victim's social relationships, such as spreading rumors, social exclusion, cyberbullying).
Pattern	Type of aggression and places(s) where it occurs.
Persistence	Length of time the behavior persists (e.g., weeks, months, years).
Impact	Teen's impairment, and harm to others.

---

he didn't feel anything. He found an alley and lay down to sleep. Hours later, police shook him awake, arrested him, and brought him to detention.

Not all aggressive behavior is psychopathic or even pathological or abnormal. Most of us have had moments when we've been aggressive in self-defense, or when we were pushed to the point of screaming, yelling, or cursing at someone; throwing something; or even hitting someone. Aggressive behavior in teens is also very common; up to 50% of parents report that their children have shown some antisocial behaviors or conduct problems, ranging from oppositionality and verbal threats, to physical violence with a weapon, sexual assault, or homicide.[1,2] These behaviors are extremely costly at the personal, familial, and societal levels. Aggressive youth are often socially isolated and can be held back in (or kicked out of) school, placed in foster care or residential treatment programs, or end up incarcerated. Understanding where aggressive behavior comes from, and helping teens make safer choices, can prevent these negative outcomes.

Because not all aggression is the same, when talking about aggressive behavior, it is best to be very specific in describing the level, pattern, persistence, and impact of the behavior (Table 3–1).

It is also important to distinguish *reactive* from *proactive* or *instrumental aggression*. Aggressive behaviors, like all other behaviors, are either a reaction to something (reactive aggression) or a means to an end (proactive aggression). Reactive aggression is an impulsive, almost automatic reaction to a perceived threat. Proactive aggression is planned, premeditated, and goal directed, sometimes to get something tangible, such as someone's new sneakers or wallet, or something intangible, such as personal satisfaction or revenge. The plan may be loose and not well thought out, and may even be somewhat impulsive, but continues to be motivated by a goal and is not in reaction to a threat. It is important to look at the context of any aggressive behaviors to figure out whether they are reactive or proactive. For example, a kid's saying "I'm gonna kill you" after someone punches him is reactive, whereas saying "I'm gonna kill you" to scare someone into handing over a wallet is proactive. Kids can show one or both types of aggression. Youth diagnosed with conduct disorder show a more severe and persistent pattern of aggressive behavior, but not all youth with aggressive behavior meet criteria for conduct disorder. In fact, within the general population, the incidence of conduct disorder is quite low, with 1-year prevalence estimates ranging from 2% to more than 10%, with a median of 4%.[1]

Most people think that premeditated violence is perpetrated only by cold, unemotional, or "evil" individuals, and that only psychopaths, serial killers, and "superpredators" would ever plan or conspire to violate the rights of another. But premeditated aggression can also come out of desperation, or might be the way that a child learned to solve problems in his family or community as he grew up. *Most youth who engage in repeated aggressive or criminal behavior have experienced childhood trauma, ranging from family and community violence to abuse to attachment disruption from foster care placements.*[3,4] Researchers have found that a large number of violent individuals whom clinicians would call "psychopaths"—someone unable to feel empathy, someone who enjoys hurting others, someone beyond help—have experienced severe trauma.[5,6] Researchers have even started to distinguish between two variants of psychopathy: *primary psychopathy*, which is thought to be genetic, and *secondary psychopathy*, which emerges out of childhood abuse and trauma.[7] This distinction is important. When aggressive teens and young adults are labeled as conduct disordered or psychopathic, they are written off as having no hope of rehabilitation. They do not receive trauma-focused treatment that might address the underlying symptoms and change their behavior. If we recognize that aggression—and even psychopathy—can be secondary to childhood trauma, we can find treatments that help.

> *Most youth who engage in repeated aggressive or criminal behavior have experienced childhood trauma.* Prevention, early recognition, and appropriate treatment of early childhood trauma and attachment-related issues can have a profound impact on both aggressive behavior and the overall well-being of these youth. Effective interventions for aggressive youth also have widespread impact on their families, communities, and society as a whole (e.g., costs of incarceration, lost productive years for young people, poverty, community violence, intergenerational transmission of trauma).

Youth with aggressive behavior (particularly those with behaviors severe enough to meet criteria for disruptive behavior disorder or to lead to incarceration) have high rates of trauma exposure and posttraumatic stress disorder (PTSD). Up to 70% of incarcerated youth report exposure to trauma,[8] compared with 25% of the general population.[9] Exposure to community violence has been shown to increase the odds of developing conduct disorder by two to four times.[10,11] Sexual abuse,[12] physical abuse,[13] and domestic violence[12] have all been shown to predict conduct disorder. For youth who have been diagnosed with conduct disorder, the likelihood of also receiving a formal diagnosis of PTSD ranges from 13% to 27% in females and from 3% to 7% in males.[8] These prevalence rates illustrate that, as discussed in Chapter 1 ("Teens and Traumatic Stress"), the effects of childhood trauma are broader than classic PTSD. Following childhood trauma, youth do not "look" like classic PTSD sufferers, and many are never diagnosed with PTSD, even if their symptoms are rooted in their experiences of trauma. This can be particularly true for boys, who often show externalizing behaviors (aggression, oppositionality) after trauma, whereas girls tend to show the internalizing problems (anxiety and depression) that people associate with trauma.

Most of the aggressive, criminally involved teens in the juvenile justice system come from communities affected by poverty, community violence, and intergenerational trauma. Historically, race, culture, politics, and socioeconomics were not given enough credit for the role they played in mental health and mental illness, especially in young people. There is no group of youth for whom this is truer than those who present with disruptive behavior, aggression, and criminality.

Understanding "Juvie"

Juvenile detention ("juvie") is the equivalent of *jail* or *prison* for youth, where youth are housed after being charged with a crime, either before being found guilty (before conviction and sentencing) or, in some states, after sentencing. In the adult correctional system, *prison* is the term used in the United States to denote where a convicted person goes to serve time. For youthful offenders these facilities are often called *placements, youth correctional facilities,* or *youth development centers.*

Asking Why: How Trauma Can Lead to Aggression and Criminality

For the first 3 years of his life, Kevin was raised by his mother, Sheila. She was 17 years old when Kevin was born. She had a history of drug use and was in an abusive relationship with Kevin's father, Jose. Jose was a drug dealer who, shortly after Kevin's birth, was sentenced to 25-to-life for murdering a rival gang member. Sheila was uncertain if she wanted a baby but was afraid to disobey Jose, who wanted a child. Sheila also liked the idea that a child would love her unconditionally, something she had never felt growing up. But when Kevin was born, it wasn't what Sheila expected. She struggled with the constant crying. She tried to soothe Kevin but felt rejected when he continued to fuss. She felt like a failure as a mother, and his angry screaming reminded her of Jose. To cope, she began drinking and smoking, first marijuana then crack cocaine, and before long she was addicted, spending any money she had on drugs instead of diapers. By the time Kevin was a toddler, their one-room apartment was dirty and disorganized, with barely any safe space for Kevin to play. Men were in and out of the apartment, and sometimes Sheila had sex with them for money. A few of them would hit her. She often felt depressed, sometimes wondering if she had made a mistake by having Kevin.

Sheila loved Kevin, but didn't know how to handle him, especially when he got sad or angry. When he cried, she didn't know how to comfort him effectively. At other times she would ignore him, fed up that a toddler required so much attention. Sometimes she felt like he hated her or did things to spite her, like poop in his diaper immediately after she'd changed him. Sometimes his crying made her angry, and she would yell or hit him. For Kevin, Sheila became an unpredictable source of safety and fear. When he was scared he would freeze, unsure whether to run away from or toward her, never certain which "mom" she would be today. Around his third birthday, a neighbor called child protective services (CPS) after noticing a quarter-size bruised welt on Kevin's cheek. CPS found out about Sheila's drug problems and prostitution. Kevin was removed from Sheila's care and placed in kinship foster care with his paternal grandmother, Felicia, a woman he had never met before.

Risk for aggression and criminal behavior can be thought of on several levels: genetic, family, community, and societal. Before he was even born, Kevin was at increased risk because of his parents' history of substance abuse, violence, criminality, and incarceration. Kevin's early upbringing put him at increased risk as well. During early childhood, parents and caregivers teach children how to self-soothe and regulate their emotions. As the caregiver responds to the baby's needs, soothes negative emotions, and shares in positive emotions, the baby learns to understand his or her feelings. From these early caregiver experiences, an infant learns whether others can be trusted for comfort or should be feared. For example, children who are afraid of something will run to a parent or caregiver, who comforts them and teaches them skills to lessen fear and anxiety within themselves. But, as in Kevin's case, if the parent or caregiver is not consistently safe or comforting, or if the adult makes the child feel ashamed of his or her emotions, the child is forced to learn to deal with painful emotions alone. Children whose caregivers are neglectful or abusive learn to numb themselves or dissociate, or if they are unable to do so, they may fly into inconsolable rages. Once these patterns are learned, they are hard to break. Even if a safe and caring person tries to console the child, the youngster doesn't know how to feel safe with this response and may reject or even hit the new caregiver. These behaviors are called *disorganized attachment*, and without specific treatment, the inability to manage painful emotions and to trust others to help persists into adolescence and even adulthood.

> Felicia was already taking care of Kevin's five cousins (all teenagers) and resented having to take care of a toddler. She was tired of taking in her children's children. But she needed the money and knew that CPS would pay her to care for him. She wasn't worried about the home visits. She had grown up in the system, too, and knew that the caseworkers were so busy that they'd only stop by for a few minutes. The children knew better than to say anything.
>
> Felicia didn't have time to potty train Kevin, so she kept him in diapers as long as she could. To save money, she usually didn't change a diaper until she absolutely had to, so Kevin often had diaper rash. Doctors just thought he was "sensitive," as Felicia assured them that she changed him on time. Felicia usually kept the kids locked in their rooms after dark, when her friends would come over to smoke weed, drink, and hang out. The loud noises always scared Kevin, and he would spend hours hiding under his bed. If he cried, Felicia would come into the room, smack him, and tell him to "shut the fuck up." Even after he'd outgrown diapers, Felicia kept Kevin locked in his room at night and wouldn't let him out to use the bathroom, so he was forced to urinate or defecate on the floor. Felicia was infuriated by this behavior, and would punish him with a smack and by locking him in the dirty room for ever longer periods of time, often without food or water. The youngest of his cousins would sometimes try to help by slipping him slices of American cheese under the door.
>
> As Kevin got older, he grew more and more withdrawn, and by the time he entered grade school, he barely spoke. His first teachers described him as painfully quiet, unable to focus or sit still. Report cards noted that Kevin struggled with social development. He had no friends, and he would laugh when a peer fell down on the playground, then show no emotion when that child started to cry. One guidance counselor wondered if Kevin was autistic, because he was so behind socially and verbally and engaged in weird behav-

iors like hiding in the classroom or stealing food from the trash. She recommended that Kevin be "tested," but Felicia refused, saying she didn't want him to be "labeled." As he got older he started acting out in school, getting into fights, disrespecting teachers, and refusing to do his work.

Kevin's difficulties continued into third grade, when he became an easy target for bullies. Outside the earshot of teachers, kids would make fun of Kevin for wearing the same clothes every day. Another recurrent taunt—"You're so stupid, you can't even read"—was in part true, as Kevin lagged behind in both reading and writing. These insults would make Kevin feel angry and humiliated. Sometimes he would lash out, but other times he felt so mad that he couldn't move or speak. Teachers perceived his reactions as mood swings and unpredictable aggression and recommended that Felicia take Kevin for a psychiatric evaluation. Kevin was diagnosed with bipolar disorder and started on antipsychotic medication, which made him feel slow and disconnected and always, always hungry. The medication did little to change his behavior, though. Eventually Kevin was transferred to a middle school for students with behavior problems. There, fights were a daily occurrence, and any kids perceived as weak immediately became targets for abuse. Kevin kept to himself socially and never demonstrated any emotion that might make him seem weak. He quickly learned to fight anyone who provoked him so he wouldn't be seen as an easy victim. After a year of constant "infractions" at school, Kevin was transferred to his first residential treatment program.

The ongoing abuse and neglect that Kevin experienced at Sheila's house, as well as the bullying and community violence in his school, are further risk factors for later aggression and criminal behavior. Each of these traumas and adverse childhood experiences—which also include poor supervision by and separation from primary caretakers, lack of family cohesion, community and school violence, and poverty—can lead to "classic" trauma-related symptoms such as flashbacks, nightmares, and mood changes. They can also lead to aggression. Traumatized youth who remain in abusive or neglectful households, are exposed to violent or delinquent peers, and are institutionalized are at particular risk for developing aggressive and criminal behavior.

Once Kevin was placed in the residential treatment program, Felicia said she "couldn't handle his behaviors anymore." He was discharged from the residential program to foster care with an older couple, Sam and Betty, who "seemed nice," as Kevin said. However, CPS didn't share any of Kevin's history or any advice on how to handle him outside of "call 911." Despite their best intentions, Sam and Betty were ill equipped to manage Kevin's behaviors. One day, after Betty criticized Kevin for leaving a mess in the kitchen, Kevin ran away from the house. When the police found him, he tried to fight the officer; he was placed in a hospital after just 2 weeks at Sam and Betty's home.

Kevin was discharged from the hospital to another residential program for adolescents, and it was there that he first encountered kids who embraced "street life." He saw how acting out got the other kids what they wanted, so Kevin started to "turn it up." He was oppositional and demanding with staff, and refused to follow the rules. He saw that the socially powerful teens bullied the weaker ones, so he started doing so as well. Bullying others made him feel powerful and in control for the first time in his life. He started "AWOLing" (running away from the facility) with the older boys. When he smoked weed offered by one boy, Kevin felt more relaxed than he had in years. He started AWOLing often to get high and numb himself against the sadness, fear, and pain that were otherwise always roiling inside him. His AWOLing meant that he fell further behind at school, but academics already felt impossible to him. Kevin had missed a lot of school when he lived with Felicia, so he had missed out on the basics, which made more advanced concepts really difficult. He also struggled to pay attention with so many other thoughts running through his mind. He wondered about Felicia and Sheila, sometimes daydreaming in class to the point that he forgot where he was. Teachers didn't seem to understand, and when he would try to explain that he felt like he wasn't even in the classroom, they'd reprimand him for "spacing out." Kevin wanted desperately to be a "normal" kid, but everything he felt, said, and did made him feel even more "broken." The only time he felt even the slightest bit in control of his life was when he was AWOL, high, or fighting. It was during an AWOL to his old neighborhood that Kevin was arrested, charged with a felony, and sent to juvenile detention.

Aggression, delinquency, and criminal behavior are the ultimate survival coping skills for abused teens. Behaviors that can help youth feel safe and protected in multiple ways include being cold and emotionally detached, argumentative and oppositional, verbally threatening and destructive of property, physically aggressive, and involved with the criminal justice system. Quite literally, running away from home or being in jail or the hospital takes an abused teen out of his or her traumatic environment. Being gang affiliated or having a reputation of being tough and quick to fight protects the youth from bullying and from getting jumped, mugged, or sexually assaulted. Aggression lets youth feel powerful, strong, and in control. A reputation for aggression also keeps prosocial peers and adults at bay. To adults, especially therapists, this behavior seems like a negative effect that the teen would want to change. However, for many aggressive youth, relationships with others have been a source of abuse, pain, and disappointment, not comfort. For them, keeping others at bay is a benefit, protecting the youth from feeling emotionally vulnerable or risking trusting others and then being hurt. The benefits of aggression and criminal behavior, to youth, include staving off negative feelings like loneliness, hopelessness, and despair;

feeling in charge of their own life and body; preventing further physical, emotional, and psychological injury; and being able to predict somewhat what will happen to them and in their lives on a day-to-day basis. When a child has grown up feeling like prey every waking minute, it is understandable that becoming a predator is the safer option.

Recognizing What's Happening in the Moment: Seeing the Triggers for Aggressive Behavior

Kevin's first few months in detention are really tough. He fights almost daily, and when he isn't fighting, he's waiting for the next battle. Kevin feels on edge all the time. Other kids' yelling and gestures feel like direct threats. When fights break out, Kevin either freezes like a deer in headlights or joins the brawl. He can never predict which side of himself will show up, which makes him feel out of control. Staff often have to restrain Kevin. Feeling their hands on his body triggers flashbacks to his earlier abuse, and he often kicks, punches, and bites detention staff. Whenever the staff tries to talk to Kevin about his anger, he closes up and acts like he doesn't care. "It doesn't matter to me if I hurt anyone; it doesn't matter to me how they feel." Truth is, Kevin often doesn't even remember what he has done, and rarely does he really understand what has set him off.

For Kevin, the worst part of detention is being locked in his room at night. Kevin has frequent nightmares, and when he wakes in the middle of the night, he is often unsure of where he is or what is happening. In the morning, staff sometimes find milk cartons full of urine in his room. Not knowing his trauma history, they laugh at him and say, "He must be crazy. Why didn't he just ask to use the bathroom?" Kevin sometimes wonders if they were right.

Aggressive behaviors in youth like Kevin often appear to come "out of nowhere," leading adults to worry that the aggression is unprovoked and either psychotic or psychopathic. But most, if not all, aggressive behavior is prompted by some trigger. For traumatized youth, triggers are often connected to their trauma history. Triggers can be literally anything—a smell, a song, someone who looks like their perpetrator, a setting similar to where the abuse occurred. The trigger can be a benign or neutral thing, such as an adult's supportive hand on the teen's shoulder, which can be misinterpreted by the traumatized teen's overactive threat detector (amygdala) and cause a fight-or-flight response. The trigger can even be an event that seems positive, such as praise or a reward for good behavior, or another teen getting a visit from family, or an adult making a caring gesture. Such events can remind traumatized youth of what they didn't have before, or what they're afraid to get used to because they know the caring person will eventually leave them too. Although it can be hard to identify triggers, helping teens to identify them can alleviate symptoms and let the youth feel more in control of themselves. Knowing Kevin's background, we can recognize reasons underlying some of his triggers in detention: being locked in his room (reminding him of being locked away at Felicia's), staff saying he must be "crazy," being restrained, and being around a lot of other dysregulated youth.

Finding the Frame: Understanding and Connecting With Youth With Aggressive Behavior

Taking on cases like Kevin's can feel daunting and at worst hopeless. Adults working with traumatized youth often begin to feel helpless in the face of so much adversity and such intense behaviors. These adults often ask common questions: Where do I begin? How can I ever understand her? How can I work with him when I'm afraid of him? What do I do with my own feelings? Why would this kid trust me of all people?

We have reason to be hopeful, however. The study of resilience tells us that there is one major difference between those youth who overcome hardship and thrive in the face of adversity, and those who don't. That difference is *connectedness*—to school, community, family, and prosocial peers.[14] It may take only one person who shows an interest, one person who goes the extra mile, one person who remains a consistent support. Finding a way to connect with aggressive traumatized youth like Kevin can make a lasting impact.

Connecting with youth like Kevin starts with *empathy*. When we discuss having empathy for our youth, we do not just mean having the ability to put oneself in their shoes; we mean having a true sense of nonjudgmental curiosity about their experience. We can never begin to truly "know" a youth's personal experiences, but we can curiously approach each individual, in a detective-like way, without judgment, and without giving the impression that we know more than the youth does. By initially meeting youth in this way, we help them to let down their defenses and start to explore their experiences together with us. We move from a place of wondering "What's wrong with this youth" to "What happened to this youth?" Especially for aggressive youth, who are accustomed to people staying away or making up their own interpretations of their behavior, this shift in approach can be incredibly powerful.

To understand and connect with a youth, start with simply asking questions. When a youth has an outburst, once he or she has calmed down, you can ask, for example, "I wonder what that was about?" (Do not ask "What were you thinking?" which sounds judgmental and assumes the teen was "thinking" when he or she was likely on trauma autopilot or in the midst of a flashback.) This type of questioning accomplishes many things: not only are you nonjudgmentally asking the youth for his or her opinion, but you're also encouraging the youth to reflect on his or her behavior, which fosters a process called *mentalizing*,[15] or making sense of the thoughts and feelings of ourselves and others. Mentalizing can be challenging for traumatized youth, but especially for those with developmental trauma or disorganized attachment. Empathy and curiosity *must* come from an authentic place, because teens have a special radar for adults whom they feel are "bullshitting" them. Traumatized youth will immediately recognize someone who is not being "real" with them. If you are not being honest, or are trying to "sugarcoat" things, you will disillusion these youth rather than build the trust they fear but desperately need.

Aggressive youth also need to know that you are in control and are not afraid of them—either their behavior or their trauma history. You can empathize with them and help them understand the triggers and emotions behind their aggression without condoning the behavior. In a nonjudgmental way, let them know what your limits are, and which behaviors are acceptable and which are not. Asking about their trauma history shows that you won't be horrified or frightened by what has happened to them. Too often, adults can't handle the truth of what has happened to kids, and this makes kids feel broken and ashamed. Shame is often a silent force behind much aggressive behavior. Shame leaves us feeling powerless. The antidote to feeling powerless is to try to engender power in any way possible, and violence is a great shortcut to power.

> Remember there is a big difference between shame and guilt. *Guilt* is a reflection of our behavior, meant to show us that what we *did* was wrong. *Shame* tells us that who we *are* is wrong. Guilt makes us want to fix what we did; shame makes us want to disappear. Youth who have experienced trauma have often been shamed throughout their lives.

When teens have done something wrong, how do we correct them without shaming? Although we can't shy away from addressing their behavior, we should be careful to make clear that we are disappointed at *what* they did, not about them as people. They are not "bad," even though they messed up this time, and we want to help them learn a different way to act. Support them using strategies that help minimize shame and that discourage any potential feeling of "I am bad." Engage them in positive interactions, laughing together, making eye contact with them, and resuming usual activities as appropriate. When discussing their behavior and setting consequences, remain empathic and help them think of what they can do to correct the behavior, make amends, or repair a relationship (e.g., apologize, write a letter, fix or replace something broken; see discussion of *restorative justice* in Chapter 11, "School Systems and Trauma"). Help them with problem solving around preventing future negative behavior, and if you see them avoid a negative reaction at some later date, be sure to acknowledge it and provide positive feedback!

If you yourself are feeling triggered, threatened, or angry, and are not yet ready to work on the correction, give yourself some time to calm down and regulate your own emotions. Authenticity is key when working with teens, and role-modeling self-care can be just as valuable as teaching them that correction does not mean criticism. Feedback can and should be delivered without shame, so be sure you are in the right mindset, and the right time and place, to help youth learn from their mistakes.[16]

In working with aggressive youth who have experienced trauma, we'll often notice days when they act friendlier to us than others; one day a youth will sit next to us and discuss some deep issues, and other times the youth will ignore us. Some of this is normal teenage behavior, but also traumatized youth often have significant ambivalence around trust and relationships. It is important for the adults to remain *consistent*. Again, shame is important here. It can be very easy to shame someone when their behavior is unpredictable and frequently changing (e.g., "Justin, what's wrong with you? You didn't act this way yesterday!"). The notion that something is "wrong" with them is a concept these youth know all too well—so again, avoid asking, "What's wrong with you?" and instead try to get answers to these questions: "What happened to this youth that might make him act this way?" or "What's different today that might have triggered her, when yesterday she was fine?" Don't take the teen's behavior personally. This is particularly hard when working with aggressive youth, whose verbal or physical actions can evoke fear, anxiety, or anger in the adults around them, but it is vitally important.

Tony is a direct care staff member at the detention facility. For some reason, Tony doesn't find Kevin as "scary" or "crazy" as the other staff make him out to be. To Tony, Kevin just seems like a kid who has had it rough, a kid who is scared and needs his help. During Kevin's first few months in detention, Tony does what he can to support him. He checks in on him daily and tries to engage him with playing basketball or chess or rapping. Tony praises Kevin when he sees the boy keep his emotions in check or avoid a fight. When Kevin begins opening up about his past, Tony listens and doesn't judge. Instead, he just asks, "What was that like?" For Kevin, Tony was one of the first male role models he had ever had—one of the first men in his life who hadn't left him, hurt him, or made him feel like something was wrong with him.

Tony feels pretty good about his relationship with Kevin. But one day, Kevin gets into an argument with another youth over a video game. Tony tries to deescalate the situation so that it doesn't get any worse. "Man, you're so mad, I see that," he says to Kevin, empathizing with and putting words to Kevin's emotions. He gets Kevin's attention and is starting to walk him away from the conflict when the other teen shouts something about Kevin "not having a family." Kevin turns and lunges at the other boy. Tony and another staff grab them and put both youth into physical restraints. As Tony holds the screaming, thrashing Kevin, all of a sudden Kevin turns and bites Tony's arm, hard—so hard, in fact, that Tony has to leave in the middle of his shift to go to the ER. When asked about it later, Kevin says that he had "blacked out" and didn't remember biting Tony at all.

That evening, after learning how badly he'd hurt Tony, Kevin feels sick with guilt and shame. He is sure that Tony will never speak to him again. He hates himself for hurting Tony, hates himself for getting attached to Tony, and hates Tony for making him feel this way.

When Tony returns several hours later from the ER and comes to talk to Kevin, Kevin is distant, even hostile. This surprises Tony; he thought he and Kevin had a connection and expected some kind of remorse. Tony tells Kevin that he understands why Kevin reacted the way he did and that he is trying hard not to take it personally. He tells Kevin that even though he feels angry about having been bitten, it doesn't mean that he doesn't still care about Kevin. Kevin visibly softens as Tony speaks. Kevin shares his feelings of shame and how he feels that if he hurt Tony, the first person in a while to be nice to him, then he must be too "fucked up to be with people." Tony doesn't dismiss this feeling by saying "no, that's silly," but he doesn't agree with it either. He validates Kevin's feelings and points out how the bad things Kevin has experienced could make him feel that way. Tony tells Kevin about other kids he had worked with in the past who had struggled with anger and aggression and who had been helped by therapy. Tony takes the opportunity to remind Kevin about the therapist working in detention. Kevin, who had been refusing therapy for months despite his lawyer telling him it was a prerequisite for his release, agrees to try it out.

One of the hardest parts of working with aggressive kids is managing aggressive behavior acutely "in the moment." With a few techniques and a little luck, we can deescalate the situation: help the kid calm down, take a breath, and return to baseline—and maybe even learn from the experience.

If you are working with a youth whom you can see is just *starting* to get triggered, or who has begun some minor aggressive behavior (e.g., throwing things), then basic verbal and environmental deescalation techniques can go a long way. When a situation becomes truly dangerous, such as when there is a physical fight between youth, more formal crisis intervention plans may need to be implemented. Many crisis prevention programs have been developed for use with law enforcement and in prisons or juvenile detention centers. Remember, though, that these interventions may not take trauma into account, and therefore may further trigger the aggressive teen. Formal training in trauma-informed crisis intervention programs would benefit schools, residential centers, foster care agencies, and, we would suggest, even parents and caregivers of aggressive youth with histories of trauma. Many begin with verbal and environmental deescalation, but they also include physical techniques to intervene and sometimes therapeutically hold or restrain someone who is at risk for causing serious harm to self or others. Therapeutic Crisis Intervention (TCI)[17] and the Crisis Prevention Institute's Nonviolent Crisis Intervention[18] are two evidence-based programs that involve multi-day instruction. Note that no intervention can be safely or effectively implemented unless all team members are fully trained and practicing the techniques regularly; this is especially true for any program that involves therapeutic holds or physical restraints to intervene during an episode of acute aggression.

Remember from Chapter 1 that when kids are triggered, their frontal cortex—the region that neuroscientist Dan Siegel calls the "upstairs brain,"[19] which is responsible for reasoning, logic, and planning—goes offline. Trying to reason with them or talk to them is usually ineffective. What we need to do first is *connect* to their "downstairs brain" (the limbic system, especially the amygdala) that has become activated by the trauma trigger, while trying to help their upstairs brain to turn back on. Here are some tips for doing that:

First, and above all, give the kid space

- Avoid touching unless it is absolutely necessary (i.e., if the kid is an immediate danger to self or someone else). If the teen is just going to throw some books at the wall and is not hurting anyone, giving space is probably more effective (and safer) than trying to restrain him or her, which can be triggering and worsen the aggressive behavior.

Keep yourself calm

- Use whatever strategies you can to keep yourself in check and keep your own upstairs brain online. Remember the safety instructions on airplanes that you should put on your own oxygen mask before trying to assist others. That applies here, too!

Connect with the downstairs brain

- Mind your nonverbal communication and body language: use a calm voice, maintain a nonthreatening stance, nod, and use eye contact to show empathy.
- Avoid getting too close—keep a distance so that the youth does not feel threatened. If the teen is sitting, get on his or her level rather than hovering above, which can feel threatening.
- Speak in short, concise phrases. Be clear and direct.
- Remind the youth that he or she is safe with you.

Try to turn on the upstairs brain

- Ask questions: "What happened?" or "How can I help?"
- Validate the experience or emotion. Remember, validation is *not* approval. It is just a reflection of what you see. Marsha Linehan, the great dialectical behavior therapy pioneer, reminds us that we do not need to get it right for it to be effective. A simple statement, such as "Justin, it sounds like you're frustrated that you got the answer wrong," helps even if Justin turns around and says, "No, I'm pissed about this other thing!" Even if you are wrong, you have shown Justin that you care enough to think about his perspective and invite him to tell his story, which hopefully turns on his upstairs brain.
- Use the youth's goals. Sometimes, reminding kids of their goals can be a really useful way to motivate them: "Justin, I know you really want to pass this class, so let's take a moment to go to the hall instead of fighting."
- Explain why you are asking the youth to do the thing you want him or her to do: "Justin, let's go to the hall so we have some privacy to talk about what happened."
- Give choices. Everyone appreciates choices. Rather than give a directive like "You need to leave this classroom now," offer a choice: "Justin, would you like to talk in the hall or in my office?" Choice implies respect, and gives the youth a sense of control. Inviting the youth to make a choice also activates the youth's upstairs brain in order to answer the question.

- Set clear limits and expectations. Be firm about what the youth *cannot* do: "I can see you're really angry, but we can't throw the books against the wall like that. Maybe we can go to my office to talk instead?"
- Identify the youth's strengths: "I know you're really frustrated right now, but you've managed to get through things like this before, so I know you can work with me and stay safe."

Invalidating, threatening, and overly simplistic reactions to aggression only serve to further escalate and make the problem worse. Some things you might want to *avoid* doing, when possible:

- Do NOT tell a youth to simply "calm down" or "relax."
- Do NOT invalidate an emotion ("Oh, that's nothing to be worried about").
- Do NOT shame the child. Saying things like "Justin, you're better than that" only makes the youth, who already feels badly about himself, feel worse.
- Do NOT threaten ("If you don't come with me, I'll have to call security/ write you up/call your mother").
- Do NOT use punitive language, insults, sarcasm, or put-downs ("Stop being such a baby; this isn't a big deal").
- Do NOT try to process or reflect upon or set a consequence for the problematic behavior when the youth is still upset. In the moment, deescalate the situation, and leave the rest for when the crisis is over.

Safety is always the first priority in a crisis. The second priority is learning. Verbal and environmental deescalation strategies teach youth to recognize their own triggers and emotions, express them safely (without violence), and think about others' perspectives. For example, when Tony is able to return to speak with Kevin, Kevin sees that relationships can have conflict and be repaired. Tony is honest with Kevin about his own feelings and empathizes with Kevin's feelings in the moment and in hindsight. This is important modeling for Kevin: showing that men can talk about feelings calmly and take responsibility for their mistakes. Tony also implicitly demonstrates that although he was disappointed in Kevin's behavior, he still believes in and cares about Kevin as a person. Remember the difference between guilt and shame, and don't underestimate the power of repairing trauma through new, nurturing relationships.

Treating More Than Just Behavior

Youth like Kevin are rarely referred for psychiatric intervention. If they are, mental health clinicians may not know the trauma history or may not bother to look beyond the immediate behaviors to consider or understand the core issues behind aggression and criminality. Often, too, earlier opportunities for prevention or early intervention for aggressive youth have been missed. Kevin's entire trajectory might have been changed had Sheila gotten parenting support and treatment for her own PTSD and addiction early on, so that she could have provided a supportive, caring home for Kevin and kept him out of foster care. Later, a more caring and therapeutic foster placement, school-based interventions, and trauma-focused therapy (instead of medications for his misdiagnosed bipolar disorder) could have reversed some of the damage of his early adversity and prevented the additional traumas he experienced in Felicia's care and at school.

Once a teen's aggressive behavior has reached the severity of Kevin's, the teen can get stuck in a useless (and expensive) cycle of repeated hospitalization, institutionalization, out-of-home placements, and incarceration. Although truly effective treatment is intensive, costly, and unfortunately often hard to come by, it can be transformative for youth like Kevin. The most evidence-based, successful treatments for delinquent behavior include Multisystemic Therapy (MST); Functional Family Therapy (FFT); and Multi-Dimensional Treatment Foster Care (MDTFC), also known as Treatment Foster Care Oregon model (TFCO). For teens who have experienced trauma, Trauma Systems Therapy (TST) is also highly effective. (See "Resources and Additional Reading" at the end of this chapter for a listing of online resources.)

Multisystemic Therapy

MST was developed for youth with severe antisocial behaviors. It is an intensive home- and community-based treatment for adolescents with a history of arrests, incarceration, aggression, violence, and criminal activity. MST focuses on keeping teens "at home, in school, and out of trouble."[20] Intensive wrap-around work with members of a teen's family, school, and neighborhood or community promotes prosocial behavior. Different therapeutic modalities are used to change the environmental factors that trigger or reinforce the youth's problem behaviors. Negative environmental factors can include conflicts or resentment in the family; lack of structure, routine, and rules; negative peer influences; alienation from school; poor conflict resolution or social skills (leading to youth turning to aggression to solve problems); and the absence of positive role models. MST therapists use a mix of cognitive behavioral therapy (CBT), family therapy, parent training, conflict resolution, and social skills/interpersonal skills training to focus on these different areas and to use the youth's (and the family's and/or community's) strengths to steer him or her toward prosocial goals.

Key Components of Multisystemic Therapy

Expand caretaker parenting skills.

Increase family functioning and improve family relationships.

Create a support network including extended family, neighbors, teachers, and friends.

Promote youth involvement with prosocial peers who do not participate in aggressive or criminal behavior.

Connect teens to school and vocational training programs.

Link adolescents to positive activities, including sports teams, school clubs, and neighborhood or community organizations (Big Brothers, Big Sisters; YMCA; Boys and Girls Club; Police Athletic League; spiritual or religious groups).

MST does not directly or explicitly address trauma, but the family- and community-level interventions within MST touch on traumatic experiences. MST addresses negative caretaker-teen interactions and parental substance use/abuse, improves family relationships through effective communication and decreased conflict, teaches parenting skills, and increases prosocial peer and community connections. These interventions can mitigate the negative outcomes of complex trauma, abuse, and neglect at the familial, relational, and community levels. Multisystemic Therapy for Child Abuse and Neglect (MST-CAN), a variant of MST developed to help families in which children are being abused and neglected, more directly addresses trauma. (For more information on MST-CAN, see "Resources and Additional Reading" at the end of this chapter.)

Once the youth is no longer engaging in acutely dangerous behaviors, transitioning from MST to a systems-based trauma treatment such as TST can further support the youth and family's recovery while providing a safe context to begin to explore trauma triggers, coping skills, and trauma exposure.

Functional Family Therapy

FFT is similar to MST in that treatment is geared toward the youth and to the family system as a whole. It is a short-term program (8–12 sessions of 1-hour duration) designed for youth at risk of being institutionalized for delinquent behavior. Like MST, FFT does not directly address trauma but is used to "assess family behaviors that maintain delinquent behavior, modify dysfunctional family communication, train family members to negotiate effectively, set clear rules about privileges and responsibilities, and generalize changes to community contexts and relationships."[21] Although less comprehensive than MST, FFT can also target education and job training/placement.

Multi-Dimensional Treatment Foster Care

MDTFC, now known as TFCO, is another effective intervention for adolescents with chronic antisocial behavior, emotional disturbance, and delinquency. Rather than providing services to a youth while he or she remains at home, MDTFC places youth with highly trained foster parents for approximately 6–8 months. Based on social learning theory, which posits that we learn how to "be" based on our social environment, MDTFC aims to reshape youth's behaviors by placing them in an environment that allows for change to occur more naturally. The biological/birth family receives parent training, support, and treatment, but does so with the child out of the home. Core components of MDTFC include "behavioral parent training and support for foster parents, family therapy for biological parents, skills training and supportive therapy for youth, and school-based behavioral interventions and academic support."[22]

Trauma Systems Therapy

Unlike the three modalities described above, TST is designed to directly target trauma. Similar to MST (another "systems" therapy), TST is a comprehensive, wrap-around treatment targeting what the authors call the "trauma system": both the traumatized child and the social environment (i.e., school, neighborhood, family, peer group[23]). The focus on the social environment is what makes TST different from other child-based trauma treatments (e.g., Trauma-Focused CBT). Because TST considers the social environment broadly (not just the immediate family), it can be used in residential programs, foster homes, even refugee centers. TST targets four main areas to help both the child and the family/social context: "the child's capacity to self-regulate, the family or social environment's ability to help him do that, the clinical team's ability to support the child and family, and the organization and service systems' ability to support the clinical team." TST can be used on the level of an individual child or family, and also on the level of an organization or service system looking to better serve traumatized youth broadly.

Choosing Among the Therapies

How do you choose among MST, FFT, MDTFC (TFCO), and TST? First, consider the youth's *presenting problems*. Is the youth aggressive? If so, how aggressive, and does the aggression lead to criminality? If the youth has a history of trauma, and the aggression is not too severe, TST may be effective. However, if the youth's aggression is severe or has expanded to other delinquent behavior (e.g., stealing, robbery), MST or FFT may be more appropriate. If the family environment is very problematic, or the youth may benefit from a brief stay outside the home to give parents time to work on their own personal issues, MDTFC (TFCO) may be appropriate.

Second, determine what therapies are *available* in your area. Resources in many areas are stretched, and these interventions are often costly, in terms of the time required for delivery to the family and youth, the level of training of the therapist or therapeutic team, and of course the financial cost of wrap-around services. Evaluate what is feasible, given the available resources, and go from there.

Lastly, evaluate the youth's and family's *desire to change*. How ready is the family or system for change? Are other things needed first, before a system-wide treatment can be effective? For some families struggling with addiction, for instance, sending a parent to rehabilitation may be an effective first-line intervention before involving one of the broader, systems-based treatments. Or maybe the family is struggling with food scarcity or unstable housing and will not be able to regularly attend sessions or focus on the content of treatment until these basic needs are met.

> Ensuring physical and psychological safety is a prerequisite to any meaningful treatment. Sometimes, providing resources for basic needs, such as food, clothing, shelter, or health insurance, can be the most important initial intervention for youth with conduct problems.

Take inventory of what a family really needs, and go from there. Remember that in the end, any intervention that is multifaceted and that targets many areas will be better than a stand-alone treatment, so do what you can. If none of these treatments are available in your area, ponder these questions: How can I work with what I have? How can I, as a single therapist, school counselor, probation officer, teacher, or physician involve more members of the child's social environment in helping him or her? It may be as simple as starting with a phone call.

Resources and Additional Reading

Evidence-Based Treatments for Aggression and Criminality

Aggression Replacement Training: https://www.crimesolutions.gov/
    ProgramDetails.aspx?ID=254
Functional Family Therapy: https://www.crimesolutions.gov/
    ProgramDetails.aspx?ID=122
Multi-Dimensional Treatment Foster Care (now known as TFCO): http:/
    /www.ncjfcj.org/multi-dimensional-treatment-foster-care-mtfc
Multisystemic Therapy: https://www.mstservices.com
Multisystemic Therapy for Child Abuse and Neglect (MST-CAN): http:/
    /mstservices.com/target-populations/chld-abuse-and-neglect.
Problem Solving Skills Training: http://www.cebc4cw.org/program/
    problem-solving-skills-training/detailed
Trauma Systems Therapy: http://www.nctsnet.org/sites/default/files/assets/pdfs/
    tst_general.pdf

Movies

Dangerous Minds (film)
Freedom Writers (film)
13th (documentary)

Additional Reading

Bernstein BE: Conduct disorder. Medscape, June 28, 2016. Available at: http://emed-
    icine.medscape.com/article/918213-overview#a5. Accessed February 28, 2018.
Burnette ML, Cicchetti D: Multilevel approaches toward understanding antisocial
    behavior: current research and future directions. Dev Psychopathol 24(3):703–
    704, 2012 22781849
Bushman BJ, Huesmann LR: Aggression, in Handbook of Social Psychology, 5th
    Edition. Edited by Fiske ST, Gilbert DT, Lindzey G. New York, Wiley, 2010,
    pp 833–863
Davis S, Jenkins G, Hunt R, et al: We Beat the Street: How a Friendship Pact Led
    to Success. New York, Penguin, 2006

Institute for Work and Health: What researchers mean by...primary, secondary, and tertiary prevention. April 2015. Available at: https://www.iwh.on.ca/wrmb/primary-secondary-and-tertiary-prevention. Accessed February 28, 2018.

Leap J: Jumped In: What Gangs Taught Me About Violence, Drugs, Love, and Redemption. Boston, MA, Beacon Press, 2012

Loeber R, Burke JD, Lahey BB, et al: Oppositional defiant and conduct disorder: a review of the past 10 years, part I. J Am Acad Child Adolesc Psychiatry 39(12):1468–1484, 2000 11128323

Moffitt TE, Arseneault L, Jaffee SR, et al: Research review: DSM-V conduct disorder: research needs for an evidence base. J Child Psychol Psychiatry 49(1):3–33, 2008 18181878

National Collaborating Centre for Mental Health (UK); Social Care Institute for Excellence (UK): Antisocial Behaviour and Conduct Disorders in Children and Young People: Recognition, Intervention, and Management (NICE Clinical Guidelines, No 158). British Psychological Society, 2013. Available at: https://www.ncbi.nlm.nih.gov/books/NBK327832/. Accessed February 28, 2018.

Phelan TW: 1, 2, 3 Magic: Effective Discipline for Children 2–12, 4th Edition, Revised. Glen Ellyn, IL, Parentmagic, 2010

Steiner H, Dunne JE: Summary of the practice parameters for the assessment and treatment of children and adolescents with conduct disorder. J Am Acad Child Adolesc Psychiatry 36(10)(Suppl):1482–1485, 1997 9334562

Thomas CR: Evidence-based practice for conduct disorder symptoms. J Am Acad Child Adolesc Psychiatry 45(1):109–114, 2006 16327588

van der Kolk BA: The Body Keeps the Score: Brain, Mind, and Body in the Healing of Trauma. New York, Viking, 2014

Weisz JR: Psychotherapy for Children and Adolescents: Evidence-Based Treatments and Case Examples. New York, Cambridge University Press, 2004

References

1. American Psychiatric Association: Diagnostic and Statistical Manual of Mental Disorders, 5th Edition. Arlington, VA, American Psychiatric Association, 2013

2. World Health Organization: World Report on Violence and Health: Summary. Geneva, World Health Organization, 2002

3. Aebi M, Mohler-Kuo M, Barra S, et al: Posttraumatic stress and youth violence perpetration: a population-based cross-sectional study, Eur Psychiatry 40:88–95, 2017 27992838

4. Becker SP, Kerig PK: Posttraumatic stress symptoms are associated with the frequency and severity of delinquency among detained boys. J Clin Child Adolesc Psychol 40(5):765–777, 2011 21916694

5. Dargis M, Newman J, Koenigs M: Clarifying the link between childhood abuse history and psychopathic traits in adult criminal offenders. Personal Disord 7(3):221–228, 221–228, 2016 26389621

6. Farina ASJ, Holzer KJ, Delisi M, Vaughn MG: Childhood trauma and psychopathic features among juvenile offenders. Int J Offender Ther Comp Criminol March 1, 2018 (ePub ahead of print) 29598432

7. Kimonis ER, Frick PJ, Cauffman E, et al: Primary and secondary variants of juvenile psychopathy differ in emotional processing. Dev Psychopathol 24(3):1091–1103, 2012 22781873

8. Bernhard A, Martinelli A, Ackermann K, et al: Association of trauma, posttraumatic stress disorder, and conduct disorder: a systematic review and meta-analysis. Neurosci Biobehav Rev S0149–7634(16):30341–30344, 2016 28017839

9. Copeland-Linder N: Posttraumatic stress disorder. Pediatr Rev 29(3):103–104, discussion 104, 2008 18310469

10. Fowler PJ, Tompsett CJ, Braciszewski JM, et al: Community violence: a meta-analysis on the effect of exposure and mental health outcomes of children and adolescents. Dev Psychopathol 21(1):227–259, 2009 19144232

11. Kersten L, Vriends N, Steppan M, et al: Community violence exposure and conduct problems in children and adolescents with conduct disorder and healthy controls. Front Behav Neurosci 11:219, 2017 29163090

12. Fergusson DM, Horwood LJ: Exposure to interparental violence in childhood and psychosocial adjustment in young adulthood. Child Abuse Negl 22(5):339–357, 1998 9631247

13. Malinosky-Rummell R, Hansen DJ: Long-term consequences of childhood physical abuse. Psychol Bull 114(1):68–79, 1993 8346329

14. Lösel F, Farrington DP: Direct protective and buffering protective factors in the development of youth violence. Am J Prev Med 43(2, Suppl 1):S8-S23, 2012 22789961

15. Bateman A, Fonagy P: Mentalization based treatment for borderline personality disorder. World Psychiatry 9(1):11–15, 2010 20148147

16. Hill D: Affect Regulation Theory: A Clinical Model. New York, WW Norton, 2015

17. The Residential Child Care Project: Therapeutic Crisis Intervention: A Reference Guide, 6th Edition. Ithaca, NY, Cornell University, 2009

18. Ryan J, Peterson R, Tetreault G, van der Hagen E: Reducing the use of seclusion and restraint in a day school program, in For Our Own Safety: Examining the High-Risk Interventions for Children and Young People. Edited by Nunno M, Day D, Bullard L. Washington, DC, Child Welfare League of America, 2008, pp 201–215

19. Siegel D, Bryson TP: The Whole Brain Child: 12 Revolutionary Strategies to Nurture Your Child's Developing Mind. New York, Delacorte Press, 2011

20. Blueprints for Healthy Youth Development: Multisystemic therapy. 2018. Available at: http://www.blueprintsprograms.com/fact-Sheet.php?pid=cb4e5208b4cd87268b208e49452ed6e89a68e0b8. Accessed February 28, 2018.

21. Blueprints for Healthy Youth Development: Functional family therapy. 2018. Available at: http://www.blueprintsprograms.com/evaluationAbstracts.php?pid=0a57cb53-ba59c46fc4b692527a38a87c78d84028. Accessed February 28, 2018.

22. Blueprints for Healthy Youth Development: Treatment Foster Care Oregon. 2018. Available at: http://www.blueprintsprograms.com/evaluation-abstract/treatment-foster-care-oregon. Accessed February 20, 2018.

23. Saxe GN, Ellis BH, Brown AD: Trauma Systems Therapy for Children and Teens. New York, Guilford, 2016

CHAPTER 4

Suicide and Self-Injury

Gabrielle Carson, Ph.D.

Kelsey, now age 14, was sexually abused at ages 3 and 4 by a worker at her day care center. The woman who abused Kelsey threatened that Kelsey better keep the abuse a secret or the woman would hurt Kelsey's mother. It wasn't until Kelsey started kindergarten and stopped going to the day care center that she was able to tell her mother what had been happening. Her mother knew how to help and support Kelsey and found her a therapist. Kelsey seemed to like the therapist, but she was nonetheless frequently irritable and acted out often as a young child, and then seemed vulnerable to depression as a preteen and adolescent.

Kelsey struggles with relationships. She has trouble trusting adults, and her friendships with peers (and her romantic relationships) have been intense but short-lived and frequently end in intense conflict. By age 12, Kelsey started taking increasingly concerning risks, staying out late at night, experimenting with alcohol and marijuana, and cutting her forearms with a broken tip of a pencil or the blade from a pencil sharpener.

Suicide is the second leading cause of death for adolescents ages 10–24 in the United States[1] and is the leading cause of death worldwide for adolescent girls ages 15–19.[2] Self-injurious or self-harming behaviors such as cutting, scratching, or burning oneself are also increasingly common among teenagers and even preteens. Sometimes teens cut themselves because they're feeling suicidal, and at other times the behavior is a way for them to cope with painful emotions or feelings of numbness. Teens who have experienced trauma are at particular risk for these dangerous thoughts and behaviors.

For parents, families, and professionals working with adolescents, finding out that a child has experienced a trauma is extremely upsetting and over-whelming. To additionally discover that a teen is engaging in self-injury or feeling suicidal following trauma can be terrifying. Adults frequently feel at a loss for how best to intervene. At other times adults write off suicidal or especially self-harming behavior as being "a cry for help" or "just for atten-tion." However, teens who consider or attempt suicide, even if they imme-diately regret it, are at extremely high risk for hurting or killing themselves. This is especially true for youth who have experienced trauma. Even teens who are engaging in self-injury without suicidal intent in the moment need immediate intervention, because cutting and other self-harm increases a teen's risk of later suicide attempts.[3] Parents like Kelsey's mom often recog-nize that they should be concerned when their teen is cutting, but they don't know why it's happening or how to help.

The first step to figuring out how to help is gaining as much informa-tion as possible regarding the level and type of suicidality or self-injury. It is important to precisely describe severity of suicidality and self-harm to com-municate clearly about risk and to decide the right level of treatment. The Centers for Disease Control and Prevention has defined specific categories for these thoughts and behaviors as laid out below.[4]

**Centers for Disease Control and
Prevention's Categories of
Suicidal Thoughts and Behaviors**

Suicidal ideation

1. Passive

2. Active, method but no intent or plan

3. Active, method and intent but no plan

4. Active, method; intent; and plan

Suicidal behavior

1. Preparing for suicide attempt

2. Aborted attempt

3. Interrupted attempt

Centers for Disease Control and Prevention's Categories of Suicidal Thoughts and Behaviors *(continued)*
Suicidal behavior *(continued)*
4. Suicide attempt
5. Completed suicide
Self-injury, no suicidal intent (also called *nonsuicidal self-injury*)

Suicidal ideation refers to thoughts of suicide, from fantasies about dying to urges to commit suicide. *Passive suicidal ideation* refers to thoughts about dying without any intent to act on these thoughts and without any plan for how to commit suicide. Passive suicidal ideation includes thoughts and statements such as "I wish I didn't exist," "I'd be better off dead," or "I wish I could just not wake up in the morning." *Active suicidal ideation* includes thoughts about dying or killing oneself but with the added element of planning action—either a means for committing suicide ("I wish I could just shoot myself"), some intent to act on the thought ("I'm going to shoot myself"), or a full plan for how to commit suicide ("Tonight when my parents are out, I'll get the gun from my dad's lockbox in the garage…").

Suicidal behavior refers to any step the person has taken toward acting on suicidal thoughts. This could include saving medication in preparation for a potential overdose, walking along the river considering places to jump in, or making actual attempts such as trying to hang oneself, taking an overdose, or, with immature or cognitively limited teens, even running into traffic.

Self-injurious behavior such as cutting, scratching, or burning can be suicidal or nonsuicidal, depending on the individual's intentions when engaging in the behavior as well as the person's understanding of the consequences of these behaviors. Often adolescents self-injure without any intent or desire to die (nonsuicidal self-injury). *Nonsuicidal self-injury* is rarely just "for attention" and usually serves another purpose, such as release of overwhelming emotions, an attempt to alleviate numbness and "feel something," or a means of communicating distress. In other cases, teens might cut, burn, or otherwise harm themselves with a wish or belief that they will die from the injury. In these cases, the self-injury *is* considered suicidal in nature.

Asking Why: How Trauma Is Connected to Suicidal and Self-Injurious Behavior

Adolescents who have experienced trauma are at increased risk for suicidal ideation and behavior and for self-injurious behavior. This is true both for teens who have just experienced a traumatic event and for those who were abused or otherwise traumatized earlier in childhood. The association between trauma exposure and risk for suicidality has been shown repeatedly in clinical research and is consistent across countries and cultures.[5,6] Traumatic experiences in childhood even increase risk for suicide decades later in adulthood.[7,8] When working with an adolescent who is suicidal or engaging in self-injurious behavior, the therapist should always ask about and assess for history of trauma.

Parents and providers can *normalize* the experience of trauma to allow the child a safe space to disclose any abuse. They can begin by saying, for example, "Many children have had at least one scary or upsetting thing happen to them at some point, and it can be hard to talk about or even think about these things. I'm going to ask you about a few scary things that can happen to kids, and you tell me yes or no if it has happened to you."

Asking suicidal youth about trauma is critical, and so is asking traumatized youth about suicide. Traumatic experiences increase risk for suicide, and also increase risk for psychological and social problems that additionally increase suicide risk. Trauma-exposed youth are at increased likelihood of developing mental illness, of using or abusing substances, and of engaging in risky behaviors and problematic patterns of interpersonal interaction that lead to unstable relationships.[9,10,11]

Trauma-exposed youth are more likely than their peers to experience depression, anxiety, posttraumatic stress disorder (PTSD), and disruptive behavior problems. In addition to suffering with these often debilitating mental illnesses, youth may attempt to self-medicate with illicit drugs, alcohol, and other substances of abuse. Marijuana, alcohol, opiates, and other drugs can provide short-term relief from symptoms of depression, anxiety, and PTSD, including flashbacks, fear triggered by trauma reminders, and increased stress and worry. However, these drugs also increase risk for both self-injury and suicide.[12] Substance use contributes to impulsive decision making and also lowers the threshold or inhibitions for acting on self-injurious or suicidal thoughts. Youth who are intoxicated are also at risk for assault, accidents, and other traumatic experiences, which worsen the very symptoms they were trying to avoid.

Traumatized adolescents also frequently struggle with issues of trust and self-worth, which can make building and sustaining healthy and supportive relationships more difficult. Those who are feeling depressed or anxious might not reach out or seek support because they feel they can't trust others or believe they are "damaged" or somehow undeserving of caring and support. They might even feel they don't deserve respect and kindness in relationships and might engage with unhealthy (or even violent) romantic or sexual partners. Some turn to promiscuity to feel connected with others, but don't get real emotional support from those contacts. Others end up isolated, lacking social supports when they are most in need. All of the above contribute cumulatively to increased risk for both self-injury and suicide.

When thinking about which children and adolescents are most at risk for self-injury and/or suicidality, keep in mind some additional risk factors. In recent years, numerous tragic deaths of teens and young adults by suicide following severe bullying have been highly publicized. These sad events have directed the focus of both clinicians and the general public onto the connection between bullying and suicide. Bullying can be traumatic for youth, and teens who have experienced prior trauma can become targets for bullying because of trauma-related symptoms and interpersonal difficulties that make them seem "odd" or vulnerable. Bullying (both in-person and cyber) is associated with increased risk of suicidal thoughts and behaviors. It is important to recognize that this is true not only for children who are bullied. Teens who bully others and those who are bullies/victims (youth who sometimes bully others and sometimes are targets of bullying) are also at increased risk of suicide.[13] Caregivers, clinicians, school personnel, and community members should be attuned to signs of bullying, both in person and online, and should approach kids who are involved in bullying to discuss the impact it is having and has had on them. This discussion should include frank and direct questions about any thoughts these kids have had of harming themselves in any way, and any thoughts about wanting to die or just not wanting to live anymore.

> Bullying is a major risk factor for suicide and self-injurious behavior. Bullying can be traumatizing in itself, or retraumatizing to teens who have experienced earlier abuse or maltreatment. The following are warning signs that teens are involved in bullying or cyberbullying[14]:

- *Warning signs for being a victim of bullying:* avoiding school or social situations, complaining of frequent headaches or stomachaches, changes in eating or sleeping, poor self-esteem, repeatedly lost or stolen phones or other valuables, unexplained bruises or injuries

- *Warning signs for being a perpetrator of bullying:* getting into fights or increased disciplinary problems at school, aggressive behavior, blaming others or refusing responsibility for actions

- *Warning signs for cyberbullying:* seeming anxious or distressed when using their phone or accessing social media, unexpectedly avoiding their phone or using it at all hours of the night, avoiding discussion of what they are doing online, withdrawing from family or friends, hiding their phone or quickly switching screens when an adult is nearby

As noted in Chapter 12 ("Child Welfare and Juvenile Justice"), adolescents in juvenile detention as well as those in the foster care system have high rates of trauma exposure. In addition to having significant trauma exposure, all of these children are separated from any support system they may have had in place prior to placement in detention or foster care, and many have learned to avoid forming meaningful relationships at all. Cumulative adverse childhood experiences in this population have been shown to be predictive of suicidality[15,16]; therefore, suicidality should be assessed on an ongoing basis for trauma-exposed children in these settings, particularly given the frequent increase in hopelessness among teens placed in detention and foster care.

Lesbian, gay, bisexual, transgender, and questioning and/or queer (LGBTQ) youth are at increased risk of both trauma exposure and suicidality. Identifying as part of a sexual minority group is a significant stressor for children and teens, both as an added challenge to confront as they develop their identities, and as a result of the stigma and discrimination they are likely to face. LGBTQ youth are often targets of bullying and violence as well as rejection by peers and family members, as discussed in Chapter 8 ("Implications of Trauma for Sexual and Reproductive Health in Adolescence"). LGBTQ teens are four times as likely as their straight peers to make a suicide attempt.[17,18,19] Family rejection, bullying, and abuse have all been shown to significantly increase the rates of suicide attempt in this population.[20,21]

Certain types of trauma, specifically sexual abuse, seem to increase risk for suicidal thoughts and behaviors. Research has shown that posttraumatic symptoms specifically following sexual abuse are predictive of later suicidality, even after controlling for depression and previous suicide attempts.[22] This association suggests a need for particularly careful monitoring of survivors of sexual abuse for whom PTSD symptoms are active, prevalent, or impairing.

Understanding Suicide Risk: Asking What's Happening in the Moment

Parents, teachers, and even clinicians who notice a youth's self-injury scars or suspect that a teen might be feeling suicidal often want to ask the teen about it but don't know how. They may hesitate to ask for fear of upsetting teens or "giving them ideas." These fears are unfounded; asking about suicide or self-harm does not put the idea in a teen's head or increase risk in any way. Although it can still be uncomfortable for an adult to ask, asking about suicide is critical. The adolescent will probably be defensive or guarded initially. This is especially true for teens who have experienced trauma or abuse, because they may have difficulty trusting others or feeling that others will understand, believe, or support them. With the right approach, however, teens will almost always open up. When asking about suicidal or self-harming behaviors, ask calmly and directly to show that you are not shocked or afraid of what they might tell you. Showing clear empathy and concern without getting overtly emotional also shows the teens that you can "handle" their pain and distress and that it is safe for them to share with you. Give the teens the space to express how they are feeling. If they say everything is fine or deny everything but their responses do not feel credible, ask again in a nonjudgmental, curious way.

How to Ask About Suicide

Validate the child's or teen's feelings by expressing understanding that things have been really hard or painful.

Ask calmly and directly whether the youth has had thoughts about dying or wishing to be dead. This could include questions like these:

- "I know things have been really hard and painful for you. Have you had any thoughts about wanting to die or wishing you were dead?"

- "Have there been times you wished you could just disappear or didn't want to wake up in the morning?"

How to Ask About Suicide *(continued)*

Ask about specific methods or plans

- "Have you thought about how you would die?"

- "Have you considered a way you might try to hurt or kill yourself?"

If the teen has considered taking action, ask if he or she has taken any steps to prepare:

- "Have you done anything to prepare to hurt or kill yourself?"

Consider asking questions that are specific to the teen's actual thoughts about suicide, such as in the following example:

- "You mentioned thinking about taking an overdose. What would you take? When and where would you do it? Do you have access to pills? Have you done anything to collect or save extra pills?"

Assess for protective factors

Assess for protective factors for the teens, such as their reasons for living, important relationships in their lives, aspects of their future they are hopeful for or invested in, what has stopped them from acting on suicidal thoughts thus far, and what might change about their life to make it feel worth living. The following are examples of questions to ask about protective factors:

- "What has/would stop you from acting on these thoughts?"

- "Are there things in your life that make life worth living?"

- "Is there anyone in your life who is important to you?"

- "Is there anyone in your life who would be affected if you died? How would they feel?"

- "Is there anything about your future you want to stay around to experience?"

When teens do admit to suicidal thoughts, adults often have an impulse to immediately try to comfort or reassure them. Adults may even argue with the teens about the value of their life or the senselessness of suicide. But this can backfire in two ways: First, although this response is well intentioned, it often leaves teens feeling invalidated or like the adult doesn't understand their suffering. Second, it misses an important opportunity to ask further questions to gain a full picture of a teen's level of thinking and/or planning regarding suicide as well as the teen's level of intent to act on those thoughts. Once you have a full picture of the teen's thinking and feelings and of any steps he or she has taken toward self-harm or suicide, it is still best to stay emotionally neutral and not argue with the teen about his or her thoughts or intentions. Rather, *validating* that the suicidal thoughts or self-harm behaviors come from a place of deep suffering and *empathizing* with that suffering will let the teen feel supported and understood and know that you want to help.

When you are trying to assess the level of risk for a potentially suicidal teen, adults who know the teen should reflect on any important insights they might have about the teen's thinking and behavior. Any information about previous self-injury, statements about death or suicide, suicide attempts, research on suicide methods (e.g., searching online or asking others), recent stressors or triggers, or steps taken toward acting on suicidal thoughts should be clearly communicated to the emergency mental health team or outpatient mental health professional who will be evaluating the adolescent.

> Adults are often hesitant to ask children or teens directly about suicidality for fear of giving them the idea to commit suicide or somehow encouraging them to act on suicidal thoughts. This is actually a dangerous misperception. Teens who are thinking about suicide often feel an immense sense of relief when they are able to share this burden with a caring adult, especially when it means they will receive validation, help, and support. There is no evidence that asking about suicide prompts anyone to act on suicidal thoughts or plans or triggers suicidal thinking that didn't exist previously.

Kelsey's mother feels confused and overwhelmed by Kelsey's increasingly scary behavior and doesn't know what else to offer or provide for her daughter. She brings Kelsey back to the therapist she had seen when she was younger. The therapist talks with Kelsey weekly over a few months. The therapist leaves the sessions open-ended, letting Kelsey talk about what feels important to her in the moment. Sometimes Kelsey is quiet and distant, and on other days she talks a lot, mostly about conflicts she has had recently with friends or family. Kelsey says that she typically cuts herself after conflicts like these when she feels rejected by peers or family members, and also that her cutting is often accompanied by intense feelings of worthlessness. She also admits that sometimes in these moments she wishes she could "just disappear" but says she hasn't thought about trying to kill herself. Despite these insights, Kelsey keeps cutting and keeps engaging in more and more risky behavior, staying out late drinking and smoking, sometimes with friends but increasingly with older kids she doesn't know well. Kelsey eventually tells her mother she doesn't want to keep seeing the therapist "because what's the point."

Unfortunately, simply discussing a behavior or symptom is not enough to stop it, especially if it is related to unaddressed trauma. Although Kelsey had a good relationship with her therapist, who was supportive and well meaning, her treatment did not focus on or directly address the trauma she had experienced. Nor did it specifically target the cutting and risky behaviors that were evidence of Kelsey's ongoing struggle.

> Most therapy is not trauma specific or trauma informed. Such treatment is unlikely to be very helpful to survivors of childhood abuse. Finding a provider trained in evidence-based trauma treatment is crucial.

Teens who are cutting or engaging in other dangerous or suicidal behaviors are often ambivalent about the behaviors. Though on the surface they are resistant to changing, it is often because they don't know how to change and want help. When treatment is supportive but does not specifically focus on self-harm or suicide, teens often become frustrated, thinking "Why are you asking me about this all the time if you're not going to do anything about it?"

Finding the Frame: Understanding Suicidal and Self-Injurious Behaviors in Traumatized Teens

Treatment for self-injurious or suicidal behavior in traumatized teens must in some way address the trauma. Treatments that attempt to target depression, self-injury, or suicidality in traumatized youth without consideration of the contribution of traumatic experiences will not be very effective or helpful. This outcome was demonstrated, for example, in the results of one of the key research studies in child psychiatry, the Treatment for Adolescents with Depression Study (TADS).[23] Although most of the depressed teens in that study experienced significant benefit from cognitive behavioral therapy for depression, youth who had experienced trauma in their lives did not. This was because the therapy designed for depression alone did not address the traumatic experiences that were causing their depressive symptoms. Teens who have experienced trauma very commonly experience depression and other psychiatric illnesses (anxiety disorders, substance use disorders, externalizing disorders, etc.) that can lead to suicide and self-harm. To be effective, their treatment requires a clear and explicit understanding of how the traumatic experiences and current symptoms are connected.

A good understanding of the adversity the child has faced is key to providing effective intervention. Good treatment always starts with a thorough assessment, which should include assessment of trauma exposure even when there is no indication that a trauma has occurred. Assessment of trauma exposure is particularly important in the context of high-risk symptoms and behaviors such as self-injury, suicidal ideation, or a suicide attempt.

Sometimes adults working with suicidal youth hesitate to ask about trauma, fearing it will upset the child or worsen suicidal thoughts. But asking in a gentle, empathic way has the opposite effect. Helping teens see the connection between what happened to them and why they are suffering now lets them see that you understand and that they are not alone.

When asking about trauma, ask about each specific form of trauma, and provide an opportunity for the adolescent to indicate whether he or she has experienced any of those events. Having the adolescent complete a questionnaire assessing for trauma can be an effective way to start, but this should always be followed up with questions by the provider during a clinical interview, even if the youth answered "no" to everything on the questionnaire. Teens who are cognitively or developmentally delayed should simply be asked verbally about trauma, in a way that is direct but appropriate for their cognitive or developmental level.

Treating More Than Just Behavior: Trauma-Informed Treatment for Suicidal and Self-Injurious Behavior

Kelsey's mother talks to their pediatrician for advice on a different therapist, someone who works with kids who are cutting and those who have been through trauma like Kelsey's. The pediatrician recommends a new therapist, Jackie, and Kelsey and her mother go together to the first session. Jackie meets with Kelsey first, Kelsey's mother next, and then with Kelsey and her mother together. Jackie asks about Kelsey's history, feelings, and current functioning and asks specific questions of both Kelsey and her mother about exposure to traumatic experiences. She asks about reminders of the traumatic experiences and questions what Kelsey tends to do when the reminders come up. Jackie tells Kelsey and her mother that she'd like to take a Trauma-Focused Cognitive Behavioral Therapy (TF-CBT) approach with Kelsey. Jackie gives Kelsey and her mother an overview of how the treatment will proceed: education about trauma and how it affects feelings and behavior, followed by skill building to provide coping skills to manage challenges and Kelsey's reactions to stress, followed by exposure therapy through the development of a trauma narrative. She also talks about what symptoms and difficulties are common for kids who have had traumatic experiences. She explains that many of the issues Kelsey has struggled with—depression, anxiety, substance use, acting out, and risk taking—are very common after abuse, even years after, as kids try to come to terms with what they've been through.

In the next few weeks, Jackie meets with Kelsey and her mother each individually for 45-minute sessions. She is able to help Kelsey recognize some patterns. For example, when Kelsey is reminded of the sexual abuse, she feels ashamed, empty, and hopeless and then cuts to try to feel in control and to feel some connection to herself and her emotions. Once Jackie an Kelsey have identified these patterns, Jackie transitions to teaching Kelsey adaptive coping skills for feelings of shame and hopelessness, to help her stop cutting. She checks in weekly with Kelsey about cutting and suicidal thoughts, but Kelsey denies both. Jackie works with Kelsey's mother as well. She helps Kelsey's mom to understand Kelsey's behavior in the context of the trauma Kelsey experienced. She teaches Kelsey's mom how to validate Kelsey's feelings. They discuss how the mother can set clear expectations for Kelsey's behavior (including that drug use and breaking curfew are not okay), while still being empathic that certain things (e.g., going to big family social events) are too hard for her to do right now. Kelsey's mother learns the same coping skills that Kelsey does, so that she can both use them when she herself is stressed (e.g., during moments of normal parent-teen conflict) and serve as a coach and support for Kelsey when Kelsey needs it.

Just as the right antibiotic is necessary to treat an infection, only the right kind of treatment will be truly effective to help traumatized youth like Kelsey. The current gold standard treatment for children and youth who are exposed to trauma is TF-CBT.[24] This trauma-specific treatment for children and adolescents is an evidence-based approach with robust research support, including several randomized controlled trials (the highest standard to evaluate the efficacy of treatment approaches). TF-CBT is a trauma-specific treatment for children and adolescents developed by Drs. Judith Cohen, Esther Deblinger, and Anthony Mannarino. This approach starts with *psychoeducation* for both the youth and the caregiver about common symptoms and difficulties following traumatic experiences. Psychoeducation not only helps youth and families understand what to expect, but also normalizes some of the difficulties they are experiencing so they feel less alone and ashamed. The rationale for the treatment and what to expect in sessions are also discussed. Next is a *skill building* phase in which youth and their caregivers learn adaptive skills to manage difficult emotions and situations. The third phase is the development of a *trauma narrative*. The youth tells the story of what happened in his or her own words with support from the therapist. Whenever there is a "hot spot" or sticking spot in the story, which hints at feelings of guilt or shame, the therapist points it out to explore it more thoroughly. Through repeated processing and discussion of the traumatic experience(s), the power of the event is reduced. The youth no longer needs to try to avoid memories or reminders of the event, and ideally feels more able to manage the feelings associated with what happened. Many youth who complete a TF-CBT treatment feel pride in having been able to write their narrative and feel they gave gotten back a sense of empowerment and control that had been taken from them by the trauma.

TF-CBT is an appropriate choice for some trauma survivors who self-injure or who are suicidal; however, safety and stabilization come first. Some teens are stable enough to complete the initial modules (psychoeducation and skill building) but might still be too unstable to undertake the process of developing a trauma narrative or processing the traumatic experiences directly. For others, the skill-building phase needs to be adapted and extended to ensure that the teen (and family) have the right tools to keep the teen safe should suicidal thoughts return. This is a challenging clinical decision that should be made on an individual basis, together with parents and treatment providers. Even if the child is unable to initiate a trauma narrative or other forms of exposure specific to the trauma, treatment should be trauma informed, with consideration for the ways trauma affects behavior and the ways children relate to others. Often the first two phases of TF-CBT can be initiated and extended until the teen's suicidality has abated enough to safely move into exposure and development of a narrative.

For teens with severe or persistent suicidal or self-injurious behaviors, Dialectical Behavior Therapy (DBT) can be a literal lifesaver. DBT was developed by Dr. Marsha Linehan and adapted for adolescents by Drs. Alec Miller and Jill Rathus, based on a combination of cognitive behavioral therapy and mindfulness approaches. DBT has been used successfully to treat adolescents with suicidal ideation, suicidal behavior, and self-harm.[25] DBT overlaps somewhat with the psychoeducation and skill-building modules of TF-CBT (as both are based in cognitive behavioral therapy) but is much more intensive. Participants in DBT attend weekly individual therapy plus a weekly multifamily group, both focused on learning and practicing skills. Participants work on a range of specific distress tolerance, emotion regulation, interpersonal, and mindfulness skills, as well as skills for finding compromise with adult caregivers and other authority figures. This type of treatment can target many of the problematic behaviors that are common in adolescent trauma survivors, including self-injury, suicidality, risk taking, and substance use. DBT can provide a good foundation and skills base to address more high-risk and immediately concerning behaviors. DBT will not, however, replace the need to address the underlying trauma directly for most youth. Sometimes youth will need to complete DBT first and then transition to TF-CBT to address the trauma directly. Parents and anyone referring a teen for treatment should talk up front with potential providers focused on the kind of treatment they provide and what they are unable to provide, to ensure the teen gets the right treatment for his or her symptoms and needs.

A few months go by. Then one evening Kelsey's mother comes home from work and finds empty Motrin and Tylenol bottles on the kitchen counter next to a half-empty bottle of vodka. Kelsey is passed out on the bed in her room. Kelsey's mother calls 911. At the hospital Kelsey has her stomach pumped in the ER before she is transferred to the pediatric ICU. Luckily Kelsey is medically stable within a few days. She is then transferred to a different hospital with an inpatient adolescent psychiatric floor. Kelsey spends 2 weeks receiving treatment on the psychiatric unit. She is started on an antidepressant and participates in therapy groups with other teens and has some individual sessions with her doctor. She tells her mother and her doctors that a few days before her suicide attempt, she was drinking with some friends when one of them sexually assaulted her. She felt guilty about having put herself in a dangerous situation but also as though she "had a target on my back" or that there must be something wrong with her that now she'd been sexually abused again.

Jackie comes to visit Kelsey in the hospital, and also meets with her mom while Kelsey is admitted to help Kelsey's mom cope with her own feelings of guilt, anger, and sadness. They talk about how best to support Kelsey and keep her safe when she returns home. In the hospital Kelsey continues to talk to her therapists, doctors, and the other kids. She feels better when another girl on the unit confides that she too had been sexually assaulted in the past. After 2 weeks, Kelsey's doctors determine that she is no longer an immediate risk to herself and discharge her to continue treatment outside of the hospital.

Choosing the appropriate level of care or type of treatment setting is important for any youth experiencing suicidal thoughts. Suicidal youth may need an inpatient level of care if the suicidal ideation is active, meaning that they have considered methods of suicide or taken steps to prepare for suicide. They may also require hospitalization if the suicidal ideation is increasing in intensity, in duration, or in the teen's level of intent to act on the thoughts. Safety considerations are primary, and each teen should be evaluated by a mental health professional to determine where treatment will be both safe and effective (an inpatient psychiatric program, residential treatment facility or center, day-treatment program, partial hospital program, intensive outpatient program, or more standard weekly outpatient treatment). Treatment may need to occur in stages as described below.

If a teen's suicidal thoughts and behavior are very intense or acute, the treatment should focus on safety and stabilization while remaining trauma informed. This should include recognition of the role of the trauma in the teen's acute symptoms and educating the teen and family about how trauma and suicidal thoughts and behavior are connected. You should normalize symptoms and difficulties following trauma and highlight the teen's immense strength and resilience in having survived the trauma. The next step is identifying triggers for suicidal thoughts (especially those that are trauma reminders) and learning coping skills to manage stress. These coping skills are helpful immediately and also prepare the teen to manage the challenge of addressing the trauma when he or she is ready to do so. The teen may also need to learn interpersonal skills to navigate issues with peers or family, to reach out for help and support, or to recognize and communicate his or her own emotions. Families should be involved whenever possible to learn and reinforce these same skills, as this will let families support and help the teen between therapy sessions. Families should also be given education about trauma and the connection between trauma exposure and ongoing difficulties.

Once the teen's suicidality is no longer so acute, immediate, or persistent—usually once the youth is no longer on an acute psychiatric inpatient unit—you should reassess whether the teen is ready for trauma-focused treatment. In Kelsey's case, her high-risk symptoms stabilized sufficiently to allow for her to return to trauma-specific treatment with Jackie in an outpatient setting. Some teens, however, have suicidal thoughts and behaviors even on discharge from an acute care program and require DBT or a modification of TF-CBT as described above. Whatever modality of treatment is used, it is important to continue to monitor the teen for suicidal thoughts and urges. Assessing the frequency and intensity of suicidal thoughts and the level of intention to act on these should continue to be a regular part of all sessions.

Many providers are uncomfortable initiating a trauma narrative, prolonged exposure, or other exposure-based approach with patients who are actively suicidal. Addressing the trauma through exposure can be stressful and may initially increase symptoms for some individuals. Sometimes, however, a clinician may feel that trauma is the primary trigger for suicidality and that therefore the suicidality is unlikely to resolve until the trauma has been directly addressed. In such a case, the teen may benefit from processing the trauma while simultaneously receiving intensive support around suicidal thoughts and behavior. Ideally this could be done in the safe confines of an inpatient unit, but inpatient program staff rarely have training in providing TF-CBT, prolonged exposure, or cognitive processing therapy (see Chapter 2, "Recognition and Treatment"). Additionally, the typical inpatient length of stay has shortened to an extent that makes completing this type of treatment difficult if not impossible. Instead, outpatient providers may be in the position of having to organize intensive outpatient care and support for their patient, which often will require increased family involvement, multiple sessions per week, and often additional modalities of therapy (e.g., group or family therapy).

> When Kelsey returns to weekly outpatient treatment, she and Jackie agree on some changes to their treatment plan. They will actively monitor Kelsey's suicidality with the use of a DBT-style diary card, on which she will rate her suicidal thoughts and urges, self-harm, substance use, and risk-taking each day on a scale of 1–10. They will review the card together at the start of each session, so that if Kelsey has been feeling suicidal or cutting again, Jackie will know right away and they can make it the focus of the session. If Kelsey reports that she has engaged in an unsafe behavior such as cutting or drinking, Jackie and Kelsey will spend part of the session doing a *chain analysis* of what led up to that behavior. Jackie helps Kelsey develop a safety plan, and they agree to review and update it periodically. The *safety plan* has several parts: First, Kelsey and Jackie list things that are triggers for negative feelings or distress, such as not sleeping enough the previous night, hav-

ing an argument with a friend, or seeing a building with an entrance reminiscent of Kelsey's daycare center. Second, Kelsey and Jackie list ways Kelsey herself, and others around her, can notice that she's starting to feel worse (e.g., becoming quiet and withdrawn, getting a headache, losing her appetite). Third, Kelsey and Jackie list coping skills that help Kelsey (e.g., listening to favorite music, calling her best friend Maggie, watching cat videos on YouTube), people who can help (Mom, Grandma, the school counselor, Jackie), and emergency resources in addition to the people she listed (calling 1-800-LifeNet, 911, or a crisis text line; going to the hospital). The last thing on the safety plan is a list of Kelsey's reasons for living ("I love Mom," "I want to be a journalist when I grow up," "I'm loving my photography class"). Kelsey agrees to post the safety plan on her bathroom mirror and also takes a photo with her phone to always have it with her. Once Kelsey feels more solid and is using some adaptive skills and strategies when things get tough, she and Jackie plan to start her trauma narrative. Kelsey's mom continues to meet individually with Jackie and sometimes joins in Kelsey's sessions, such as to review Kelsey's safety plan. She starts to feel more confident in how to help Kelsey when her daughter is having a tough day.

Completing a Chain Analysis

In the case example, Jackie, Kelsey's therapist, uses a technique called a chain analysis, which is a key component of DBT, to help Kelsey better understand all the factors that led up to an unsafe behavior such as cutting or a suicide attempt. The purpose of the chain analysis is to break down all the steps that led up to or contributed in making the unhealthy choice and to illuminate all the opportunities to use adaptive coping skills during that course of events.

Steps for developing a chain analysis:

1. Identify the problem behavior. Be detailed and specific in describing the behavior. Someone else hearing the description should have enough details to picture the event as if watching it on television.

   • Example: "I cut my left forearm with a broken razor blade while I was taking a shower on Saturday afternoon. The cut bled a little bit for about 10 minutes and left a dark red scratch."

Completing a Chain Analysis *(continued)*

2. Identify all the thoughts, feelings, and behaviors that occurred at the time.

- Example: "I felt sad, embarrassed, and a little bit angry. I was thinking, 'No one even notices if I'm not around, no one cares, I'm such a mess.' Then I looked at the razor and grabbed it, and before I knew it I was cutting my arm."

3. Describe the event(s) that led to the problem behavior.

- Example: "I went online last night and saw that everyone was at a party for Tatiana's birthday and I wasn't invited."

4. Describe any vulnerabilities that contributed to the problem behavior.

- Example: "I went to bed at 3:00 A.M. and only slept for 4 hours. I hadn't eaten anything since breakfast the day before."

5. Describe in excruciating detail the chain of events that led to the problem behavior.

6. Describe the consequences of the behavior.

7. Go back through the chain of events identifying each place where you could have done something different to find solutions.

8. Describe a detailed prevention strategy—at each point, state what could have been done differently, what coping skills could have been used, or how the teen could have reached out for help or support.

9. Describe the plan to repair the significant consequences of the problem behavior.

Once the adolescent is no longer suicidal, treatment can shift to focusing on other goals and topics including additional trauma work. First, however, you should review with the teen what has worked to reduce the suicidality and make a plan to continue those strategies and behaviors. You should always continue to assess suicidality. For example, you could do a brief weekly check by asking the adolescent whether he or she had any thoughts about suicide and what the intensity of those thoughts were on a scale of 1–10. If the teen had thoughts of suicide, you should question the likelihood that the teen would take any action to hurt himself or herself on a scale of 1–10. It is helpful for you to ask proactively and routinely about suicide, even if—and perhaps especially if—it has been a while since the teen felt suicidal. Often if teens have been doing well but then suicidal thoughts return, they are embarrassed to share these thoughts with a therapist because they feel they have failed or are backsliding. If you regularly ask about suicide, it is easier for the teen to answer honestly. When suicidality is absent or is only fleeting, reinforce what is working by asking the teen what coping skills, tools, and resources they've used to manage stress, disappointment, sadness, and anger. Highlight that they have been successfully managing the stressors or urges that had previously been so difficult, and praise their use of adaptive coping, engagement with supportive peers and adults, and choices of healthy environments and activities. The goals are for the adolescents to internalize their success, to feel a sense of empowerment, and to remember to use the approaches that work for them going forward. Good trauma-informed care for adolescents who have experienced trauma and suicidality or self-injury can be highly effective, healing, and give hope to kids and families in the midst of crisis.

Online Resources

Association for Behavioral and Cognitive Therapies: http://www.ABCT.org
Dialectical Behavior Therapy (includes "Find a Therapist" page as well as resources for families): http://www.behavioraltech.org
National Child Traumatic Stress Network: http://www.nctsn.org
Trauma-Focused Cognitive Behavioral Therapy: https://www.musc.edu/tfcbt2

References

1. Sullivan EM, Annest JL, Simon TR, et al: Suicide trends among persons aged 10–24 years—United States, 1994–2012. MMWR Morbid Mortal Wkly Rpt 64(8):201–205, 2015 25742379

2. World Health Organization: Global health estimates 2015: deaths by cause, age, sex, by country and by region, 2000–2015. 2016. Available at: http://www.who.int/healthinfo/global_burden_disease/estimates/en/index1.html. Accessed March 1, 2018.

3. Guan K, Fox KR, Prinstein MJ: Nonsuicidal self-injury as a time-invariant predictor of adolescent suicidal ideation and attempts in a diverse community sample. J Consult Clin Psychol 80(5):842–849, 2012 22845782

4. Crosby AE, Ortega L, Melanson C: Self-Directed Violence Surveillance: Uniform Definitions and Recommended Data Elements, Version 1.0. Atlanta, GA, Centers for Disease Control and Prevention, National Center for Injury Prevention and Control, February 2011. Available at: https://www.cdc.gov/violenceprevention/pdf/Self-Directed-Violence-a.pdf. Accessed June 2018.

5. Cluver L, Orkin M, Boyes ME, et al: Child and adolescent suicide attempts, suicidal behavior, and adverse childhood experiences in South Africa: a prospective study. J Adolesc Health 57(1):52–59, 2015 25936843

6. Jeon HJ, Lee C, Fava M, et al: Childhood trauma, parental death, and their co-occurrence in relation to current suicidality risk in adults: a nationwide community sample of Korea. J Nerv Ment Dis 202(12):870–876, 2014 25370752

7. Bruffaerts R, Demyttenaere K, Borges G, et al: Childhood adversities as risk factors for onset and persistence of suicidal behaviour. Br J Psychiatry 197(1):20–27, 2010 20592429

8. Guendelman MD, Owens EB, Galán C, et al: Early adult correlates of maltreatment in girls with attention-deficit/hyperactivity disorder: increased risk for internalizing symptoms and suicidality. Dev Psychopathol 28(1):1–14, 2016 25723055

9. Cash SJ, Bridge JA: Epidemiology of youth suicide and suicidal behavior. Curr Opin Pediatr 21(5):613–619, 2009 19644372

10. Pirard S, Sharon E, Kang SK, et al: Prevalence of physical and sexual abuse among substance abuse patients and impact on treatment outcomes. Drug Alcohol Depend 78(1):57–64, 2005 15769558

11. Whitesell M, Bachand A, Peel J, et al: Familial, social, and individual factors contributing to risk for adolescent substance use. J Addict 2013:579310, 2013 24826363

12. Esposito-Smythers C, Spirito A: Adolescent substance use and suicidal behavior: a review with implications for treatment research. Alcohol Clin Exp Res 28(5 Suppl):77S–88S, 2004 15166639

13. Brunstein Klomek A, Sourander A, Gould M: The association of suicide and bullying in childhood to young adulthood: a review of cross-sectional and longitudinal research findings. Can J Psychiatry 55(5):282–288, 2010 20482954

14. Hinduja S, Patchin JW: Bullying Beyond the Schoolyard: Preventing and Responding to Cyberbullying, 2nd Edition. Thousand Oaks, CA, Sage, 2015

15. Bielas H, Barra S, Skrivanek C, et al: The associations of cumulative adverse childhood experiences and irritability with mental disorders in detained male adolescent offenders. Child Adolesc Psychiatry Ment Health 10:34, 2016 27688799

16. Pilowsky DJ, Wu L-T: Psychiatric symptoms and substance use disorders in a nationally representative sample of American adolescents involved with foster care. J Adolesc Health 38(4):351–358, 2006 16549295

17. Bouris A, Everett BG, Heath RD, et al: Effects of victimization and violence on suicidal ideation and behaviors among sexual minority and heterosexual adolescents. LGBT Health 3(2):153–161, 2016 26789401

18. Centers for Disease Control and Prevention: Sexual Identity, Sex of Sexual Contacts, and Health-Risk Behaviors Among Students in Grades 9–12: Youth Risk Behavior Surveillance. Atlanta, GA, U.S. Department of Health and Human Services, 2016

19. Coker TR, Austin SB, Schuster MA: The health and health care of lesbian, gay, and bisexual adolescents. Annu Rev Public Health 31:457–477, 2010 20070195

20. Mustanski BS, Garofalo R, Emerson EM; IMPACT: Mental health disorders, psychological distress, and suicidality in a diverse sample of lesbian, gay, bisexual, and transgender youths. Am J Public Health 100(12):2426–2432, 2010 20966378

21. Ryan C, Huebner D, Diaz RM, et al: Family rejection as a predictor of negative health outcomes in white and Latino lesbian, gay, and bisexual young adults. Pediatrics 123(1):346–352, 2009 19117902

22. Brabant ME, Hébert M, Chagnon F: Identification of sexually abused female adolescents at risk for suicidal ideations: a classification and regression tree analysis. J Child Sex Abuse 22(2):153–172, 2013 23428149

23. March JS, Silva S, Petrycki S, et al: The Treatment for Adolescents with Depression Study (TADS): long-term effectiveness and safety outcomes. Arch Gen Psychiatry 64(10):1132–1143, 2007 17909125

24. Cohen JA, Deblinger E, Mannarino AP, et al: A multisite, randomized controlled trial for children with sexual abuse-related PTSD symptoms. J Am Acad Child Adolesc Psychiatry 43:393–402, 2004 15187799

25. Mehlum L, Tørmoen AJ, Ramberg M, et al: Dialectical behavior therapy for adolescents with repeated suicidal and self-harming behavior: a randomized trial. J Am Acad Child Adolesc Psychiatry 53(10):1082–1091, 2014 25245352

CHAPTER 5

Risky Behavior and Substance Use

Sophie de Figueiredo, Psy.D.
Moises Rodriguez, Ph.D.

Ana, age 18, and Alex, age 19, arrive at a drop-in center for homeless youth, both looking distressed. Alex, appearing worn out, carries a tattered backpack and reusable grocery bags stuffed with clothes. Ana also looks exhausted with dark circles under her eyes, but seems somewhat more alert and put together than Alex. She carries a large purse with a child's doll and a pack of cigarettes sticking out of it. The communication between them is brief and tense. Ana pushes Alex through a check-in area where personal items are inspected, and both are "wanded" for weapons. Alex is overheard telling Ana, "Nobody better take my shit here." Ana replies, "You need to relax. You're basically out of options and you're lucky I agreed to come here with you."

Alex completes a medical screen, during which the on-site nurse practitioner notices multiple scratch marks on his arms and treats them with disinfectant cream. Alex then meets with Nancy, a case manager, for intake. Alex is short in his responses but admits that he regularly uses drugs and alcohol, frequently has unprotected sex with multiple partners, and has been arrested several times for shoplifting, assault, and selling drugs. Alex tells Nancy that he and Ana have a 2-year-old daughter, Emily, together but that they aren't technically "together" as a couple right now because they "fight too much."

While Alex completes the intake, Ana is overheard on her phone arranging child care for Emily. "I'm trying to help Alex get his shit together. Yes, I know, he doesn't deserve anyone's help, but what am I going to do?" she exclaims to the person on the other end of the call. A staff member notices Ana looking more upset as the call goes on. She comes over to help and notices rows of faint cuts and several bruises on Ana's forearm, and the unmistakable smell of alcohol. Before the staff member can say anything, Ana abruptly hangs up the phone, pulls car keys out of her purse, and announces that she has to get her daughter and can't wait for Alex. The staff member runs after Ana to ask if she is okay and to offer her services, as well. Ana responds, "I'm all good. He's the screwup, not me," and rushes out.

Risk taking is normal in adolescence. Exploration and experimentation are central to adolescents' growth and psychological maturation. These experiences foster teens' identity development and help teens gain a better sense of who they are, what they like, what they're capable of, and how to handle tough decisions. As teens gain independence, taking on new challenges and taking risks helps them understand the world and their own identities. Most risk taking is benign; asking someone on a date, trying a new sport, driving for the first time, and applying for a new job or for college all involve taking risks. But if this developmentally normative risk taking goes too far, it can be dangerous and lead to serious, negative health outcomes, including accidents, illness, and even death,[1] and traumatized teens are particularly at risk. Unfortunately, teens who have experienced trauma or abuse are particularly vulnerable to engaging in more dangerous risky behaviors.

Adolescent experimentation exists on a spectrum of risk. Teens may not realize when their behavior has moved past typical risk taking to something more concerning (Table 5–1). Many factors contribute to whether a teen's risk taking will become dangerous. Trauma is one of those factors, enough so that the DSM-5[2] lists risky and self-destructive behavior as a core symptom of posttraumatic stress disorder (PTSD). Generally, risk behaviors most often seen in adolescence include substance use, unsafe sexual practices, violence among peers or in romantic relationships, dangerous driving and car accidents, self-harm, and running away/homelessness, among others.

Alcohol is the most often used and abused substance among youth in the United States. According to the 2015 National Survey on Drug Use and Health (NSDUH), 20% of youth ages 12–20 years reported drinking alcohol and 13% reported binge drinking in the past 30 days.[1] Binge drinking can have academic (increased truancy, poor grades), social (intimate partner violence, social isolation), and legal (DUI arrest, accidents, physical assault) consequences and can disrupt brain development.

Alcohol use goes hand in hand with unsafe sexual practices. In a 2015 survey of U.S. high school students, 30% reported having had sexual intercourse in the past 3 months, and of these, 43% did not use a condom the last time they had sex, 14% did not use any method to prevent pregnancy, and 21% had sex while drunk or high.[1] The combination of substance use and

TABLE 5–1.   Adolescent behaviors: risky or not?

Typical	Not typical/Risky
Increased sexual maturation; heightened focus on body image and self-consciousness	Sexual promiscuity; bingeing, purging, or restricting eating; social withdrawal
Sexual experimentation	Multiple partners; unsafe sexual practices; pregnancy
Increased parent-adolescent conflict	Verbal or physical aggression; running away
Experimentation with drugs, alcohol, and cigarettes	Substance abuse; selling drugs; having heavily substance-using peer group
Increased sensation seeking and risk taking	Multiple accidents; encounters with firearms; excessive risk taking
Stressful transitions to middle and high school	Lack of connection to school or peers; school truancy, failure, or dropout
Increased argumentativeness, idealism, and criticism	Excessive defiance of social rules and conventions; causing trouble with family members, teachers, or other authority figures
Becoming overwhelmed with everyday decisions	Becoming paralyzed with indecision

Source.   Adapted from Miller et al. 2007.[3]

risky sexual behavior increases the likelihood of unplanned pregnancies, sexually transmitted infections, sexual assault, and/or teen dating violence.

Intimate partner violence (also called *dating violence* or *domestic violence*) occurs among teens surprisingly often. Defined as psychological, emotional, physical, or sexual violence (including stalking) within a dating relationship, intimate partner violence can occur in person or electronically between current or former dating partners.[4] In the 2013 and 2015 surveys, 10% of high school students reported physical victimization and 10% reported sexual victimization from a dating partner each year.[5,6,7] Teen girls are equally as likely as teen boys to be violent toward a partner.

> Alex tells Nancy, the case manager, that he and Ana met 3 years ago when they were both in high school. They went to the same school, but they were very different. Ana was quiet and studious, whereas Alex was loud and rowdy; he knew everyone and was always talking to girls. He frequently got in trouble for skipping school and talking back to teachers. Despite their differences, Alex

found Ana intriguing. He noticed that Ana looked sad a lot and he wondered why. One day, Ana stopped coming to school. Months later, they ran into each other at a party. Ana looked different. She was dressed provocatively and was smoking a joint, which surprised Alex since she had always seemed so innocent and introverted. He asked for a hit and they talked for a while. They started dating, and a year later Ana discovered she was pregnant.

As mentioned, experiencing trauma is a significant risk factor for a teen's involvement in risky behaviors. The more trauma a teen has experienced, the greater the risk. Experiencing different types of traumatic events also significantly increases the odds of high-risk behaviors.[8] To complicate matters further, risk taking may further put youth into dangerous situations that may expose them to even more trauma.

Working with high-risk youth can be intimidating or scary. Watching teens we care about put themselves at risk is painful. But understanding that trauma is often underlying and driving these behaviors lets us approach teens with more compassion, empathy, patience, and a better understanding of how to help them.

> Ana thinks about Alex as she drives to pick up Emily. She regrets drinking so much last night, but she was so upset after her fight with Alex. She loves him and knows he tries his best to be a good dad to Emily, to be a different man than his own dad was to him. But Ana is so tired of how much they fight and how easily he gets "set off." She understands that he has had a rough life and has been through a lot, just like she has. Sometimes this helps them to "get" each other, and other times they trigger each other. She feels stuck: she wants Emily to have a father in her life but doesn't want Emily to see the kind of fighting that she and Alex both saw growing up. She has been thinking of checking out a program for young mothers that her friend Jessica attends. Jessica's baby's father is not in the picture; she broke up with him after he became too violent. When Jessica first suggested Ana come to the program, Ana flipped out. "You have no idea what you're talking about—Alex and I are nothing like you and your baby daddy! I don't need to talk to some therapist." Deep down, however, she knows that they are similar and that she does need help.

Asking Why: How Trauma Can Lead to Risky Behaviors in Teens

Adolescents engage in risky behaviors in part because their prefrontal cortex—the rational-thinking, problem-solving part of the brain responsible for steering teens away from dangerous behaviors—is not yet fully developed. Adding the toxic effects of traumatic stress puts trauma-exposed teens at especially high risk for engaging in risky behaviors.

The Teenage Brain Is Susceptible to Risky Behaviors

Brain development occurs in a hierarchical fashion. The most basic area (i.e., the brain stem, which is responsible for breathing, heart rate) develops in utero. Next to develop in early childhood are the areas responsible for getting physical and emotional needs met, such as the limbic system. The most complex areas develop last, including the prefrontal cortex, which is responsible for executive functions such as decision making, judgment, abstract reasoning, and impulse control. The prefrontal cortex starts to "come online" around age 12 and only reaches full maturity in the mid-20s to early 30s.[9,10,11] The following is very important to remember when working with adolescents: *The prefrontal cortex—the part of the brain responsible for making safe, reasonable decisions; for learning facts about safe sex or the dangers of drunk driving, and then applying this knowledge when deciding whether to use a condom or drink and drive; and for using logic to think through what is "right or wrong"—is not fully developed in adolescence, and won't be for at least a decade.* Meanwhile, the impulsive, emotional parts of the brain developed much earlier, so they are strong and quick to respond. Teens might be able to problem solve or show sophisticated reasoning when things are calm, when the weaker, slower, less-developed prefrontal cortex doesn't have any competition. But when emotions are high and the impulsive brain areas kick in, the rational brain often gets overruled.[9,12]

Remember that teens can look and even act like "mini adults." This sometimes tricks adults working with teens into thinking that what's going on outside matches what's going on inside. However, although the adolescent body is rapidly changing, teens' emotional awareness and cognitive abilities are still relatively immature. Skills such as foresight and judgment are just starting to develop.

Be mindful of falling into the "you should have known better!" trap when working with teens, even if they sometimes talk or act like they do know better. Remind yourself: teens were children not long ago and are very much still learning.

The toxic effects of traumatic stress make it even harder for the teenage brain to consistently make safe choices. Instead of moving through developmental milestones as expected, the brains of trauma-exposed youth remain in "survival mode," prioritizing networks and pathways needed for survival rather than those needed to learn language, math, manners, and so forth.[13] Chronic exposure to traumatic experiences puts brains into a constant state of fight, flight, or freeze. Whether teens seem to fight, flee, or freeze more often depends on the nature of the trauma they experienced and when the trauma occurred.[14] Girls, teens who experienced neglect, and teens who experienced trauma during early childhood may be more likely to freeze, whereas boys typically fight or flee.[14] Some teens alternate between the hyperarousal of the fight-or-flight response and the underarousal of the freeze response.

Teens having the freeze response can appear flat, shy, nervous, avoidant, unresponsive, depressed, "checked out," inattentive, or as if in a daydream, although they'll generally tell you they feel fine. They might find themselves often dissociating as a way of avoiding the pain of trauma or memories, or they might use drugs or alcohol in an attempt to "feel something." The freeze response can also make it harder for teens to recognize or escape dangerous situations.

Teens who respond to trauma by developing the hyperarousal associated with the fight-or-flight response can demonstrate agitation, aggression, defiance, extreme alertness or awareness of surroundings, talkativeness, fidgetiness, or the general appearance of being "keyed up." The fight response can lead to physical fights, relationship violence, and impulsive behaviors that can lead to unwanted negative consequences (e.g., getting arrested or in trouble), as well as substance use (as the teen tries to self-medicate to avoid feeling out of control) or homelessness (if the teen is kicked out of the home by adults sick of the fighting or runs away from home to escape violence or trauma triggers).

Ana and Alex both grew up in families where yelling and fighting was the norm. Even as a baby, Alex was forced to scream to get his parents to notice him, feed him, or change his diaper, so he learned that was what he had to do to get his needs met. If screaming didn't work, aggression always did, especially as he got older. These reactions became so automatic for him that he now often starts yelling without even realizing it himself. Ana's father and stepmother also fought frequently, and her family environment was very chaotic. But in her family, speaking up was met with physical violence or punitive responses. When her stepmother spoke up to her father, he would hit her. When Ana fussed or talked back, her stepmother would take away her next meal. Ana learned to make herself as invisible as possible; the less attention she drew to herself, the safer she'd be.

Alex and Ana both experienced neglect and violence growing up, but their experiences translated into very different patterns of interacting with others and getting their needs met. These patterns are evident in how they engage with each other now. The strategies they use today are those that were reinforced in the trauma-filled environments in which they were raised.

Risky Behaviors Can Be Learned Responses to Trauma

Traumatic experiences involve a profound loss of safety, power, and connection to others. Trauma alters people's ability to trust others, themselves, and the world around them. Children exposed to chronic trauma, and especially interpersonal or developmental trauma, learn from an early age that the world and the people around them are not safe or trustworthy. Many, if not all, reactions to trauma can be thought of in one way or another as efforts to survive (to ensure physical and emotional safety or basic needs). Risky behaviors are no exception. Alex, for example, is quick to throw the first punch because aggression is his way of establishing safety in a world he has learned is dangerous. Similarly, a teen who gets arrested for theft might have developed this behavior by stealing from stores or people as a means of basic survival.

Behaviors considered risky now may have been crucial in helping a teen escape or survive past danger. Alternatively, the risk taking may be useful now by helping traumatized youth cope with ongoing physical and emotional effects of trauma, regain a sense of control over their lives, and create much needed social connections. Asking teens to stop these behaviors without giving them something else to serve these vital functions is like asking people to take off their life vests without first teaching them how to swim.

Nancy, Alex's case manager, feels unsure about how to work with him. Overwhelmed, she seeks guidance from a senior case manager, who e-mails her a link to a National Child Traumatic Stress Network (NCTSN) Web site called "What Is Complex Trauma? A Resource Guide for Youth and Those Who Care About Them."[15] Reading it, she finds herself thinking in a new way about many of the youth and young adults she has worked with. She learns that teens who have experienced several traumatic events over many years, especially if they were abused or neglected from a very young age, fit the profile of what is called "complex trauma." *Complex trauma* describes both the exposure to and effects of traumatic events, and Nancy realizes that many of the young people she has worked with fit this profile, having difficulties with attachment, emotion regulation, behavior, thinking, and relationships, among others. She is ashamed to recall that she hadn't even thought to ask many of them about experiences of trauma. To make sure she doesn't forget, Nancy tapes a quote on the wall above her desk:

Just as an earthquake can cause deep foundation cracks that are the hidden cause of a building's instability even decades later, Complex Trauma can disrupt healthy development and is often the unseen cause of many problems and difficulties youth face years later that are not obviously connected to early childhood experiences.[15, p. 6]

The risky behaviors of high-risk youth can seem like earthquakes, which are threatening and destructive. But in reality, the trauma exposure preceding these behaviors is the earthquake, leading to "foundational cracks" in development that often go unseen. The effects of complex trauma create deep vulnerabilities in a child's developmental foundation. These points of tension and vulnerability can lead to the risky behaviors, which are better thought of as the "aftershocks," smaller earthquakes occurring along stressed fault lines caused by the initial earthquake of trauma. Aftershocks are triggered by changes in stress levels and function to release pressure or tension in the earth created by the original event. Much in the same way, risky behaviors seen in adolescence are direct responses to early traumatic experiences and serve as a means of releasing and managing traumatic stress.

Risky behaviors can be a response to trauma in several ways. As noted above, traumatized teens might be drawn to risky behaviors in an effort to escape painful sensations in their bodies, to dull intense emotions, or to avoid traumatic thoughts or memories. Physiologically, exposure to danger desensitizes the nervous system to be either more or less reactive to internal arousal. Traumatized youth, especially those who experienced traumatic events prior to developing language, feel the effects of trauma deeply in their bodies. Risky behaviors may be a way to regulate what they feel inside, either increasing physiological input in a controlled way ("turning up the volume of experience") through thrill seeking, pain, or sex, or decreasing sensation ("turning down the volume of experience") through isolating or using drugs. For example, Ana has always felt depressed and isolated, and also very confused about how to interact with men. Sex brings affection and helps her feel less alone, but the sex itself either made her dissociate or filled her with shame. Alex uses drugs to numb painful feelings triggered by intrusive thoughts. His parents had always told him he was a "bad kid," so eventually he started to believe it and stopped trying to be "good." Substances helped him get the courage to do even more risky things, which helped him feel alive inside in ways he did not feel when sober. Some teens may turn to substances as a way of accessing and talking about traumatic memories or experiences from which they may otherwise guard themselves. The immediate gratification afforded by risk behaviors can serve as a "break" from intense and painful trauma-related symptoms.

Every behavior has meaning and serves a function for the teen. Before assuming that a teen who is engaging in risky behaviors is irresponsible or rebellious, ask yourself these questions:

- What might the behavior symbolize or communicate given the teen's trauma history?

- What feelings or experiences is the teen trying to cope with by using the behavior?

- How are the behaviors helping this teen get his or her needs met at this time?

Even if you don't have the answers yet, when working with traumatized teens it is the safer, compassionate, and more trauma-informed approach to trust that there is a deeper reason for the behavior that you just aren't yet aware of. Stay curious and open.

Adolescents exposed to trauma are more likely to turn to risky behaviors as a way to cope with the painful aftermath of traumatic stress if they lack healthy coping skills and supports. Many traumatized teens, especially those who have experienced early abuse or neglect, never had the positive, safe, consistent caregivers to teach them how to cope with distress in healthy ways. Left to fend for themselves, teens turn to risky behaviors to cope with the physical, emotional, and cognitive effects of complex trauma.

Risky behaviors can also provide a sense of social connection and belonging. Substance use, risky sexual behaviors, and gang affiliation can provide a sense of community, connection, and/or safety that to an isolated or frightened teen makes the potential risks worthwhile.

Some adolescents engage in risky behaviors as a way of reenacting or repeating past traumatic experiences, whether consciously or unconsciously. Repeating these experiences can feel familiar or known and thus safe, or the teen may be trying to "do it differently" and therefore gain a sense of control or mastery over previous traumatic events. Engaging in risky behaviors can also be automatic or reflexive; some teens engage in high-risk behaviors because these are what they were exposed to growing up and therefore are all they know. Repeated risky behaviors may reflect what teens have witnessed, endured, and learned by example from abusive homes, neglectful parents, or violent neighborhoods. Once these experiences are triggered, trauma-tized teens instinctively operate from "survival mode" with automatic reactions they learned from early experiences.

It is important to keep in mind that when teens are engaging in risky behaviors, the behaviors may not seem risky or dangerous to them. This is especially true for teens who have experienced trauma, because their perception of safety versus danger can be skewed by their trauma exposure. A teen raised in a neighborhood where shootings occur frequently, among families where violence is common, or within a gang-affiliated community where fighting or other criminal activity is the norm, will perceive these as standard and expected behaviors. Trauma-exposed teens may actually experience calm environments or particularly uneventful periods in their lives as scary, threatening, or uncomfortable.

Even if teens do recognize that their behavior is risky or carries unwanted consequences, it can be difficult to change. Trauma makes people feel powerless, so teens who experienced trauma often lack a sense of self-efficacy and doubt their abilities to change. Or they may worry that giving up gang life, substance use, or stealing may make them more vulnerable to further danger, and sometimes they may be right, especially in the short term. Living in "survival mode" forces teens to live life day to day with little attention to long-term consequences. Complex trauma exposure also inhibits teens' perceptions of the future; they may have negative expectations of what is to come or anticipate no future at all.

That said, teens *can* heal from complex trauma and go on to have rich, productive lives. Caring adults play a key role in this healing, and knowing how to effectively connect and engage high-risk youth is essential.

> Positive stimulation helps promote healthy brain development. In particular, positive attachment experiences with caregivers help build trust, strong emotional connections with others, and self-regulation skills. Often, teens exposed to complex trauma lack consistent, reliable, and safe caregivers to help them develop the emotional and interpersonal skills they need to be happy and successful. *But it is never too late.* Because adolescence is a period of tremendous brain growth, it is an opportunity to make changes to the brain in a positive direction. Healthy attachments to positive adults help traumatized teens heal. Just by being a safe, reliable adult in a teen's life, you are helping to rewire his or her brain in healing ways.

Behavior in Context: Understanding and Connecting With Traumatized Youth

When confronted with a teen engaging in risky behaviors, consider the behaviors in the context of the teen's unique trauma history. Looking at the behavior alone can lead to making false assumptions about the adolescent and his or her character. Teens who engage in risky behaviors are often labeled as oppositional, defiant, irresponsible, rebellious, or dangerous. Classmates used to call Ana "crazy" and said that she "just wanted attention" after seeing the cuts on her arms, and neighbors called her a "slut" after finding out she was pregnant. Judging the behavior in isolation this way misses what is actually going on for traumatized teens.

> A few weeks later, Ana gets a phone call from Alex. He says he has been trying to "do good": attending the drop-in center regularly, trying to cut back on drinking and drugs, and even considering meeting with a therapist. He asks to speak to Emily and says hi to her on the phone. Before saying goodbye to Ana, Alex tells her that he loves her and is trying to "get on the right path" so they could be a family again. Ana has heard this before, but somehow this time feels different. She decides to check out the program her friend Jessica attends to get help for herself too.
>
> Ana packs Emily's favorite toys and snacks and heads to the clinic. Emily senses Ana's nerves and asks, "What's wrong, Mama?" Ana reassures her daughter but inside feels terrified that the clinic staff will ask about her history. She rarely shares details about her life. Even when she is trying to open up to others, she can't get the words out. How do you tell someone that your own mother abandoned you and never looked back, or that your father molested and raped you for years, and that running away was the only way to escape? How do you admit that you've had to have sex with men just to feel connected or have a place to stay, or that you stayed with several boyfriends who hit you because you had nowhere else to go? How do you share this without making others think you're damaged or crazy? Telling her story has only ever pushed people away.
>
> Over the course of her life, Ana has learned that asking for help was rarely beneficial. Teachers didn't believe her when she told them about what her dad was doing to her, and when police were called to her home to investigate a report of "suspected abuse," officers reprimanded her for "making up stories" before shaking her father's hand and leaving. Even her friends didn't know what to say when she told them small bits of her life. She looks down at Emily's hopeful face and pushes through the doors of the clinic. She wants a better life for Emily, and she knows she won't be able to achieve this without dealing with her own "stuff" first.
>
> While filling out paperwork, Ana pauses at the questions about her period. It was around the time she began puberty that her father began sexually abusing her. He used both physical strength and "charm" to coerce her

to give in to the sexual acts. He would start by telling her how beautiful she was, how he liked her curvy body, and how he was only trying to take care of her. After raping her, he would become angry and yell at her, blaming her and threatening to kill her if she ever told anyone. She started cutting to distract herself from the fear and feel some sense of control, relief, and oddly even a sense of pleasure. She also began binge eating to dissociate from the shame and powerlessness. The binge eating made her gain a lot of weight, which cut down on unwanted male attention, though the sexual abuse by her father continued. Eventually she started bingeing so heavily that she threw up, which was painful but somehow also a relief. Purging was pain she could control. When she was 15, she ran away from her father to live with an older boyfriend. When that boyfriend became abusive too, she lived on the streets or with friends for a while, doing whatever she needed to do to get by. After becoming pregnant with Emily, Ana got a second job at night so she could afford to rent a room from her aunt.

Teen girls exposed to trauma are likely to engage in self-harming or disordered eating behaviors or to have tumultuous romantic relationships, which can put them at risk for sexual exploitation.[8] Self-injurious behavior may provide relief from painful emotions or from emotional numbing; bingeing and purging may have the same effect. Risky sexual behaviors, as discussed above, may provide a sense of connection or may be seen as an effective tool to solve practical issues such as housing, food, or money.

Teens who have experienced trauma are at significantly increased risk of becoming homeless or being runaways. Teens may opt to leave and live on the streets to escape ongoing danger or abuse by their family or in foster homes. Living on the street puts teens at risk for further abuse or exploitation. Homeless youth may turn to "survival sex" or prostitution, selling drugs, gang affiliation, or other risky behaviors in order to earn money, food, or housing. Living on the streets, staying in shelters, or "couch surfing" increases the risk for sexual assault. Homeless teens may turn to drugs and alcohol to momentarily ignore their dire circumstances. Drugs and alcohol may make a teen feel warmer in the cold, less hungry when food is lacking, or less isolated when alone. "Self-medicating" with drugs and alcohol can also numb painful feelings related to PTSD or other symptoms of traumatic stress. Teens who have experienced trauma are three times more likely to use substances than those without histories of trauma.[16]

Although he is generally not open about his personal life or history, Alex often candidly speaks with several staff members and other youth at the drop-in center about his substance use. Alcohol helps him to party with friends, he says, and lets him feel happy and distract himself from problems. Marijuana helps with hangovers, and also lets him "forget things" and fall asleep when nightmares keep him up. Stimulants such as cocaine and meth help him get "keyed up" to do things that would be hard to do sober. He has tried hallucinogens out of curiosity but had "bad trips." He shares that he was "forced" to get substance use counseling in the past but that "it was a joke" and that he mostly came high to sessions.

> Maintain a neutral, curious, and nonjudgmental approach when learning or asking about high-risk behaviors. Alex was able to share details of his substance use largely because staff and youth at the drop-in center were open and accepting. No one assumed that Alex considered his polysubstance use to be problematic, and no one "lectured" him about the negative health effects of using drugs. Understanding that Alex perceived benefits related to his substance use was essential to his establishing positive and collaborative relationships with specific staff members, as well as the agency as a whole.

Treating More Than Just Behavior: Engaging Teens in Mental Health Services

Finding a Trauma-Informed Frame

Addressing risky behaviors in a trauma-informed way requires first ensuring that teens know we are not judging their behaviors but instead are genuinely trying to understand the behaviors in the context of their unique trauma histories. Intentionally approach each teen keeping in mind the question "What happened to you?" as opposed to "What's wrong with you?" It can be easy to be distracted by and focus on a teen's behaviors, because these are more tangible and visible than the underlying painful emotions driving these behaviors. But remember, these are not the earthquakes!

> Despite our best intentions, sometimes our own "stuff" gets in the way of our being nonjudgmental. We all have our own stories and worldviews. Spend time thinking through your own morals, values, and beliefs and considering how hearing teens' stories about trauma and risky behaviors could trigger you. In the interest of building collaborative and trusting relationships with traumatized teens, take some time to check in with yourself, practice being mindful of your own reactions, and utilize self-care.

There may be times when a teen becomes dysregulated and displays risky behaviors that need to be addressed in the moment—perhaps to maintain a safe environment, or to uphold your program's guidelines or rules, or to model appropriate limit setting for the teen. In such situations, you may feel compelled or even be expected to apply consequences for the behaviors, assert yourself as an adult in a position of authority, and "correct" the behaviors. In situations like this, if you respond to the teen impulsively, emotionally, or punitively, your reaction has the potential to trigger and possibly retraumatize the teen. That said, when implemented with trauma-informed sensitivity and awareness, setting limits and enforcing consequences do not necessarily have to conflict with trauma-informed care. For example, the Hollywood Homeless Youth Partnership (HHYP) encourages the use of trauma-informed consequences (TICs) rather than punishment when responding to problematic behaviors among traumatized youth (Table 5–2). TICs reflect a collaborative, trauma-informed way to effectively and compassionately assist youth in gradually addressing behaviors of concern. More recently, the HHYP shifted to using the term *trauma-informed consciousness* (A. Schneir, personal communication, December 1, 2017) within staff trainings to emphasize the importance of taking the time to understand the core underlying causes of teens' behaviors and choices and to explore ways to generate, facilitate, and support more adaptive approaches. Responding from a place of trauma-informed consciousness has the potential to enhance a teen's sense of overall safety and trust in his or her relationship with you and the agency as a whole.

Ana feels surprisingly safe talking with Olivia, the social worker with whom she meets for intake. Olivia is warm, but also honest and direct, and doesn't sugarcoat things. Olivia explains the program, services, and policies clearly, and describes each step of the appointment in advance so that Ana knows exactly what to expect. Olivia tells Ana that she can opt out of answering any questions and can take breaks at any time. She gives Ana the choice of telling her story in whatever order she wants, instead of Olivia asking questions. Ana appreciates being able to choose and is more able to open up without fearing that she might be asked to talk about something she isn't ready to share. Nonetheless, Ana feels familiar waves of panic as she touches on the "bad parts" of her story. Her heart beats faster, she feels hot and dizzy, and she struggles to breathe as the words get stuck in her throat. Olivia seems to notice, asking if Ana is okay, offering water, and changing the topic to talk about lighter things like music. Olivia also keeps checking in with Ana about whether she wants to continue the intake or stop for the day. These pauses help Ana focus on the here and now, and with a few deep breaths, her breathing and heart rate return to normal. Olivia talks for a bit, sharing that it's normal for our bodies and brains to need

TABLE 5–2. Trauma-informed consciousness: punishment versus trauma-informed consequences

Punishment	Trauma-informed consequences (TIC)
Punishment is used to enforce obedience to a specific authority and it uses words that escalate conflict.	TICs are intentionally designed to teach, change, or shape behavior, and to offer options within firm limits.
Punishment is usually used to assert power and control and often leaves a young person feeling helpless, powerless, and ashamed.	TICs are logical consequences that are clearly connected to the behavior, given with empathy and in a respectful tone.
Punishment is for the benefit of the punisher and not for the individual whose behavior needs to be corrected.	TICs are reasonable and use words that encourage thinking and preserve connections between people.

Incident: Youth becomes agitated, gets "in your face" and begins calling you "stupid" and "annoying," requesting to speak to your boss because you're "not helping me at all."

Punishment	Trauma-informed consequences (TIC)
Staff interpretation: Youth is being disrespectful. Youth doesn't appreciate the services we are offering. I need to set a firm example that we don't allow this type of verbal abuse.	*Staff reflection and interpretation:* Did something trigger this youth or bring up uncomfortable feelings or memories? What else could I do to help her feel safe?
Reaction: Staff threatens to ask youth to leave the program if behavior continues.	*Response:* Staff can address youth outside of waiting room to find out what happened. Let the youth know that safety (for her, you, and others in the waiting room) is most important. Validate that the youth seems to feel upset. Ask her if she would like a minute to herself. You can ask her if she wants to talk to someone about any feelings she might be experiencing.

Source. Adapted from Hollywood Homeless Youth Partnership 2009, 2010.[17,18]

a break when talking about emotionally intense situations. When Ana is ready to talk again, she shares about her cutting, and when Olivia doesn't wince or seem disturbed, Ana decides to tell her about being raped. Olivia still doesn't seem to pity or be disgusted by her, so Ana shares more and more. Olivia responds in a calm, quiet, and kind way, reflecting on how awful it must have been and observing aloud how strong Ana has shown herself to be. Ana feels understood and respected, and like maybe she isn't a crazy or terrible person or "too much" for Olivia. Olivia encourages Ana to consider a referral to mental health services. Ana is reluctant, but since she feels like Olivia gets her, she accepts.

> Be curious and stay curious. Traumatized teens may present initially as provocative, uninterested, mistrusting, or "hard." They may push you away, reject your attempts to help, and push to see if you can "handle them." Sometimes this may manifest in the teen telling you all the "bad stuff" (e.g., risky behaviors, details of trauma histories) up front. Other times, they may avoid sharing much personal information with you until they are able to fully trust you and your authentic interest in them. Either way, stay the course and trust in the power of connection.

Psychoeducation can be a powerful and validating intervention. Risky behavior should be framed as an understandable reaction to overwhelming and painful thoughts, feelings, and memories, or as a way to cope with the symptoms of traumatic stress. However, this does not mean that you should encourage risky behavior. What feels useful or inevitable in the short term can have long-term unwanted consequences. Balance validation of the teen's behaviors with gentle guidance toward change. Parents, caregivers, or any other important adults in the adolescent's life should be given the same psychoeducation, and should also be coached on balancing empathy and validation with clear limits and expectations for change.

> Consider giving teens the choice to join while you provide psychoeducation to important adults in their lives. Given that much of trauma is enveloped in secrecy, mistrust, and shame, being open, honest, and transparent are key elements of trauma-informed care.

After her first appointment with Dr. Torres, the therapist that Olivia recommended, Ana feels a strange mix of relief and deep anxiety. On the one hand, telling her story made her feel lighter, like she had been able to leave pieces of her past behind. On the other hand, she worries about having shared as much as she did with Olivia and Dr. Torres. But Olivia had warned her she might experience these feelings, which she jokingly called "disclosure remorse," so Ana decided to trust her intuitive sense that therapy could be useful to her and continued to see Dr. Torres.

Screening

It is equally important to screen youth with high-risk behaviors for exposure to trauma or abuse, and to screen youth who have experienced trauma for high-risk behaviors. Screening high-risk teens for trauma exposure will help to identify whether they have been exposed to traumatic events and to put their risky behaviors into this important context. Whenever possible, screen repeatedly to assess for exposure to ongoing trauma or maltreatment. If a teen is currently in a dangerous or unstable situation, safety must be addressed before proceeding with anything else. This focus on safety communicates to the teen that he or she is important and worth keeping safe, and that you can be counted on to help. This approach can be considered "therapeutic case management." Assessing safety also includes determining whether a teen's basic needs are being met. For example, when Alex first presented to the drop-in center, his case manager Nancy identified that he needed food, resources for housing, and vocational training, as well as medical and mental health services, parenting classes, and substance use treatment. Helping with these concrete needs builds trust and engagement. If basic needs are not being met, a teen is unlikely to show up for weekly therapy, let alone address issues such as risky sex and substance use.

> You might be in a position where you read documents or hear stories from other people about a high-risk youth before meeting the individual. Take these with a grain of salt. Hold off on making any conclusions until you spend time with the youth, build a trusting relationship, and get a first-hand understanding of the adversities he or she has experienced.

Screening for risky behaviors should assess a teen's type, severity, and frequency of behaviors; immediate needs and safety concerns; the function of the behaviors; and the teen's readiness to change. You might not get this information all at once. The teen may slowly open up over time as his or her trust and relationship with you strengthen. For a more thorough assessment, screening tools can help us. The HEEADSSS psychosocial interview, with questions related to each letter of the acronym (Home environment, Education and employment, Eating, peer-related Activities, Drugs, Sexuality, Suicide/depression, and Safety from injury and violence), is one commonly used screening tool for trauma and risky behaviors.[19,20] There are several versions available, including for typically developing adolescents, runaway and homeless youth, and transgender youth.[21] Don't just ask about negatives; it is equally important to get a good sense of the teens' resilience factors by focusing on strengths, positive qualities, and examples of adversity they have overcome.

> Nancy, Alex's case manager, e-mails a psychologist friend for ideas about getting to understand Alex better. The psychologist sends Nancy a copy of HEEADSSS 3.0[22] with a note saying, "This interview focuses on assessing a kid's Home environment, Education and employment, Eating, peer-related Activities, Drugs, Sexuality, Suicide/depression, and Safety from injury and violence. It was developed for doctors, but anyone can use it. I typically follow the order of letters in the acronym, and teens seem to like that, but sometimes kids who have been homeless feel uncomfortable starting with the H. In that case start with whatever area you think a teen is most open to." Nancy tries out the HEEADSSS at her next meeting with Alex, asking about Education and employment, Eating, and peer-related Activities. She tries to focus on his strengths in these areas, and encourages Alex's interest in drawing and graffiti. Later, asking about Alex's home and living circumstances, Nancy learns that Alex experienced chronic neglect and physical and emotional abuse growing up, as well as other abusive experiences at school and in foster care. Alex has lived with his biological mother and father, with his maternal aunt, in multiple foster care and group home settings, in the homes of fellow gang members, and most recently on the street. He was briefly in a shelter but was kicked out for threatening another resident. Alex describes multiple sexual partners and boasts about frequent unprotected sex, but Nancy is surprised that he knows little about sexually transmitted infections and has never been tested. Alex said he couldn't remember all of his previous mental health diagnoses but recalled reading records stating that he had been diagnosed with attention-deficit/hyperactivity disorder, bipolar disorder, and antisocial personality disorder. He seems much less comfortable talking about these diagnoses than about his drug and alcohol use, and admits that no one ever explained to him what those "labels" were about.

> Use open-ended questions with teens to help avoid assumptions. When inquiring about the home environment, provide prompt by saying "Tell me about your living situation" instead of asking "Did you grow up with your mother and father?" Similarly, use gender-affirming and LGBTQ-inclusive terminology when asking about gender identity, sexual orientation, and sexual practices.

Treatment

Several treatments can help reduce risky behaviors; regardless of treatment type, safety is the first and primary target. Talking about safety concerns up front serves several purposes. Of course, assessing safety is important for practical reasons. Also, as discussed above, it shows teens that you care and aren't just looking to punish or judge them. Genuine, caring adults who overtly prioritize the teen's safety in an understanding way help a teen to begin to chip away at the negative perceptions of others and the world that are the legacy of their early traumatic experiences. Conversations about safety should happen throughout treatment to ensure that there is no new danger and reinforce the importance of safety. For teens who have perhaps experienced little safety in their lives, this focus is tremendously powerful.

> Traumatized teens may initially have a negative reaction to compliments, acts of kindness, or expressions of care and support. Many have never heard positive feedback about themselves. For others, kind gestures or positive comments have been precursors to abuse, or unsafe adults may have used nice words and compliments to engage the teens. Be mindful of teens' reactions to your expressions of concern and adjust as needed. Proceed cautiously, but continue showing kindness so teens can begin associating kindness with safety instead of danger.

If you are trying to link a teen to mental health treatments focused on reducing high-risk behaviors, look for agencies or providers who provide trauma-informed care, and specifically those who offer evidence-based treatments such as Trauma-Focused Cognitive Behavioral Therapy (TF-CBT)[23]; Dialectical Behavior Therapy (DBT)[24]; Motivational Interviewing (MI)[25]; Attachment, Self-Regulation, and Competency (ARC)[26]; Integrative Treatment of Complex Trauma for Adolescents (ITCT-A)[27]; or Multisystemic Therapy (MST)[28] Keep in mind that even the best treatments take time to work. Expecting that teens will give up all coping behaviors simply because they are being told of the dangers is unrealistic. Instead, remember that it can be really scary for teens to give up risky behaviors that have been very functional over the years for escaping pain and danger. Change will take time, support, and perhaps even forgiveness. Teens' urges to engage in risky behaviors may even increase during treatment, especially during potentially painful parts of treatment, such as the trauma narrative. Knowing this in advance lets you and the adolescent make a plan in advance to cope with these urges and anticipate potential setbacks.

Web sites for the National Child Traumatic Stress Network (NCTSN) and the Substance Abuse and Mental Health Services Administration (SAMHSA) offer resources that may be helpful in obtaining additional information regarding trauma treatments and trauma-informed care. The Hollywood Homeless Youth Partnership Web site is a helpful resource for information focused on youth experiencing homelessness and complex trauma, trauma-informed care, and low-barrier engagement approaches for working with high-risk youth. (See "Resources and Additional Reading" at the end of this chapter.)

> Teens may be more open to a *harm-reduction approach* when discussing the possibility of giving up risky behaviors. This approach focuses on reducing negative consequences of a behavior by supporting any steps toward "safer" choices and suggesting alternative behaviors that are less risky. Examples of this approach include encouraging a teen to practice safe sex rather than to stop having sex altogether or helping a teen to problem solve around how to drink alcohol safely (e.g., sleep at a friend's house instead of driving home). Any steps toward reducing risk are positive and important.

"Emily, music, and not letting my dad 'win.' Those are the things that make my life worth living." Ana has been attending therapy with Dr. Torres for 4 months now, the longest she has ever stayed in therapy. Dr. Torres specializes in trauma therapies and other treatments for improving emotion regulation and improved coping, including DBT. When Dr. Torres first described DBT to Ana, they talked about DBT's goal of "building a life worth living." Ana likes this idea and appreciates that DBT largely focuses on building skills. She hopes these skills will help her deal with the symptoms of PTSD that are making life painful. She also likes that DBT is about understanding how the behaviors we engage in "make sense" in light of our histories. She has always felt so ashamed of herself—her past and the decisions she made after—so this approach is very validating. Ana continues to struggle with flashbacks and panic at times during the treatment, and sometimes still has urges to cut or smoke weed. Dr. Torres is always there to coach her through these moments and reminds her to use her "distress tolerance" skills and to "think effectively, not emotionally."

Meanwhile, Nancy is able to convince Alex to try therapy too. She sets him up with a therapy team that uses the ARC model.

The Attachment, Self-Regulation, and Competency (ARC)[29] model is a way of working with high-risk behaviors in youth who have experienced trauma. It focuses on enhancing and promoting resiliency by targeting three core areas in which traumatized youth often struggle.

Attachment: Focus on promoting positive attachment. Consider these questions:

- What quality of relationship does this youth form with his or her peers?

- How does this youth relate to adults, program staff, and authority figures?

Self-Regulation: Focus on developing and maintaining the ability to notice and control feelings such as frustration, anger, and fear. Consider these questions:

- What does it look like when the teen is experiencing unpleasant feelings?

- What situations trigger unpleasant feelings, and what skill does the teen use to cope?

Developmental Skill Competency: Focus on mastering the developmental tasks of adolescence and developing abilities to plan and organize. Consider these questions:

- Does the teen accurately perceive his or her current life circumstances?

- Is the teen able to think about his or her past, present, and future?

- Is the teen able to problem solve, organize and prioritize time, and plan ahead?

- What specific skills does this youth possess and still need to acquire?

The team works with Alex for more than a year. They provide case management, mental health, medical, occupational/vocational, and other services, including basic needs (food, clothing, mobile health clinic) and help with housing. Alex's treatment team collectively uses the ARC framework to guide his overall care. Dr. Musa, Alex's psychiatrist, uses ARC in his individual therapy and holds regular team meetings to coordinate everyone's work with Alex and support the team's integration across ARC domains. Therapy with Dr. Musa initially focuses on better understanding Alex's attachment/relational history to help Alex connect with others. Dr. Musa and the team prioritize engaging Alex on his own terms, with a collaborative and mutually respectful approach. Over time, Alex becomes acquainted with most of the team, including security, case managers, medical providers, and educational and vocational specialists, as well as other young people receiving services at the drop-in center. At first, Alex's attendance and level of engagement fluctuates, but his team engages him by tapping into his interests in art (graffiti workshops or local events) and exercise ("walk and talk" or throwing a football). They always leave a message when Alex doesn't attend a session, and that simple outreach helps to build trust. The consistency, sincerity, and continuity of treatment in a noninvasive fashion are crucial in helping Alex to build a healthy attachment to this support system.

Slowly, Alex becomes more receptive to learning emotional regulation skills in therapy. He starts to open up about his gang involvement, abuse history, and sexual experiences. One day he tells Dr. Musa that he likes that the staff at the drop-in center "actually care about helping me and making me feel less stressed out." He continues to engage more with services at the center, especially educational services such as the GED program and a training program in set design for film. Staff members help him with his resume and assist him to set up medical care. Although he's hesitant to entirely disengage from the gang and "leave my homies behind," he notices that he has become less motivated to participate in gang activities and instead prefers to spend time with Emily. He starts to have a more hopeful and positive outlook for his future, something he had never thought possible.

Conclusion

Like so many youth, Ana and Alex experienced chronic neglect, abuse, and other horrific traumatic events that no youth should have to experience. Neither had the appropriate emotional support or guidance to prepare them and keep them safe during the trials and tribulations of adolescence. It is no surprise, then, that they struggled to meet the societal and developmental growth expectations for teens and emerging young adults. Understanding their difficulties through the lens of trauma lets us understand how the neurobiological and psychological effects of trauma are at the root of their high-risk behaviors.

When working with high-risk, trauma-exposed teens like Ana and Alex, we must remember that chronic, complex trauma creates "cracks" in teens' psychological foundations and drives them to participate in risky behaviors. It is crucial to remain consistently mindful of the profound and often invisible effects of trauma in order to truly meet teens where they are developmentally. Developing and maintaining a healthy and positive relationship with teens is the first step toward any behavioral change. Remember too that although cracks may give rise to an unstable foundation, cracks are also "how the light gets in," as the late singer-songwriter Leonard Cohen sang. With much adversity comes much opportunity for growth. A teen's life can be changed by digging beneath the surface, nurturing the roots, and fostering a safe and caring environment with strength-based approaches, positive intentions, and resilience-building practices. Remind yourself of the transformative power of positive connections and the important role we can have in teens' healing. Neither Alex nor Ana would have been able to engage effectively in services or begin to make progress had it not been for relationships with caring, safe, and trusted adults. Through safe, consistent, and compassionate relationships, "cracks" can be patched, teens' foundations can be strengthened, and the negative effects of complex trauma can start to be reversed and slowly healed.

Resources and Additional Reading

Online Resources

National Child Traumatic Stress Network: http://www.nctsn.org
Substance Abuse and Mental Health Services Administration: https:// www.samhsa.gov/nctic/trauma-interventions
The Hollywood Homeless Youth Partnership: http://hhyp.org

Additional Reading

Cook A, Blaustein M, Spinazzola J, et al: Complex trauma in children and adolescents. National Child Traumatic Stress Network Complex Trauma Task Force, 2003. Available at: https://nursebuddha.files.wordpress.com/2011/12/complex-trauma-in-children.pdf. Accessed March 2, 2018.
Knight JR, Sherritt L, Shrier LA, et al: Validity of the CRAFFT substance abuse screening test among adolescent clinic patients. Arch Pediatr Adolesc Med 156(6):607–614, 2002 12038895
Spinazzola J, Habib M, Blaustein M, et al: What is complex trauma? A resource guide for youth and those who care about them. National Center for Child Traumatic Stress, 2017. Available at: http://www.nctsn.org/sites/default/files/assets/pdfs/ct_guide_final.pdf. Accessed March 2, 2018.

Substance Use and Mental Health Services Administration: Key substance use and mental health indicators in the United States: results from the 2013 National Survey on Drug Use and Health (HHS Publ No SMA-14-4887, NSDUH Series H-49). 2014. Available at: https://www.samhsa.gov/data/sites/default/files/NSDUHmhfr2013/NSDUHmhfr2013.pdf. Accessed March 2, 2018.

References

1. Center for Behavioral Health Statistics and Quality: Key substance use and mental health indicators in the United States: results from the 2015 National Survey on Drug Use and Health (HHS Publ No SMA-16-4984, NSDUH Series H-51). 2016. Available at: https://www.samhsa.gov/data/sites/default/files/NSDUH-FFR1-2015/NSDUH-FFR1-2015/NSDUH-FFR1-2015.pdf. Accessed March 2, 2018.

2. American Psychiatric Association: Diagnostic and Statistical Manual of Mental Disorders, 5th Edition. Arlington, VA, American Psychiatric Association, 2013

3. Miller AL, Rathus JH, Linehan MM: Dialectical Behavior Therapy for Suicidal Adolescents. New York, Guilford, 2007

4. Centers for Disease Control and Prevention, National Center for Injury Prevention and Control, Division of Violence Prevention: Understanding teen dating violence (fact sheet 2016). 2016. Available at: https://www.cdc.gov/violenceprevention/pdf/teen-dating-violence-factsheet-a.pdf. Accessed March 2, 2018.

5. Kann L, Kinchen S, Shanklin SL, et al: Centers for Disease Control and Prevention (CDC): Youth risk behavior surveillance—United States, 2013. MMWR Suppl 63(4):1–168, 2014 24918634

6. Kann L, McManus T, Harris WA, et al: Youth risk behavior surveillance—United States, 2015. MMWR Surveill Summ 65(6)(Suppl. 4):1–174, 2016 27280474

7. Vagi KJ, O'Malley Olsen E, Basile KC, et al: Teen dating violence (physical and sexual) among U.S. high school students: findings from the 2013 National Youth Risk Behavior Survey. JAMA Pediatr 169(5):474–482, 2015 25730143

8. Layne CM, Greeson JK, Ostrowski SA, et al: Cumulative trauma exposure and high risk behavior in adolescence: findings from the National Child Traumatic Stress Network Core Data Set. Psychol Trauma 6(S1):S40, 2014

9. Child Welfare Information Gateway: Understanding the effects of maltreatment on brain development. Washington, DC, U.S. Department of Health and Human Services, Children's Bureau, 2015. Available at: https://www.childwelfare.gov/pubs/issue-briefs/brain-development/. Accessed March 2, 2018.

10. National Scientific Council on the Developing Child: Excessive stress disrupts the architecture of the developing brain: working paper 3, updated edition. 2014. Available at: http://developingchild.harvard.edu/wp-content/uploads/2005/05/Stress_Disrupts_Architecture_Developing_Brain-1.pdf. Accessed March 2, 2018.

11. Perry BD: The neurosequential model of therapeutics: applying principles of neuroscience to clinical work with traumatized and maltreated children, in Working With Traumatized Youth in Child Welfare. Edited by Webb NB. New York, Guilford, 2006, pp 27–52

12. Chamberlain L: The amazing adolescent brain: what every educator, youth serving professional, and healthcare provider needs to know. 2009. Available at: http://www.documentcloud.org/documents/468776-the-amazing-adolescent-brain. Accessed March 2, 2018.

13. Perry BD, Beauchaine T, Hinshaw S: Child maltreatment: a neurodevelopmental perspective on the role of trauma and neglect in psychopathology, in Child and Adolescent Psychopathology. Edited by Beauchaine TP, Hinshaw SP. New York, Wiley, 2008, pp 93–128

14. Perry BD, Pollard RA, Blakley TL, et al: Childhood trauma, the neurobiology of adaptation, and "use-dependent" development of the brain: how "states" become "traits." Infant Ment Health J 16(4):271–291, 1995

15. National Child Traumatic Stress Network: What is complex trauma? A resource guide for youth and those who care about them. 2018. Available at: http://www.nctsn.org/sites/default/files/assets/pdfs/ct_guide_final.pdf. Accessed March 2, 2018.

16. National Child Traumatic Stress Network: Making the connection: trauma and substance abuse. 2008. Available at: http://www.nctsn.org/sites/default/files/assets/pdfs/SAToolkit_1.pdf. Accessed March 2, 2018.

17. Hollywood Homeless Youth Partnership: Trauma informed consequences for homeless youth. 2009. Available at: http://hhyp.org/wp?content/uploads/2012/02/Trauma?Informed?Consequences.pdf. Accessed March 2, 2018.

18. Hollywood Homeless Youth Partnership: Trauma informed consequences for homeless youth: putting theory into practice. 2010. Available at: http://hhyp.org/wp-content/uploads/2012/02/HHYP_TIC_Theory_into-Practice.pdf. Accessed March 2, 2018.

19. Goldenring J, Cohen E: Getting into adolescent heads. Contemp Pediatr 5(7):75–90, 1998

20. Goldenring J, Rosen D: Getting into adolescent heads: an essential update. Contemp Pediatr 21:64–90, 2004

21. Cohen E, Mackenzie RG, Yates GL: HEADSS, a psychosocial risk assessment instrument: implications for designing effective intervention programs for runaway youth. J Adolesc Health 12(7):539–544, 1991 1772892

22. Klein DA, Goldenring JM, Adelman WP: HEEADSSS 3.0: the psychosocial interview for adolescents updated for a new century fueled by media. 2014. Available at: http://contemporarypediatrics.modernmedicine.com / contemporary-pediatrics/content/tags/adolescent-medicine/heeadsss-30-psychosocial-interview-adolesce?page=full. Accessed March 2, 2018.

23. Cohen JA, Mannarino AP, Deblinger E: Treating Trauma and Traumatic Grief in Children and Adolescents. New York, Guilford, 2006

24. Linehan M: Cognitive-Behavioral Treatment of Borderline Personality Disorder. New York, Guilford, 1993

25. Naar-King S, Suarez M: Motivational Interviewing With Adolescents and Young Adults. New York, Guilford, 2011

26. Kinniburgh KJ, Blaustein M, Spinazzola J, et al: Attachment, self-regulation, and competency. Psychiatr Ann 35(5):424–430, 2005

27. Briere J, Lanktree CB: Integrative Treatment of Complex Trauma for Adolescents (ITCT-A): A Guide for the Treatment of Multiply Traumatized Youth, 2nd Edition. Los Angeles, CA, USC Adolescent Trauma Treatment Training Center, National Child Traumatic Stress Network, U.S. Department of Substance Abuse and Mental Health Services Administration, 2013

28. Henggeler SW, Borduin CM: Family Therapy and Beyond: A Multisystemic Approach to Treating the Behavior Problems of Children and Adolescents. Pacific Grove, CA, Brooks/Cole, 1990

29. Blaustein ME, Kinniburgh KM: Treating Traumatic Stress in Children and Adolescents: How to Foster Resilience Through Attachment, Self-Regulation, and Competency. New York, Guilford, 2010

CHAPTER 6

School Refusal and Other Behavioral and Academic Problems at School

Rachel Mandel, M.D.

Ms. Shah, the dean at Westside Middle School, is surprised to hear that two of her students, brothers, have been uncharacteristically absent from school for more than a week. Josh is a small and gregarious 13-year-old in sixth grade, and his 15-year-old brother Tyler is a gentle giant in the smaller eighth-grade classroom for kids with learning disabilities. Ms. Shah has met their adoptive mother, a kind older woman whom many at the school know well. Their mother often walked the boys to and from school, both to make sure that Josh did not get into trouble on the way, as he was prone to minor mischief, and to check in with Tyler's teachers, as he tended to be embarrassed about his academic struggles and asking for help. She reliably called the school if one of the boys was sick and staying home, or if she needed to have Tyler go to an appointment with her as her stamina began to decline with age. As their absence reaches almost 2 weeks, Ms. Shah gets more concerned; she tries calling their home, but no one picks up. Finally Josh and Tyler return to school. Tyler seems his usual self, perhaps even more quiet than usual, but within an hour of their first day back Josh is out of control. He spends most of the morning running through the halls, turning over furniture, and jumping down stairwells. Josh has always been a bit of a class clown but never so wild, and Ms. Shah and the other staff worry he might hurt himself. The school nurse sees the commotion with Josh and comments that perhaps he missed his medication, a treatment for attention-deficit/hyperactivity disorder (ADHD) to help control his hyperactivity and impulsivity. She asks Josh about his medication, and he says that he has not taken his medicine since he went into foster care. Ms. Shah is shocked—foster care? She tries to ask Josh what happened, but he runs off again.

School is a cornerstone in the lives of children and adolescents, and the immense value of caring and responsive school staff cannot be overstated. At school, students learn and grow not only academically but also socially and emotionally. It should be a place of safety and nurturance. School may also be the only place outside the home where teens regularly experience structure and authority. Because teens spend years with the same peers, teachers, counselors, and administrators, schools are also in a unique position to observe and understand individual teens as they grow and develop over time. For adolescents whose lives are upended by traumatic life events, schools may be the only source of consistency in an otherwise unpredictable world. But traumatic experiences and the symptoms that follow can also make it difficult for a teen to function in school, academically or socially, or even to attend school at all. This is a cruel twist, because trauma and its effects can separate teens from crucial supports and resources at school just at the time when they need them most.[1]

> Sudden unexplained absence, academic decline, or marked behavioral change in school is a red flag for a traumatic event or other stress in a child's life, and warrants investigation. Major stress, change, or trauma occurring outside of school can greatly impact a teen's educational experience.

For some teenagers the effects of trauma will be obvious to school staff, and for others they will be more subtle. Every individual responds to trauma differently; one teen may even respond differently to various traumatic experiences depending on the nature of each event, the teen's age at the time, and how the event affects the teen. There is no right or wrong way for a student to process trauma. Some experience its effect briefly and then return to their normal state of function, whereas others are affected by trauma well into adult life. Teachers and other school staff may know the teen better than anyone and are often the first to notice a change. As discussed in Chapter 1 ("Teens and Traumatic Stress"), trauma can present with externalizing symptoms, like Josh's hyperactive and oppositional behaviors, or internalizing symptoms, like Tyler's being quiet and isolative. Externalizing and internalizing symptoms do not necessarily indicate trauma in and of themselves, but astute school staff who notice these symptoms as a marked change from a child's baseline would be wise to consider that the child may have experienced a traumatic event.[2] The most important thing that school staff can do in the face of trauma is to be supportive and to keep in mind that a teen may be struggling with trauma but may not be able to identify or fully articulate it.

Asking Why: How Trauma Can Lead to Problems in School

The next day, Josh is again hyperactive and impulsive and quickly gets kicked out of class for being disruptive. The principal, who is unfamiliar with Josh, calls 911. However, when the school social worker, who knows the brothers well, hears the commotion in the halls, he invites Josh into his office to talk. He calls Ms. Shah and enlists a school aide to find a snack and a drink for Josh. Ms. Shah asks Josh about his medication, and Josh again says he hasn't taken it. When EMS arrives at the office door, Josh appears aggravated and scared. He is still full of energy, but the school social worker and Ms. Shah agree that Josh doesn't need to go to the ER as they can continue to contain his behavior in the office and they seem to have found an explanation (being off his medication) for his behavioral crisis. The EMS workers ask a few questions before agreeing that the situation can best be handled within the school without a complicated and potentially scary trip for Josh to the ER. After the EMS workers leave, Ms. Shah asks Josh if he knows the name or phone number of his new foster family. He has it written in his notebook, and Ms. Shah calls the foster mother to get more information about the foster care agency and caseworker for the family. The caseworker informs her that the boys had been placed into foster care last week after their adoptive mother died suddenly in her sleep.

Calling 911 should be reserved for emergencies, when a teen is in immediate danger to self or others. Although a teen who is destroying property can be disruptive, surprising, and even scary in the course of a standard school day, the teen will often calm down in a more one-on-one setting, especially with familiar staff. Music, a snack, and even paper and markers can be useful for distraction and deescalation. Some teens will be able to sit and talk when in a private space away from peers, the pressures of academics, and other triggers. Josh's behavior was not acceptable in the classroom setting, but once he was removed to a more quiet area with fewer demands and with more individualized attention, it was clear that he was not dangerous and did not need to be taken to the ER from the school. Keep in mind that when children are taken from school to the ER, they are taken in an ambulance on a stretcher, and they will likely be in a hospital setting for hours while several unfamiliar health care personnel evaluate them. Being taken to the ER is a strange and potentially scary process for students, especially those who may have already experienced trauma. If calling emergency services can safely be avoided, school staff have an opportunity to understand what is behind the behavior and help the adolescent feel heard, which can be useful for staff and deeply therapeutic for the teen.

> When the foster mother arrives at the school, she admits to Ms. Shah that she had no idea Josh was supposed to be taking medication. Then Ms. Shah and the school nurse find the name of Josh's clinic and the names of his providers in their files, and they assist the foster mother in arranging an urgent appointment for later that day. The school social worker speaks to Josh's psychiatrist to discuss the recent major events in his life and his behavior today, and they agree to keep in contact as needed regarding further issues at school. Because Josh doesn't have a guardian to consent for treatment, the foster care agency worker makes an expedited request for the director of the foster care agency to consent for Josh's usual medication to be prescribed and for Josh to continue treatment with his psychiatrist. Later that day at the clinic, Josh's psychiatrist recognizes Josh's behavior as similar—worse but not dangerously so—to when he has not had medication in the past. He writes a new prescription for Josh's usual medication. He spends the rest of the session listening, providing support, and offering reassurance to Josh as he anxiously recounts about foster care and getting in trouble at school. They agree to schedule more frequent appointments to check in.

Stressors, traumas such as traumatic loss of a loved one, and changes in living environment as occur during placement in foster care can directly and indirectly impact an adolescent's academic performance and behavior in school. Safety and expedient housing are of utmost importance, as they should be, but other important elements of students' lives outside of the school also impact their ability to attend school, participate, focus, learn, remember, perform, socialize, and cooperate. Medications, appointments, clothing, phones with key numbers, schoolwork, textbooks, and keepsakes can all disappear during transitions, causing frustration or difficulty in completing assignments. Intangible aspects of life, such as changes in neighborhoods and relationships, can have dramatic psychological impact as well and can be difficult for a teen to understand and accept.[3]

For Josh, the death of his adoptive mother, adapting to a new foster family and a new neighborhood, and inconsistency with his medications directly contribute to his sudden and noticeable change in behavior at school.

> Adjusting to major changes, such as removal from one home and placement in another, is a process in which safety, adjustment, and stabilization are the primary goals. More often than not, personal and important belongings are lost or forgotten along the way. Do not take for granted that a child in foster care has everything he or she needs!

Josh's foster mother is not able to fill the prescription for several days because prior authorization is required now that Josh's insurance changed when his adoptive mother died and he entered foster care. She lets Ms. Shah know it will be a few days before Josh can get his ADHD medication. Ms. Shah arranges with Josh's teachers and the school social worker for Josh to have some breaks throughout his day until he resumes taking his regular medication. During the breaks he meets with the social worker. They walk around the gym, they both share their memories about Josh's adoptive mother, and Josh talks about missing her. Once Josh restarts the medication, his teachers note with relief that he seems back to himself. Josh continues meeting with the social worker, transitioning to regular weekly meetings as things settle down.

They meet weekly for several months, and then Josh requests not to come as frequently because he does not want to miss the experiments in science class and he is eager to get a big part in his school play. The social worker agrees that Josh can check in as needed.

While Josh initially requires a lot of attention, his brother Tyler seems to be doing alright from the beginning. He's a bit quieter than before, keeping to himself at lunch and free time, and he quits the school basketball team, even though he seemed to be enjoying it before. His teacher, coach, and some other staff check on him periodically, but Tyler only responds with a few words like "I'm fine" or "thank you." He seems not to want to talk about his loss, so everyone just lets him be. He stops doing homework and finishes little work in class, but his teacher wants to be sympathetic to what he has been through, so she continues to pass him and only briefly mentions the issue to Tyler's foster family at parent-teacher conference.

One day, about 2 months after his adoptive mother's death, Tyler doesn't show up for fourth period after lunch. A few students report they had seen him going upstairs instead of downstairs, but he didn't respond when they asked where he was going. School security finds Tyler standing near the ledge of the roof of the school building, despondent. They ask what is wrong and try to get him to come downstairs, but Tyler remains still and silent. They call down to Ms. Shah, who grabs Tyler's former basketball coach and heads up to the roof. The coach is nervous and not too sure what to do, but he walks over to where Tyler is standing and sits down. "Hey Tyler, I'm just going to sit here next to you." The coach waits for some kind of sign from Tyler. Once Tyler looks up at him, the coach continues: "I'm not sure what's going on, but I'm here for you. I know things have been tough lately." Tyler admits that he has been thinking of jumping from the roof in order to end his life. The coach empathizes with how bad things have been and expresses that he wants to help. He reaches his hand out to Tyler and convinces Tyler to come away from the ledge and go back downstairs. Ms. Shah calls 911 and Tyler's foster mother, and gathers Tyler's most recent relevant records and staff contact numbers to take to the ER. She accompanies Tyler in the ambulance to the hospital and waits until she can talk to the ER team who is evaluating him, knowing that the more information she gives the ER clinicians, the better decision they can make about Tyler. She also gives the ER clinicians the phone numbers for Tyler's foster mother and foster care agency worker. The social worker in the ER is able to talk with all of them, and given Tyler's suicidal intent, suicide plan, and suicidal behavior all in the context of the sudden death of his adoptive mother, Tyler is hospitalized on an inpatient psychiatric unit for 2 weeks.

Just because students are quiet and cooperative does not mean that they are not suffering. It is human instinct to pay more attention to students who present with externalizing symptoms because they can be disruptive and more obviously potentially dangerous. However, students who present with internalizing symptoms are often more vulnerable precisely because they can go unnoticed for so long, holding in their pain and not seeking help.[4] These teens need adults to be aware of trauma and its effects and understand trauma-informed approaches; simply being a consistent or supportive presence will not be enough. For example, the school staff occasionally asking Tyler if he was okay did not do much good. His teacher's well-intentioned decision to let Tyler get away with not turning in work and ignore his slipping grades was not helpful either. A decline in school performance should be an indicator of concern, even for a teen with learning disability. Similarly, Tyler's dropping off the basketball team should have been a red flag. Thankfully, Tyler maintained trust and positive regard for his former coach, which was enough for the coach to be able to talk Tyler down off of the roof to get help.

> Don't ignore the quiet kids! Checking in with the teens is a good start, but "I'm fine" does not guarantee that a teen is fine. Adults can learn more by getting to know a teen; maintaining a positive relationship; noticing subtle changes in attitude, mood, energy level, and level of participation; and having more open-ended and casual conversations.

Considering What's Happening in the Moment

In the hospital, Tyler is able to open up to a therapist about what he has been going through. Tyler misses his adoptive mother profoundly and feels responsible for her death. Her death also brings up other painful memories he works desperately to keep away. Although Josh was very young, Tyler was old enough to recall how bad things were before they entered into foster care when he was age 5. Living with his biological mom, he was often left alone with baby Josh while his mother partied, and at times he witnessed substance abuse, violence, and sex in the home. Tyler and Josh were in several foster homes over a few years, and intermittently put back with their biological mother, before she finally lost her parental rights due to ongoing drug use. Things finally settled down once the boys were placed with the woman who would adopt them. As Tyler got bigger, he developed a sense of responsibility and pride in being able to look after his little brother and help his adoptive mother with physical tasks and errands. In the weeks before her death, Tyler recalls noticing that she was moving more slowly and eating less. He worried that something was wrong, but whenever he asked her, she would laugh him off. He adds that when he hears the laughter of kids in his class, even friendly ones, he has that memory of his adoptive mom's laugh and his heart aches. It was Tyler who found her dead that morning. Tyler tells his therapist that he should have known how sick she was and insisted that she go to the hospital. Tyler thinks about her constantly now, and he frequently experiences flashbacks and nightmares of finding her body. He doesn't feel like he can connect to his new foster family or the kids and teachers at school because they don't understand what he has gone through. Tyler is relieved that Josh is adjusting well, but he also feels guilty for not recovering Josh's medication and some of their other belongings from the home before they were removed.

> Inpatient psychiatric hospitalization might be needed for safety and stabilization if a teen is a danger to self or others in the home and/or school setting. Intensive therapy may be initiated in the hospital, and sometimes medication is prescribed. The information that is disclosed from the hospital to schools depends on the child, parent, or foster care agency. Nevertheless, coordination of care between the hospital and the school is essential and can facilitate an easier transition back to school and reintegration into the community. Often, it is helpful for teens who have experienced traumatic events that resulted in mental health issues to follow up with a counselor in school for additional support, to make sure that the teens are adjusting well and getting what they need. Through collaboration with the mental health professionals at the hospital, the school counselor can gain greater insight into a teen's behavior. Information and insights from the hospital staff can also help to assist school personnel in understanding and responding to the teen's behavior, and inform how the school will work with the teen moving forward.

Death and illness of family members can be traumatic for adolescents.[5] These, like any other traumatic experiences, are hard for teens to understand, which can lead to confusion, frustration, worry, and guilt. These reactions can be especially problematic for teens who take on a caretaker role in their family, or those with intellectual or developmental disabilities. It can mean a lot for teachers, coaches, and counselors to check in with students when they have lost someone, and even if the student doesn't want to talk right away, to continue approaching the teen to keep the lines of communication open. It is also important to note that when adolescents experience a loss or other trauma that results in a change of caregiver, distressing emotions and painful memories linked to previous trauma can reemerge. Although Tyler and Josh were adopted into a secure and loving home as young children, they experienced years of neglect, abuse, and overall instability that shaped their early lives. Although they adjusted well in the years during which they were in their adoptive mother's home, feelings of abandonment and guilt resurfaced following the sudden loss of their adoptive mother. Tyler's more profound reaction to this trauma as compared to Josh's may have to do with their different ages and developmental levels now, the different ages at which initial life traumas occurred, their different relationships with their adoptive mother, their different exposures to the trauma, and the way they managed and coped with the previous traumas. Again, no two people respond to trauma in the same way. There is no way to know what individuals have gone through other than by providing the space and time for them to tell their own story. Tyler's discovery of his adoptive mother's death, combined with his role as a caregiver to her and his younger brother, made his experience much different from Josh's.[6]

It is also important to keep in mind that adopted teens and teens in foster care have a much greater likelihood of having experienced trauma in early life than children living in their family of origin. Even if teens who have been adopted or placed in foster care have been in a stable home for years, their early traumas can still affect them later in life and can manifest themselves in the school setting. By definition, children in foster care have experienced some alleged abuse or neglect that necessitated removal from the home.[7] The removal itself and the sudden change of caregiver and home can be traumatic. School staff should take special care to support and get to know these students. For teens who have been through so much, just one adult caring for and taking an interest in them can make the difference between resilience and despair.

> Tyler returns to school after his hospitalization. His foster mother presents Ms. Shah the hospital discharge papers, which say that Tyler will be meeting every other week with a psychiatrist in a local clinic. Ms. Shah and the school social worker both check in with Tyler, but he doesn't say much, and his teachers say he remains quiet and disinterested in schoolwork. The basketball coach encourages him to join the team again, but Tyler politely declines. Noticing Tyler isolating himself during lunch and recess, the coach offers Tyler the opportunity to use the gym during recess. Tyler agrees, and they shoot hoops together

when Tyler has free time. The coach discovers that Tyler becomes more talkative and even smiles sometimes with the ball in his hands.

> Nonverbal support can be just as effective as verbal support. Many people have difficulty or discomfort expressing their emotions with words. Caring and supportive actions can be equally, if not more, important.

Although psychiatric treatment outside of school can be appropriate for teens who have developed posttraumatic symptoms, treatment (whether therapy or medication) can take weeks, months, or even longer to be fully effective. Returning from a hospitalization can be difficult to navigate for any student—catching up on missed schoolwork, readjusting to a routine, and dealing with questions and gossip among peers. When 911 is called because of an incident in school, the situation can be even more embarrassing, especially when hospitalization for an emotional or psychiatric issue results, which often entails more intimate and complicated explanations than, say, a compound fracture from skateboarding. It is crucial for all students to feel that school is a safe place and that they have a safe space within it. This is especially true for the quiet students who might not have many friends and those returning from a stressful event such as a hospitalization. This safe space may be a favorite teacher's classroom during lunch, a counselor's office, or an auxiliary room where other activities may be a source of distraction and competence (e.g., sports, technology, arts and crafts).

One day, about a month after Tyler returned to school, Tyler's coach notices that he looks sad when he enters the gym during lunch. Tyler walks past the basketball, which is unusual. The coach invites him to sit in his office, where Tyler breaks down and cries. The coach gives him some tissues and sits quietly to allow Tyler to be. Tyler continues to cry without saying anything for a while, finally revealing that it would have been his deceased adoptive mother's birthday today, and he had been thinking about her all day.

> School can serve as a positive distraction from past traumatic memories. At the same time, anniversaries of birthdays and dates of trauma, as well as holidays, can be very triggering for traumatized youth. Kids may present as more sad and withdrawn, or more angry and oppositional. If you are aware of anniversaries and holidays, check in about these as the days draw near. Acknowledge that things may be more difficult and offer that you will still be here to provide support and an eager ear.

The coach talks with Tyler for the rest of the period, mostly about missing his adoptive mother. The coach brings up missing his own mother who had recently passed away, normalizing Tyler's grief. Tyler reveals that he wants to visit his adoptive mother's grave. He didn't get to go to her funeral, because he and Josh were in the midst of changing homes at the time. Tyler doesn't know where she was buried and hasn't wanted to bother his foster family about it; besides, Josh is afraid of cemeteries. The coach shares how visiting his own mother's grave was useful for him to say good-bye and to still feel close to her. He offers to talk to Tyler's foster family about the possibility of visiting the cemetery. Tyler agrees, and when the coach calls Tyler's foster father, the foster father is more than willing to take Tyler to visit.

Rituals and routine can be very important to those who have experienced traumas, major changes, and other life upheaval. Staying in the same school or same community can provide stability. Just as many people will shy away from talking about or bringing up past traumatic experiences, many are uncertain whether to expose children and adolescents to funerals and wakes, and whether to discuss death at all. The answer depends on the child's personal preference and readiness. Josh expresses fear, so he should not be forced to go to the cemetery, but Tyler expresses appropriate interest in going to help process his grief, so he should be supported to do so.[8] The coach's disclosure of his own loss helps to provide empathy and a sense of connection with Tyler. The coach also models for Tyler that a man can talk about feelings and loss, which encourages Tyler to identify and talk about his own experience. While teachers must always remain professional and maintain appropriate boundaries with students regarding their personal lives, loss is a universal experience. Thus, it is appropriate for the coach to share his personal experience in order for Tyler to feel less alone and less "crazy." Especially with teenagers, who are naturally suspicious and doubtful, an appropriate level of disclosure may grant you permission or an opening to further explore what might be going on for the teen.

The following Friday, Tyler's last period class is unusually rowdy. A few of the kids are telling "Yo mama" jokes, which most of the class finds hilarious. The teacher intermittently gets the kids to calm down, but the jokes continue in the form of written notes passed around the class. Tyler does not find these jokes amusing and does not pass the notes along when they come across his desk, instead taking them up to the teacher. The other kids get irritated, and after class they taunt Tyler for not participating, saying that he is a "loser" and a "snitch." Tyler ignores them and does not say anything back, but he is visibly uncomfortable.

Tyler seems to have a good weekend, with an extra day off for a Monday holiday, but on Tuesday morning he wakes up complaining of a stomachache. He tells his foster parents that he threw up and asks to stay home.

They let him stay home that day, but when Tyler has the same complaints the following morning, his foster dad takes him to the doctor, who finds nothing physically wrong. Tyler agrees that he will return to school on Thursday, but then that morning he wakes up complaining of the same symptoms and not wanting to go to school. His foster dad reminds him of what the doctor said and of their agreement about going back to school. Tyler starts to yell, "You don't care about me! Nobody cares about me!" His foster dad tries to calm Tyler down. He tells Tyler that he does care about him and tries to hug him, but this seems to upset Tyler more. He pushes his foster father's arms away and starts throwing items around the room. This lasts for several minutes. Never having seen Tyler behave this way, his foster father calls 911. By the time the ambulance comes, Tyler is crying and not speaking, but once he reaches the ER, he is calm. Tyler is evaluated and sent home, as this seems to be an isolated incident and he did not pose any serious danger to himself or others. In the ER, Tyler talks a bit about what his peers said that bothered him. He admits that this kind of teasing has been going on for a few weeks. The ER doctor shares this with Tyler's foster dad, who calls Tyler's outpatient psychiatrist and Ms. Shah at school to let them know. They all agree to be more vigilant of such bullying and to intervene should it happen again. The ER doctor explains that today's outburst was not solely linked to the notes and name calling, but connected to anger and sadness fueled by painful memories. The ER doctor suggests that through therapy, Tyler could explore and process these memories to make holidays and other reminders less painful.

Finding the Frame: Putting Behaviors in Context

Tyler seems okay after the ER visit, but the morning of the next schoolday he still refuses to go to school. Wanting to avoid another major tantrum and feeling sympathetic about Tyler's loss, his foster dad acquiesces and agrees to let him stay home. Once that is decided, Tyler is notably less tense. He does chores and helps around the house, and he even completes some school-work before his brother comes home. In the evening, Tyler's foster dad speaks with him and they agree that the following day he will go to school. However, the following morning is the same. Tyler eats breakfast, washes up, and prepares to go to school, but when it is time to leave, he becomes tense and despondent, and his foster dad lets him stay home. This pattern continues through the week. Tyler seems fine on the weekend, and even during the week in most scenarios except going to school in the morning. When Tyler's foster dad talks to him about it, Tyler seems reasonable and does not know why it is so hard for him to go, but it is. Tyler feels guilty about the stress that he causes his foster family every morning, but he cannot think of any way to make things better. Tyler's foster dad wants to give Tyler a break and finish off the school year on a good note. So at their appointment with Tyler's psychiatrist later that week, Tyler's foster dad asks the psychiatrist to apply for home schooling, which seems to him like a logical and sensitive option. He is very surprised when the psychiatrist says no.

> Home schooling is *not* useful for school refusal. Counterintuitively, it can actually make things worse. Home schooling is rarely indicated. It is reserved for situations of significant but temporary disability, such as a medical illness that is debilitating but likely to heal (e.g., a fractured spine after a car accident), or to cover the time needed to secure more long-term accommodations for a more chronic problem (e.g., a specialized school program for a child with autism or deafness). It is very important for teens to attend school for their academic and social development.

Tyler's psychiatrist is wise to recommend that Tyler continue to attend his community school, especially given the teen's previous good attendance and overall good social and academic experience in school. School refusal is often based in anxiety. That means that avoiding school, the source of the anxiety, will only lead to increased anxiety about returning to school in the future. The longer a teen does not attend school, the harder it is to return to school.[9] The sooner that families, schools, and mental health providers can help the teen get back to school, the easier it will be. The foster family's impulse to let Tyler stay home a bit and have a break is understandable yet actually not helpful in the long term. Of course, the solution is not as simple as instructing Tyler to return to school. If Tyler could make himself go back to school, he would. Getting back to school takes a more gradual and supported approach, similar to the treatment for a phobia. Sometimes, in the early stages of school refusal, this can be done by the family with the support of the school. However, school refusal can be severe, even involving panic attacks, aggression, barricading the door, and so forth.[10] In these cases, a home-based mental health team can be essential. There are different types of home-based services (e.g., community mobile crisis programs, waiver services, home-based crisis intervention programs) that can be accessed in different ways. Many can be set up by the outpatient mental health providers.

In speaking privately with his psychiatrist, Tyler is able to describe some of his thoughts and feelings about being in school. Tyler understands that his peers' "yo mama" jokes were just adolescent silliness, but they still felt terrible to hear because they made him think of his deceased adoptive mother. Those thoughts led to other painful thoughts and memories: of when she used to walk the boys to school, of when she would pick him up early to accompany her to an appointment, and of when she came as a surprise in fifth grade with donuts for the class on his birthday and everyone sang to him. Everything at school seemed to remind him of her, making him feel overwhelmed with sadness. The psychiatrist expresses understanding and thanks him for sharing this so articulately. She talks to Tyler and his foster dad about involving a home-based mental health team that would help Tyler to return to school in a step-by-step, day-by-day manner, pushing him a bit but according to what he is able to tolerate. She frames it as getting control over his feelings again, and Tyler likes this idea. His psychiatrist encourages Tyler to continue to let them know when he is having thoughts and feelings about his deceased adoptive mother, and explains that letting people know what is going on in his head is the best way to let them know how they could help.

> Speak with the school counselor, a mental health professional, and the teen to determine whether the teen should in fact receive counseling or mental health services, and if so, whether services should be provided through the school counselor, a school-based mental health service, and/or an outpatient mental health clinic.

The examples of Josh and Tyler illustrate how trauma can affect a teen's entire life and how its effects can present in a school setting. School for teenagers is equivalent to work for adults—it can be a place of purpose, learning, growth, comfort, and stress. It is a necessary part of academic and social development. When an adolescent experiences difficulties in life, these will often surface in school, although the exact root of the troubles can be hard to trace. School staff can only know as much private information as a teen or family is willing to divulge. School staff can support teens going through acute stress or trauma in myriad ways. As described in this chapter, Ms. Shah and the school nurse helped Josh's foster mother identify that he was not himself and was missing his medication; Josh's counselor served as a primary supportive therapist; and Tyler's coach took the role of an older friend or family member. Ms. Shah also supports Tyler, in the following section, by serving as an intermediary player assisting in the transition between his home-based therapist and his classroom. In all of these scenarios, school staff are key in noticing the students' behaviors and whether there is a significant change from normal. It is also crucial that schools work with families, child protective agencies, and outside mental health providers to coordinate care and achieve the best possible outcomes. No child lives in isolation, and the people who take care of them should not have to function independently of each other. At times the frame for treatment of problems in school is indeed within the school, and at other times it is in the home or in a clinic. In any case, schools can provide invaluable support and insight into a teen's strengths and weaknesses; therefore, schools are a central part of the frame of treatment of children and adolescents with trauma.[11]

Treating More Than Just Behavior

The focus remains on getting Tyler back to school. Over the next several weeks, a therapist comes to the home each morning to help Tyler take steps toward returning to school. A few times Ms. Shah comes to the home as well to encourage Tyler and provide support. The therapist builds trust with Tyler by getting to know him and chatting about basketball, and gradually they talk more about school and his feelings there. Eventually, they walk to the school building, first on a weekend day and then eventually on a school day. Tyler becomes very anxious and shut down, so they sit in the park down the street. Ms. Shah comes out to meet them. Tyler talks about feeling scared to see all the kids at school. The therapist praises him for articulating the anxiety and for getting this far. She reassures him that they will continue just walking to the school building on school days until it feels a bit better, before they try to go inside. For several more days, they walk to the building, then go to the park and talk. The therapist points out to Tyler that he seems less anxious each time. Tyler shrugs but doesn't disagree. They agree that the next morning, they'll go inside and meet with Ms. Shah for a few minutes, then come back to the park. The first few times they try, Tyler says that it is "too much" and refuses to go inside. The fourth time, though, Ms. Shah and the basketball coach greet him at the front door. Tyler gets a big smile when he sees his coach, and the adults help Tyler walk to Ms. Shah's office, providing support and distraction so he doesn't feel overwhelmed. They do this again for the next few days, and Tyler is able to spend more time in Ms. Shah's office, then eventually at the gym as well, and then to return to the classroom for a period at a time. After each visit, his therapist takes Tyler to the park and coaches him on how to cope with the thoughts of his deceased mother as they pop into his head. Eventually, Tyler's foster dad joins the walks to school, and then Tyler travels with the foster dad to school, where they meet the therapist and Ms. Shah. Over time, the therapist gradually accompanies Tyler less, as the foster dad takes Tyler to school, and Ms. Shah checks in with him and walks with him to class. By the end of the school year, Tyler attends full school days again. He at times experiences symptoms of anxiety and depression, and intermittent struggles with his grief, but these are gradually improving with the help of his psychiatrist and therapist. Given his many missed days of school and difficulty completing schoolwork throughout the year, Tyler has to do summer school, but he attends without a single day of refusal. Tyler's therapist, foster parents, and teachers collaborate throughout the summer term, and they all agree that because his academic decline in school this year was related to his struggles dealing with trauma and missing school days (as opposed to isolated learning problems, oppositionality, etc.), and because he has made such significant strides, he should be allowed to progress to the next grade.

Tyler starts the fall semester without a hitch. His psychiatrist and therapist celebrate his hard work, and Tyler is shy in the face of their praise but clearly pleased. They talk about where to focus next in his treatment. Treatment had been focused on getting him back to school and on managing unpleasant feelings experienced in school, but now he is doing well with those goals. The psychiatrist and therapist suggest that they start therapy more focused on Tyler's traumatic loss, an adaptation of Trauma-Focused Cognitive Behavioral Therapy called Trauma-Focused CBT With Childhood Traumatic Grief (TF-CTG) (see "Resources and Additional Reading" at the end of this chapter). Tyler agrees, as long as the appointments don't conflict with his basketball practice, as he's proud to be back on the team.

Human beings, teenagers included, are resilient, and support from both established relationships and new ones, especially when nonjudgmental and trauma informed, helps teens act on that resiliency. No one can predict how trauma will affect youth, or in what ways, or for how long. What school staff can do, however, is consider themselves as integral parts of a child's environment and thus as a potential source of safety and support. Consistent presence, openness, care, and connection are sometimes more valuable than any evidence-based therapy or medication.

In the case in this chapter, Josh was briefly affected by the loss and transition into foster care, but he was able to reconstitute with short-term help from his school counselor. Tyler seemed okay in the beginning but ended up needing more help. Functionality is a good gross measure of an adolescent's mental health and well-being. Just as there is no way to predict how long a teen may be impacted by trauma, there is no way to predict how long a child may need additional supports. For Josh, weekly counseling sessions at school were helpful to process his grief. Given that his academic and social functioning were stable, it made sense that the frequency was decreased as his grief resolved and his interest naturally drifted back toward age-appropriate activities. Alternatively, had behavioral or academic problems emerged over the year, or had Josh refused to engage with the counselor or been unable to discuss his loss and life changes, referral to more specialized child mental health care may have been indicated. Tyler needed that more specialized treatment, but the treatment would never have worked without the collaboration from Ms. Shah and his teachers and the ongoing support and connection with Tyler's basketball coach. In the long run, it is these connections with ordinary school staff that will save Tyler's life. Adults at school can provide essential support to children who experience trauma precisely because they interact with kids on such a regular and genuine basis. The role that consistent, empathetic, caring, and open school staff play in a student's life cannot be underestimated, and their observations and collaborations should always be welcomed in the course of treatment of childhood trauma.

Resources and Additional Reading

Online Resources

Medical University of South Carolina, CTGWeb—A web-based learning course for Using TF-CBT With Childhood Traumatic Grief: http://ctg.musc.edu

National Child Traumatic Stress Network: Child Trauma Toolkit for Educators: Available at: http://www.nctsn.org/resources/audiences/school-personnel/trauma-toolkit

Additional Reading

Cohen JA, Mannarino AP, Perel JM, et al: A pilot randomized controlled trial of combined trauma-focused CBT and sertraline for childhood PTSD symptoms. J Am Acad Child Adolesc Psychiatry 46(7):811–819, 2007 17581445

Greene RW: The Explosive Child: A New Approach for Understanding and Parenting Easily Frustrated, "Chronically Inflexible" Children. New York, HarperCollins, 1998

Herman JL: Trauma and Recovery: The Aftermath of Violence, From Domestic Abuse to Political Terror. New York, Basic Books, 1997

Ko SJ, Ford JD, Kassam-Adams N, et al: Creating trauma-informed systems: child welfare, education, first responders, health care, juvenile justice. Professional Psychology: Research and Practice 39(4):396–404, 2008

Leblanc AN: Random Family: Love, Drugs, Trouble, and Coming of Age in the Bronx. New York, Scribner, 2003

Minahan J, Rappaport N: The Behavior Code: A Practical Guide to Understanding and Teaching the Most Challenging Students. Cambridge, MA, Harvard Education Press, 2012

Saxe GN, Ellis BH: Collaborative Treatment of Traumatized Children and Teens: The Trauma Systems Therapy Approach. New York, Guilford, 2012

Walkley M, Cox T: Building trauma-informed schools and communities. Children and Schools 35(2):123–126, 2013

References

1. Stempel H, Cox-Martin M, Bronsert M, et al: Chronic school absenteeism and the role of adverse childhood experiences. Acad Pediatr 17(8):837–843, 2017 28927940

2. Morrow AS, Villodas MT: Direct and indirect pathways from adverse child-hood experiences to high school dropout among high-risk adolescents. J Res Adolesc July 24, 2017 28736884

3. Linares LO, Li M, Shrout PE, et al: The course of inattention and hyperac-tivity/impulsivity symptoms after foster placement. Pediatrics 125(3):e489–e498, 2010 20123778

4. Stein K, Fazel M: Depression in young people often goes undetected. Practitioner 259(1782):17–22, 2–3, 2015 27254891

5. Griese B, Burns MR, Farro SA, et al: Comprehensive grief care for children and families: policy and practice implications. Am J Orthopsychiatry 87(5):540–548, 2017 28945443

6. Burrell LV, Mehlum L, Qin P: Sudden parental death from external causes and risk of suicide in the bereaved offspring: a national study. J Psychiatr Res 96:49–56, 2018 28965005

7. Bethell CD, Carle A, Hudziak J, et al: Methods to assess adverse childhood experiences of children and families: toward approaches to promote child well-being in policy and practice. Acad Pediatr 17(7S):S51–S69, 2017 28865661

8. Weller EB, Weller RA, Fristad MA, et al: Should children attend their parent's funeral? J Am Acad Child Adolesc Psychiatry 27(5):559–562, 1988 3182618

9. Last CG, Hansen C, Franco N: Cognitive-behavioral treatment of school phobia. J Am Acad Child Adolesc Psychiatry 37(4):404–411, 1998 9549961

10. Tyrrell M: School phobia. J Sch Nurs 21(3):147–151, 2005 15898849

11. Kasehagen L, Omland L, Bailey M, et al: Relationship of adverse family ex-periences to resilience and school engagement among Vermont youth. Matern Child Health J 22(3):298–307, 2018 28942565

CHAPTER 7

Trauma and Psychosis

Ruth Gerson, M.D.

Janelle, age 14 and a few weeks into ninth grade at a new high school, is sent to her guidance counselor because a few teachers have reported that "something is going on with her" and she seems "in another world." The guidance counselor, Mr. Charles, pulls Janelle's middle school profile but there aren't any flags, and when he seeks information from an old college friend who is a counselor at Janelle's middle school in another city, she says Janelle was known there for being smart and accomplished. Mr. Charles is surprised that Janelle's new teachers say that she often seems distant and distracted in class and that she rarely completes assignments in or out of school. But the reports that are most worrisome are that sometimes, when the bell rings and the students pack up their bags to move to the next class, Janelle has appeared to be seeing or hearing something that wasn't there— her eyes would be darting around and she would be mumbling to herself, seeming fearful and even paranoid. When teachers have tried to talk to her in these moments, she responds to them somewhat but seems confused or maybe a little cagey and guarded in her answers. When Mr. Charles tries to talk to her, she is initially quiet and polite, but as soon as he asks about these episodes, she spits with sudden irritation, "I don't remember." When he tries to ask more, she bristles at his "interrogation." Mr. Charles is worried and tries to ask about "hearing voices," but that just upsets Janelle further. "I'm not crazy," Janelle shouts as she storms out of Mr. Charles's office.

Symptoms that take people out of touch with reality can be terrifying, both to the individuals having the experience and to others around them. *Is this psychosis? drugs? What does this mean? Am I losing my mind?* It can be difficult to explain these experiences to others. How does one describe something when one doesn't know what it is? How does one articulate the experience when one doesn't know what is real?

Symptoms that follow abuse, maltreatment, and other forms of trauma can manifest as this kind of break from reality. If adults don't know that a young person has experienced trauma, and if they aren't looking at the teen's symptoms through a trauma-informed lens, then posttraumatic symptoms can look a lot like psychosis. Intrusive thoughts and flashbacks of a traumatic experience, hyperarousal, and dissociation take the traumatized teen out of the reality of here and now, and can look bizarre to others—even at times as though the teen is actually hallucinating. Hypervigilance and hyperreactivity related to traumatic events can be misconstrued as psychotic paranoia. Even avoidance and numbing can be misinterpreted as the so-called negative symptoms (withdrawal, emotional numbing, lack of motivation) of schizophrenia and seen as more evidence for the (wrong) diagnosis.

If trauma symptoms are misdiagnosed as schizophrenia, treatment is unlikely to be effective. Teens who are misdiagnosed will miss the opportunity to identify and learn to deal with trauma reminders and triggers that have been setting them off. They will never experience trauma-focused therapies that can provide long-term relief. Instead, if treated for schizophrenia or other primary psychotic disorders, they are likely to receive only medication, which may be calming in the short term but is unlikely to provide long-term relief and can carry significant side effects. And perhaps even more important, when teens are misdiagnosed, no one acknowledges the trauma and its impact. These teens may take away a message that everyone believes that what happened (both the trauma and the suffering that has followed) is all in their head.

Diagnosing Trauma or Psychosis... or Both

What does it mean when a teenager says he's "hearing voices"? Even scientific experts do not even fully understand all the different ways our brains can confuse us about what is real or not real. *Psychosis* is defined as a break from reality, typically taking the form of either hallucinations (seeing, hearing, feeling, or even smelling something that is not there) or delusions (odd beliefs not based in reality, such as a paranoid delusion that everyone is out to hurt you when they're not). But there are many reasons a person can experience a hallucination or delusion that is not part of a psychotic disorder. Hallucinations and delusions are actually fairly common in the general population[1] and even more common in traumatized individuals.[2] Many people, particularly in childhood and adolescence, momentarily see a figure or hear a voice as they're falling asleep, or think they hear someone calling their name when there is no one there, or think they have heard the phone ring when it did not. Many people talk about having heard "a voice in my head" at some point, telling them something they feel they wouldn't have otherwise grasped or thought of; typically this is intuition, our

TABLE 7–1. **Differential diagnosis of psychotic-like experiences**

Hearing voices	Imagination
	Anxiety
	Misinterpretation of own thoughts (especially if negative or shameful)
	Mood-congruent negative auditory hallucinations from depression
	Flashbacks
	Auditory hallucinations from posttraumatic stress disorder
	Primary psychotic disorder
Delusional thinking	Learned suspiciousness (of adults who have been abusive or unreliable, or peers who have been rejecting or bullying)
	Misreading faces or actions (e.g., thinking someone bumped them on purpose in the hall when it was an accident, or that someone is giving them a dirty look)
	Cognitive distortions from depression or anxiety
	Primary psychotic disorder

own thoughts, or a sudden memory. Delusions are less common, but many people experience odd beliefs or a deep sense of something that isn't based in reality. For example, many people believe in déjà vu, superstitions, or psychics, or briefly feel great certainty that a coworker has it out for them or that their spouse is cheating on them, even if there's no real evidence for this.

In clinical settings, "hearing voices" or having odd beliefs is often thought to be a specific sign of psychosis, specifically schizophrenia, but this is a false assumption, especially in children and adolescents. Schizophrenia and related disorders are very rare in childhood and early adolescence; these illnesses typically start in early adulthood, or less often in late adolescence. A teen can hear voices or have odd beliefs for many reasons that have nothing to do with schizophrenia (Table 7–1). Sometimes teens (particularly those who are younger, emotionally immature, or intellectually disabled) misinterpret their own sudden thoughts and urges as being like a voice in their head. This is especially common during emotional moments. Children and adolescents (again, especially those who are emotionally immature or intellectually limited) can have odd beliefs, and teens who are anxious can feel so certain that their worries are valid that the teens seem to be having delusions. Youth who are anxious can also experience their worries as being like a "voice" saying something bad will happen. "Voices" can also be hallucinations that are part of depression or other mood disorders. Youth with posttraumatic stress disorder (PTSD) can experience hallucinations as part of PTSD, especially when they are very angry, sad, or anxious. The hallucinations are generally related to the emotion or to PTSD in some way; for example, a teen might "hear" a voice saying "you are worthless" or otherwise degrading the teen, or telling the teen to harm him- or herself.[3] Youth with PTSD can also feel that others are looking at them or wanting to hurt them; these experiences can look to observers like paranoid delusions but are more likely hypervigilance experienced as part of PTSD.

> Don't take a teen's report of "hearing voices" at face value. Try to understand what he or she actually means. Be curious and genuine and try to understand the teen's experience. *Context* is everything! When does it happen? Does the teen hear the voice in certain situations, or only when angry or sad? What does the voice sound like, or feel like, or say? What does the teen make of it? Is the teen worried about what it means? Does it make the teen scared, angry, or sad? Does the voice feel like his or her own voice, or sound familiar or remind the teen of someone?

PTSD symptoms of dissociation and flashbacks can also look like psychosis to the untrained eye (or even a trained one) (Table 7–2). PTSD can take two primary forms,[4] both of which can mimic psychosis. In the first, keyed-up form of PTSD, children and adolescents predominantly experience flashbacks, rapid shifts in emotion or mood, and hyperarousal (being constantly keyed up or on edge and overreacting to stimulation such as loud noises, frustrating or irritating experiences, or reminders of the trauma). *Flashbacks* are the vivid reexperiencing of a traumatic experience—not simply remembering, but reliving the thoughts, feelings, and sensations of the traumatic event as if it were happening again. Children who are experiencing flashbacks are not aware in the moment that this is happening. They feel they are back in the moment of the trauma and may act in response to the sensations or memories in the flashback. A child's appearance during such an experience can vary: a child might appear to be daydreaming or "spacing out," or might seem to be talking (even screaming) to someone who is not there, or might appear to be lashing out physically for no reason.

In the second, numb or depressed type of PTSD, children and adolescents feel disconnected and may dissociate in response to trauma reminders. *Dissociation* is an experience of being separated from reality; young people

TABLE 7–2. How trauma symptoms can look like psychosis

	Symptoms include	Can be mistaken for
Keyed-up type (hyperarousal–adrenergic)	Flashbacks Hypervigilance Exaggerated responses	Hallucinations/internal preoccupation Paranoia Hallucinations
Numb or depressed type (dissociative–dopaminergic)	Dissociation Numbing Fantasy	Hallucinations/internal preoccupation Negative symptoms Delusions

Source. Adapted from American Academy of Pediatrics: *Helping Foster and Adoptive Families Cope With Trauma.* Itasca, IL, American Academy of Pediatrics, 2016. Available at: https://www.aap.org/en-us/Documents/hfca_foster_trauma_guide.pdf. Accessed February 21, 2018.

and adults who experience dissociation describe feeling unsure of what is real, and feeling like they are floating above their body, or even like they are blacking out and not being aware of their actions in the moment. Dissociation is a self-protective response that a child's brain uses during traumatic experiences to protect the child, psychologically, from the frightening experience by separating him or her from the experience. Dissociation can continue for years after trauma (often in response to trauma reminders or triggers), which makes the youth feel out of control and can be scary for the adults around the youth.

Youth who have experienced trauma, abuse, or neglect can hear or see things that aren't there for lots of reasons besides PTSD. They are more likely to be anxious or depressed or experience strong mood swings, during which they might misinterpret their own strong urges and feelings as being a "voice" inside them. The numbing and avoidance that follow trauma make teens more vulnerable to such misinterpretation: if the individual can't recognize or acknowledge that he or she is very angry, the urge to punch someone feels strange and alien. Youth who have experienced trauma have often had their emotions or reactions questioned, judged, or invalidated by adults, which also makes it harder for them to recognize uncomfortable thoughts or urges as part of themselves.

Typically, teens want to talk about these symptoms about as much as they want to talk about the trauma they experienced: not at all. How we approach asking about a teen's experiences is extremely important. Many adolescents who have been abused or maltreated have had adults not believe them, accuse them of making things up, or make them feel damaged or crazy. Asking directly about "hearing voices" without first trying to understand a teen's broader experience is likely to cause the teen to shut down. Youth who are experiencing hallucinations, dissociation, or flashbacks generally recognize that something unusual is going on. They often fear they are "going crazy" (or that others will think they are), so they are even less likely to be forthcoming, especially at school or with a therapist.

Whenever an adolescent is experiencing strange or unusual symptoms or behaviors, the counselor or clinician should try to understand the child's experience without jumping to an assumption about the cause. It is important to try to understand the youth's perspective and the contexts of the symptoms: both the context in which the symptoms or behaviors may have originated and the context in which they are flaring up now. This effort will help in identifying possible causes and making a differential diagnosis, which should always include considering trauma (recent or past) as a possible contributor to the current problems. When Janelle gets called into the guidance counselor's office, she knows she has been struggling in her new school and fears she is in trouble with this new authority figure. When Mr. Charles begins sharing the teachers' concerns about Janelle's unusual behavior, Janelle feels judged, ashamed, and frustrated, because she truly doesn't fully understand what has been going on with herself recently.

> Adolescents tend to assume adults won't "get" them, and teens who have been through trauma have often had lots of times when adults didn't believe or understand what they've been through. Try to get to know the young person in front of you—his or her strengths and likes and concerns—before you jump into asking about symptoms. When you do ask about symptoms, start with general questions, normalizing the symptoms by noting that lots of people experience these things, and then ask more specific questions. A good opener, so the teen doesn't feel judged or accused of something bad or weird, can be "A lot of people, when they're stressed, experience...." This approach can help a teen feel safer opening up so that together you can understand what he or she is experiencing.

Feeling concerned after his first meeting with Janelle, Mr. Charles asks her to come to weekly appointments. He plans to approach Janelle differently this time by taking the conversation in a different direction instead of jumping directly into the teachers' concerns about Janelle's behavior and performance. He wants to get to know Janelle better, to understand what is going on with her more broadly, how she's doing, and who she is. Janelle is wary after their disastrous first meeting, but she shows up for the first meeting and quietly listens as Mr. Charles makes conversation and asks about her life. Over the next few weeks of meeting together, Mr. Charles sees that Janelle is quiet and shy but funny, and he can see glimmers of the intelligence her middle school teachers described, though at other times she seems to be tired or in a fog. Janelle tells him she has lived with her father and stepmother for the past several months after her mother, who raised her, was killed suddenly in a car accident. Janelle shuts down when talking about her mother, and seems far away to the counselor. She says she likes the high school okay but hasn't really made friends yet. She says she had "a bad summer" and that she "doesn't like people" as a result, preferring to stay by herself. She denies any bullying or any specific problems with the schoolwork, but she admits it has been harder to concentrate this year and that she hasn't felt like herself. She says that often when she's in class, things will come to her mind and distract her, and then it's hard to catch up again. Mr. Charles asks what kind of things come to her mind, but Janelle won't say. Mr. Charles wonders how her mother's death affected her and whether Janelle might be depressed, but she doesn't describe feeling sad, exactly, and she doesn't talk about any worries or anxiety. She just seems shy, withdrawn, and sometimes sort of far away or disengaged, and he's not sure how that behavior relates to the odd behaviors her teachers described before.

Adults often don't realize how trauma can contribute to "hearing voices" or other symptoms that appear psychotic, or may not know that a youth has experienced trauma at all. Teens who are experiencing symptoms such as "voices" or "bizarre behavior" are rarely asked about exposure to trauma. There can be several reasons for this. Many adults fail to ask about trauma when youth are experiencing "voices" because the adults think trauma causes "only" PTSD, not psychosis. Others fear that the symptoms are "too acute" to risk potentially upsetting the youth by asking about traumatic experiences. This thinking is misguided. Of course, we should not be aggressively pushing youth to delve into the details of their trauma history when they do not want to. However, eliciting the trauma history from a youth by gently asking about what happened lets us understand and empathize with the child's experiences. It shows them that we care about what has happened to them, and aren't merely curious about what's wrong with them.

> When making a diagnostic assessment or trying to get to know a troubled adolescent, ask about trauma exposure in a gentle, gradual, and patient way. Start with broad questions, such as "Have you ever experienced anything really scary or frightening?" or "Has anyone ever hit you or hurt you?" This can help the teen see that these things are okay to talk about with you. Asking is unlikely to upset or trigger the teen, as long as you are gentle and respect the limits of what the teen is willing to talk about. Notice if the teen starts to look anxious or upset, and respond with support and empathy.

Another reason that clinicians might not ask about trauma exposure in young people with potential psychotic symptoms is that clinicians fear that a young person might be delusional and report a traumatic event that never really happened. Although this is theoretically possible, as the youth is talking, it is generally fairly easy to determine what is a real memory and what is a delusion (delusions tend to be bizarre, not plausible, and without cohesive or coherent details). Even if the description is not clearly a memory or a delusion, asking still brings forth clinically useful information about what the young person believes in that moment, real or not. If you aren't sure whether a traumatic experience is or is not real, you can still empathize with how scary, hurtful, or sad it sounds, which helps the young person feel heard and understood.

Asking Why: How Trauma Can Lead to Psychotic Symptoms

Mr. Charles continues meeting with Janelle, trying to understand what she is experiencing. Janelle had mentioned thoughts coming to mind and distracting her in class, so he tries to ask about these. He also asks, gently and at different points, about her "bad summer" and not "liking" people. Eventually Janelle admits that the past summer, having just lost her mother and moved here to a new city, she was feeling lost and lonely and fell in with an older crowd. One evening she had too much to drink, and one of the boys sexually assaulted her. She was afraid to tell her father and stepmother because she has never been close to them and already feels that her stepmother doesn't want her in the house. Now she feels wary of everyone, unsure about which kids at the new school to trust, and also worried they might have heard gossip about her or might somehow sense that she's damaged or dirty. She worries if she'll see the boy who raped her in the neighborhood or when she's going home from school. And when she's in school, particularly when it's loud or crowded, something she can't put her finger on will trigger a flashback and she'll feel like she's experiencing the assault all over again. She feels ashamed about having gone out drinking with older boys, like it was her fault. Mr. Charles tries to tell her it wasn't her fault, but Janelle just shrugs. In a small voice, she tells him that sometimes when she is really down she hears a voice she can't recognize saying "you deserved it," or her mother's voice calling her name.

Experiences of trauma in childhood and adolescence change the way the brain develops. In some ways, this makes sense. Our brains and bodies adapt to the world around us. If the world around us is scary and violent, our brains and bodies adapt to be more on edge, hyperreactive, and alert. Alternatively, if the threat persists or if escape is impossible, our brains and bodies adapt by going numb. These brain changes are chronic versions of the fight-or-flight and freeze responses that everyone experiences in response to threat or fear. But these brain changes can also make it harder for children and adolescents to learn, discern safe from unsafe situations, and build healthy relationships. These brain changes also contribute directly to the symptoms that occur in traumatized children and adolescents.

Traumatic experiences in childhood and adolescence impact the brain's development in several key areas, with different effects seen depending on the type of trauma and the child's age when it happens. Trauma changes the hypothalamic-pituitary-adrenal (HPA) axis, which releases the body's stress hormones cortisol and adrenaline. At very high levels, stress hormones can be harmful (e.g., causing increases in weight, blood pressure, and cholesterol), but cortisol and adrenaline are critical to the body's ability to know when a situation is safe or unsafe. The brain starts to process whether a situation is safe even before we're consciously aware of it; this is what gives us that feeling of hair standing on end. When the brain perceives a threat, the HPA axis starts releasing stress hormones, triggering an immediate fight-or-flight or freeze response (see Chapter 1, "Teens and Traumatic Stress"). If these stress response systems are damaged by too much traumatic stress, youth can find it difficult to know safe from unsafe and to react appropriately. Trauma also changes areas of the brain that respond to highly emotional situations, especially the hippocampus and the amygdala, which process memory and fear, and brain pathways that regulate attention, emotion, and perception.

> Youth who have been abused have often been told to "let it go" or that "it's in the past." This can make them feel crazy or like there is something wrong with them when traumatic events still affect them. But forgetting a traumatic event is not so easy. Talk to youth about how trauma affects our brains, and explain that our brains hold onto these memories to protect us and keep us safe in the future. Even though the flashbacks and memories are scary and painful, the reactions are normal and don't mean that the teens are "crazy." Talking about the effects of trauma on the brain can help youth see that although the scars of trauma might not be visible, they're still present, and that talking about the trauma and getting help is okay.

Depending on the individual and the nature of the trauma, each child and adolescent tends to develop different brain patterns that lead to the symptoms we see.[4] These different patterns explain the two different types of PTSD that we discussed in the previous section (see Table 7–2). Some youth fit one pattern clearly, whereas others change as they grow older or experience aspects of both. Some youth who have experienced trauma develop brain pathways and an HPA axis that are overreactive to stress. The pathways from the prefrontal cortex, which should quiet the stress response once the child consciously recognizes that the situation is safe, are confused and disrupted by traumatic stress. So even if the child "knows" consciously that the situation is safe, his or her brain can't stop the runaway stress response. This leads the youth to chronic feelings of stress and emotion dysregulation (easily becoming upset, sad, or angry for no clear reason) even when the traumatic situation has passed, and puts the youth constantly in the flight-or-fight mode. These children tend to experience the first type of PTSD that we mentioned before, marked by flashbacks, hyperarousal, and reexperiencing symptoms that at times can seem like voices or delusions. For other youth, particularly those who experience chronic abuse or repeated traumatic experiences, their body cannot sustain the high level of stress hormones, and their HPA axis and neural stress pathways become shut down or downregulated, so their bodies barely respond in stressful situations. These teens feel numb or depressed much of the time and can dissociate or freeze when they are stressed or faced with reminders of the trauma; this is the second type of PTSD.

> Remember that every experience, good or bad, changes our brains. Trauma changes our brains, but so do being understood and cared for by someone, learning new ways to think about ourselves through therapy, and practicing new ways of managing stress and getting support. Trauma's effects on the brain are strong, though, so it takes a lot of positive experiences over time to reverse the patterns of thinking and behavior set by a traumatic experience.

The ways in which trauma changes the brain can also cause children and adolescents to experience hallucinations. Those who have experienced trauma and abuse in childhood can have unusual perceptual experiences and hallucinations because of the changes in the limbic pathways that come from early trauma, especially when the youth are feeling sad, embarrassed, angry, or afraid. They might describe hearing a buzzing sound or a repetitive voice, seeing flashes of shapes and patterns, or perceiving distortions in the sizes or shapes of objects.[5]

Brain changes secondary to trauma can also increase risk for schizophrenia and other chronic psychotic illnesses.[6] These chronic psychotic illnesses can develop when individuals with a genetic or neurobiological vulnerability experience a severe physical or psychological stress that triggers the onset of the illness. For children or adolescents with a genetic vulnerability to schizophrenia (i.e., a first-degree relative with schizophrenia), a traumatic experience can be the severe stress that starts the hormonal and neurobiological changes that can develop into schizophrenia. Even if a child does not have a genetic risk for schizophrenia, if the trauma the child experiences is early, frequent, and severe, the rewiring of the brain and changes in the stress response can put the child at risk for later developing schizophrenia as well.[7] A young child who is repeatedly abused or neglected by her primary caregiver, for example, might have brain changes that put the child at risk for schizophrenia in adulthood. Youth at risk for schizophrenia, either from genetics or from severe trauma, often experience subtle or milder psychotic symptoms for several years before schizophrenia develops. These subtler symptoms can include visual illusions or paranoid thoughts that the adolescent recognizes as not real, or very brief psychotic symptoms, problems in memory and concentration, social withdrawal, and decline in overall functioning. A safe environment and the right support and therapy, especially to help the teen stay off drugs such as marijuana that can increase risk even more, can reverse these symptoms and prevent the adolescent from developing schizophrenia or other severe and lasting mental illnesses.

Recognizing What's Happening in the Moment

Trauma can make the brain vulnerable to flashbacks, dissociation, and hallucinations. But in the moment, there is something that triggers these symptoms, something either inside the teen (a thought, feeling, or memory) or in the environment. It is important for the youth to learn to identify what these triggers are to find ways to avoid or cope with them so that the frightening symptoms happen less often. Understanding the context in which symptoms occur can also help to determine what kind of symptom the youth is experiencing—a flashback or hallucination, for example—and whether the symptom is related to PTSD, depression, anxiety, or a psychotic illness. Adolescents are often unable, on their own, to identify the triggers or context in which they experience symptoms. Youth are often frightened or disturbed enough by these symptoms (which can feel like "going crazy") that they try not to think about them after they occur. And identifying triggers requires a high degree of self-awareness and mindful attention to the environment that many adolescents (and adults) lack. It can also be difficult for adults working with the youth to identify when a reminder of the trauma has triggered an acute symptom. Trauma reminders are often subtle; for example, for a teen who has been abused by his family, seeing a happy family might be just as triggering as witnessing a parent berating a child. Trauma reminders can also change the flow of blood and nutrients in the brain, cutting off nutrients to the brain's language centers. This explains why, if a teen's traumatic experience has been triggered, asking what she is experiencing in that moment is often ineffective: if the language centers of the brain aren't working, a traumatized teen cannot process your question, let alone "use her words" to describe what she is experiencing.

> For Janelle, the noise and chaos that happen when students are changing classrooms are triggering, because they are reminiscent of the loud, chaotic party where she was sexually assaulted. But she is also triggered when male peers wear shirts with a certain kind of striped pattern that is similar to the shirt worn by the older boy who raped her. Intense emotional situations for Janelle tend to trigger the "voices" that she hears. It's her mother's voice Janelle usually hears when she is feeling very sad or lonely, typically at home alone when lying in bed. This also happens when peers talk about their parents (particularly when they complain about their mothers, which makes her feel guilty about times she complained about or disrespected her own mother before she died) or when staff use the overhead announcement system to call a student to the principal (which reminds her of how she was summoned to the principal's office to be told of her mother's sudden death). She often hears the voice saying "you deserved it" when something makes her feel ashamed; for example, when she gets a bad grade or a wrong answer in class, it triggers thoughts of all the ways she fears she has disappointed her father and culminates in hearing the voice. Sometimes Janelle is consciously aware of these triggers but often she's not. Sometimes when talking with Mr. Charles, she can think back and see triggers she wasn't aware of in the moment, but sometimes it really feels like the symptoms happen out of nowhere. Janelle also has flashbacks and hears voices more often when she is tired (which is a lot, due to the nightmares she started experiencing after her mother's sudden death) or after recent conflicts or disagreements with her stepmother.

Identifying these triggers and risk factors is difficult, but adults can help youth to identify them with a process called a *chain analysis*. In a chain analysis, the adolescent thinks back to a specific time when he or she experienced the symptom (e.g., a flashback or a hallucination). Writing it out on paper, the youth and the adult who is helping work backward from the symptom to remember what the youth was thinking, feeling, and doing immediately beforehand, and then immediately before that, and immediately before that, all the way back to the prior hours or days. Sometimes others who were around at the time of the symptom can also help to fill in gaps, particularly if the youth has a flashback or dissociation and was not aware of what was happening. It is usually impossible to determine all the triggers from a single chain analysis, but going through that process over and over can identify patterns of what is going on around the teen or in his or her mind before the symptoms come. Identifying those patterns can help to determine what kind of symptom the youth is experiencing and the diagnostic context in which these symptoms are occurring, as discussed in the next section.

Janelle and Mr. Charles meet regularly over several weeks, and the counselor is able to help Janelle better articulate what she was experiencing in those moments that the teachers were worried about. They practice using the chain analysis to look closely at these moments and understand them better. Janelle appreciates that Mr. Charles is patient and understanding and doesn't make her feel judged or like she's weird. She starts to talk with Mr. Charles more about her mother's death. After learning about her mother's death, Janelle felt numb, like she was in a fog, as her aunt drove her home from school and helped her pack up a few things before her father came to get her. In the car driving to her father's house, and in the months since, the numb feeling has persisted but now alternates with periods of intense sadness and guilty feelings about things she said or didn't say to her mother before her death. At school, Janelle typically feels a little better than she does at home, where watching her stepmother interact with her young half-siblings makes her long for her own mother. But she has struggled to make friends and doesn't feel connected to anyone at school, or at home. She thinks of her mother often but doesn't talk about it with her father because she knows his relationship with her mother was "complicated," and also he's never spoken to her about her mother, though he does sometimes ask her how she's doing. (She always says she's "fine.") She hasn't been sleeping well, crying herself to sleep and waking up often with nightmares. She knows her father is disappointed in her grades, but it's hard to concentrate on schoolwork even when she isn't experiencing a flashback. When she experiences flashbacks related to her sexual assault, it feels like she is back in that moment and she loses track of her surroundings momentarily. When she comes back to the present, she feels flushed and embarrassed, uncertain of what she has done or whether others are thinking she seems crazy. She only hears the voices sometimes, when she feels intensely sad or ashamed. When Mr. Charles asks her about dissociation, Janelle seems confused. She says she loses touch with the reality of the moment during a flashback, and sometimes zones out and loses track of time when she's listening to music or on Facebook, but otherwise she doesn't ever feel out of her body or black out.

Listening to this, Mr. Charles starts to think that Janelle might need something stronger than the support and empathy he can provide. But he struggles with deciding where to refer her. He's still not sure what's going on with Janelle. Some things she has told him seem like depression, and others seem like PTSD, but it's more severe than he has seen before, and some of the symptoms she describes (like the voices and dissociation) are new to him. He wonders if it might be schizophrenia. He confers with a friend who is a social worker, and she encourages him to refer Janelle to an adolescent psychiatrist in town who specializes in PTSD. When Mr. Charles approaches Janelle about this idea, she is initially very resistant, insisting that she isn't crazy and doesn't need to be medicated. Mr. Charles agrees, emphasizing that this is just a consultation. He tells her that the psychiatrist might help with the zoning out and flashbacks that she finds so disruptive and embarrassing, and that he thinks might be related to her traumatic history. Janelle still refuses, so Mr. Charles moves on to talking about other things, and then asks about it again at their next visit, and the next. He offers to talk to the psychiatrist in advance, so Janelle doesn't have to tell her whole story from scratch. He reminds her that the psychiatrist will be able to help her get control over the flashbacks. Janelle finally agrees to give it a try.

The psychiatrist, Dr. Soo, meets with Janelle and her father separately (Janelle first) and then together. She reassures Janelle that their conversation is confidential, and assuages Janelle's fears that Dr. Soo will tell her father everything. Dr. Soo asks Janelle to describe her recent symptoms, and gently asks about both her mother's death and the rape. Having talked about it with Mr. Charles, Janelle is a little more comfortable speaking about these painful topics, and she is able to tell the psychiatrist when she is feeling overwhelmed and needs to take a break. Dr. Soo does a complete psychiatric assessment, including asking about suicidal ideation (which Janelle states she felt once after the assault but not since), self-injurious behavior, and thoughts of hurting others (both of which Janelle denies). She asks Janelle what her biggest concerns and goals are. Janelle says that she's worried she's going crazy and that she's going to fail freshman year and disappoint her father. Her goal is to get back on track and maybe to feel better, though she finds that hard to imagine. Janelle also says she doesn't want her father to know about the rape. Dr. Soo encourages Janelle to consider telling her father later, as part of the therapy, but for now they together tell her father about Janelle's grief over her mother and about her current symptoms. The psychiatrist provides psychoeducation to Janelle and her father and gives Janelle a diagnosis of PTSD. Janelle's father is surprised and visibly moved to learn that Janelle has been suffering. He admits he had taken her withdrawal to be normal teenager behavior and that he hadn't asked about the impact of her mother's death because he was still upset about it himself. He asks Dr. Soo if Janelle could be developing something like his cousin, who was institutionalized with schizophrenia. Dr. Soo suggests that the hallucinations Janelle is experiencing are worrisome and deserve treatment but that she does not have schizophrenia now, and the symptoms she is experiencing seem connected to traumatic grief. Dr. Soo also reassures Janelle's dad that therapy to process the traumatic grief and reduce her level of stress and anxiety should reduce her risk of developing schizophrenia or other problems in the future.

Finding the Frame: Putting "Psychotic" Symptoms in Context

Psychiatric treatment can be lifesaving for youth who have experienced trauma or abuse, but knowing what to treat and how to treat it is a crucial first step. Sometimes the diagnosis is not immediately clear, or the diagnosis may evolve over time if new symptoms develop. Nonetheless it is counterproductive and can even be dangerous to start treatment without understanding what we are treating and how. Making an incorrect diagnosis of schizophrenia or another psychotic disorder can have serious negative effects on a young person.

> Keep in mind that worldwide, only about 1% of the population has schizophrenia, and only some of these individuals develop symptoms in adolescence (more typically the disorder begins in young adulthood). In comparison, about 7% of the population has PTSD. As much as 68% of youth experience a traumatic event before age 16, and 13% of them experience emotional difficulties or other problems after the trauma.[8,9]

The psychological impact on adolescents of being told that they are at high risk for developing schizophrenia can be profound.[10] Given the stigma that surrounds schizophrenia, an incorrect diagnosis of schizophrenia or even being told they are at risk for this debilitating illness may cause the adolescents to feel they will be unable to achieve success at school, work, or relationships and to withdraw from these activities. A family may treat a young person with this diagnosis differently, and may start to doubt that the abuse or trauma really happened because they see the youth as "crazy." If the youth is in foster care, a diagnosis of schizophrenia may negatively impact options for placement or adoption. If a youth is erroneously diagnosed with schizophrenia and prescribed antipsychotic medications, these medications may have a sedating or anxiolytic effect, but they will not directly address the PTSD, anxiety, or depression that is underlying the symptoms. These medications can also have significant adverse effects, some of which (specifically involuntary muscle spasm or movements such as acute dystonia or tardive dyskinesia) are more likely to occur in those youth who do not have schizophrenia. Young people who are taking medication that is not truly addressing their illness can also begin to feel hopeless and disillusioned when the treatment does not really work, and then may drop out of treatment feeling nothing can help them. They also miss the opportunity to receive treatment (trauma-focused, family-oriented therapy, and sometimes medication) that addresses the effects of their traumatic experiences, teaches them how to understand their symptoms and recognize and cope with trauma triggers, and effectively treats their underlying psychopathology.

> Adolescents are developing their sense of self and their vision for the future. But one of the symptoms of PTSD that traumatized youth can experience is a feeling that they are damaged or an inability to imagine a future for themselves. When you are talking to youth about their symptoms and their diagnoses, be careful that you are clear that symptoms and psychiatric illnesses can be treated. Share that you see them getting better and being able to finish school, to work, and to have successful relationships in the future. Be honest about how recovery can take hard work, and don't give false reassurances, but show hope and confidence that treatment will work for them.

Making a correct diagnosis starts with performing a broad assessment of the child's symptoms rather than responding only to the presenting issue. Youth who have suffered trauma and are now experiencing flashbacks, dissociation, or hallucinations often manifest a complex range of symptoms, including mood swings or depressed mood, anxiety, perceptual disturbances, and problems with attention, learning, and memory. Individuals with schizophrenia can have many similar symptoms, but the pattern is generally different.

The onset of schizophrenia is typically insidious and gradual, with symptoms usually building over 1–2 years. It starts with flattening of the emotions (so a youth feels—and seems—indifferent to everything, and doesn't show happy, sad, or angry feelings). Social withdrawal and decline in functioning (especially academic functioning) also happen long before hallucinations and delusions begin. Hallucinations and delusions in schizophrenia are accompanied by changes in thinking and speech, specifically disorganized thinking and speech. Disorganized thinking does not mean that an adult can't understand the teen's thinking in the sense of "I don't understand why she does this." Teenagers constantly do things that make no sense to adults (but that make perfect sense to other teens). Disorganized thinking in schizophrenia means that the actual words and train of thought are nonsensical and do not flow logically from one word to the next. Hallucinations and delusions in schizophrenia may become stronger during periods of stress, but they are present fairly consistently. In contrast, the perceptual disturbances and flashbacks seen in PTSD are more transient and situational, triggered by a trauma reminder or a moment of intense emotion. The nature or content of schizophrenic hallucinations compared with flashbacks, dissociation, or PTSD perceptual disturbances is very different as well, as described earlier in this chapter (see "Diagnosing Trauma or Psychosis…or Both"). At the most basic level, the hallucinations, flashbacks, and dissociation in PTSD are frightening and distressing to the person, whereas the hallucinations of schizophrenia are typically ego-syntonic (meaning not psychologically distressing or uncomfortable to the person) (Table 7–3).

When you are clarifying the diagnosis, it is important to go beyond a symptom checklist to understand when and how often the experiences occur, what a teen's individual experience is like, whether the teen has noticed any patterns, and whether the teen feels that the symptoms are related in any way to the trauma or to any other experience or stress. Observing the youth over time and talking to people around the teen who know him or her well can also help to identify the patterns and triggers for the behaviors.

In trying to understand a teen's individual experience, *normalizing* the symptoms and showing genuine curiosity about the teen's experience can go a long way. "Lots of teens tell me they hear things sometimes. What exactly is it like for you? What does it sound like, and where does it come from? Is it your own thoughts or imagination or something else? Is it frightening or upsetting when that happens?" Ask if any other experiences—perhaps intense emotion such as anger or shame, certain memories, or a racing heartbeat—go along with the "voices." It may not be possible from the initial interview to be certain whether a young person is experiencing either a psychotic hallucination or a flashback or hallucination secondary to PTSD, but through repeatedly talking about these experiences with the youth in an open, empathic, and curious way, you can clarify the diagnosis and then design the correct treatment.

In the previously described meetings with her school counselor, Janelle is able to describe flashbacks as distinct from the hallucinations of her mother's voice and of the voice saying she deserved to be assaulted. The flashbacks she experiences are typical of PTSD; they occur in response to trauma reminders or triggers (although without treatment, Janelle is not always able

TABLE 7–3. Hallucinations and delusions in posttraumatic stress disorder (PTSD) versus psychotic disorders

Symptom	In PTSD they usually.	In psychotic disorders they usually
Hallucinations	Occur in moments of intense emotion, such as anger, sadness, or anxiety	Can occur at any time and tend to be more persistent
	Are related to the emotion or PTSD in some way, such as a voice saying "You are worthless" or "You should die"	Can be more varied in content, or can include hearing multiple voices mumbling, hearing "static," or other perceptions
	Can begin abruptly, even at a young age, or come and go for years after the trauma	Tend to begin in late adolescence or adulthood after a several-year period of withdrawal and decline in functioning
	Respond best to trauma-focused therapy and to medications that lower anxiety or arousal	Respond to antipsychotic medications and cognitive behavioral therapy
Delusions	Can involve feelings that others are thinking negatively toward or wanting to hurt the teen, but in a way that is based in their experience (e.g., "I can't trust my new caseworker because my prior caseworkers said they'd help me get back home, and here I am still in foster care")	Are bizarre (e.g., "The CIA is trying to get me," or "I am Jesus," or "The Russians are controlling my thoughts through a chip in my brain")
	Can be seen at a young age	Tend to begin in late adolescence or adulthood after a several-year period of withdrawal and decline in functioning
	Respond best to trauma-focused therapy	Respond to antipsychotic medications and cognitive behavioral therapy

to identify what those triggers are, so sometimes they feel as though they are random and unprovoked). She experiences hallucinations during periods of intense emotion; they are related to her experiences of traumatic loss and sexual assault, and she finds them frightening and upsetting (ego-dystonic). These are more consistent with PTSD than with schizophrenia, particularly because she does not have any of the other associated symptoms of schizophrenia (such as disorganized thinking or delusions) and the onset of the symptoms has not been gradual over 2 years, but rather fairly rapid over the months since her mother's death.

Treating More Than Just Behavior

The first step of treatment, as always, is to ensure that the teen is safe, both from potential self-harm and from ongoing trauma. Dissociation and psychosis, and to a lesser degree flashbacks, can put youth at risk for harm or abuse because their body's natural threat detection system is derailed, so talking to teens repeatedly about safety in their environment and relationships is important. Make sure that each teen's social, school, and family system is safe and that there is no ongoing abuse or violence. Help the teens identify people they can turn to at home and at school if they feel their traumatic experience being triggered. Making a *safety plan* for how they'll manage difficult symptoms or frightening situations can be helpful, so they've thought in advance about how they might cope and get help.

> Mr. Charles meets with Janelle after her initial meeting with Dr. Soo to talk about how it went. Janelle shrugs and says it was fine, a little weird, but that Dr. Soo seems nice enough. She felt reassured that Dr. Soo said she didn't think Janelle was crazy, but she is worried about what her dad said about his cousin's schizophrenia—she doesn't want to end up on medication. Mr. Charles encourages her to talk with Dr. Soo about this concern, and emphasizes that a lot of people who go to therapy never need medication.
>
> When Janelle sees Dr. Soo again, the psychiatrist shares that she has been thinking about Janelle since their last meeting and reflecting on how articulate and thoughtful Janelle was. She asks if Janelle had any thoughts about their last meeting, and Janelle brings up her concern about medication and being "locked up" like her dad's cousin. Dr. Soo agrees that this is not at all what Janelle needs. They agree to start with therapy, and then if Janelle's symptoms get worse, they can always talk again about medication in the future. They talk about how Janelle has been managing her symptoms so far, using Mr. Charles's office as a refuge at school when things get hard, and listening to music or perusing Facebook if she feels stressed at home or wakes up with a nightmare. Dr. Soo asks Janelle about friends and relationships, and Janelle laughs darkly; she says that she hasn't gone out at all since

she was raped. Dr. Soo empathizes with how common this is and offers that part of treatment might be aimed at helping Janelle feel safe and okay again about making friends and letting herself have fun.

Once the teen is in a safe environment, deciding which treatment is the best fit depends on the teen's diagnosis, most pressing symptoms, and goals and preferences for treatment. For youth with intense symptoms such as flashbacks, dissociation, and hallucinations, which can in some cases worsen when teens are under significant stress, it can be helpful to start with psychoeducation (to explain the connection to trauma and normalize symptoms) and the building of coping skills. Jumping directly to the trauma narrative and exposure to trauma reminders can risk making the youth feel worse or drop out of treatment.[4] Relaxation skills and affect regulation skills give youth the tools to manage their symptoms early on, increasing their motivation for ongoing treatment (because their goals were addressed) and enhancing their ability to tolerate the trauma narrative and exposure sessions that youth are often nervous about.

Two treatments that fit the bill for youth like Janelle are Trauma-Focused Cognitive Behavioral Therapy (TF-CBT) and Skills Training in Affective and Interpersonal Regulation (STAIR).[11] In both of these programs, treatment starts with psychoeducation to help the youth and family understand the connection between their experiences of trauma and their current difficulties. The next step in each is skills training, focusing on relaxation and coping skills such as deep breathing, self-soothing, distraction, and positive self-talk to counter negative thinking. STAIR also teaches self-care and interpersonal skills such as self-advocacy and saying no. After skills building, the next step in both TF-CBT and STAIR is for the youth and clinician to work together to develop a trauma narrative, which should ideally be shared with the parent or another trusted adult. The clinician then helps the teen practice exposure to trauma reminders or triggers, and works with youth and families on turning toward the future. In addition to treating the trauma symptoms, cognitive behavioral therapies (CBTs) like TF-CBT and STAIR can reduce overall stress and reduce a youth's risk for developing later illnesses such as schizophrenia. CBT can also be used directly for psychotic symptoms (whether they are part of depression, PTSD, or schizophrenia). This version of CBT, targeting psychosis, also starts with psychoeducation, then focuses on coping with stress and symptoms, and then uses cognitive techniques to determine whether hallucinations or delusions are real and to counter the negative things the voices may say.[12] STAIR can also work well in individuals with psychotic symptoms due to schizophrenia but who have also experienced trauma.[13]

> If you're interested in learning TF-CBT, a free training program, provided by the Medical University of South Carolina (MUSC), is available online (see "Online Resources" at the end of this chapter). The training walks you through each of the different sections of TF-CBT, from psychoeducation, to skills training, to trauma narrative and future planning, with practice scripts and handouts you can use. The program also has pages with resources, manuals, and opportunities for additional training. Once you have completed the training, you can also access free online supervision for help with difficult cases. MUSC also has a training program for TF-CBT adapted for childhood traumatic grief (see "Online Resources"), so you can help youth who have experienced the sudden or traumatic loss of a family member, friend, or loved one.

Dr. Soo tells Janelle she'd like to use TF-CBT because this will help Janelle learn how to cope with stress and process the trauma. They meet weekly for several months, working through the TF-CBT program together. Dr. Soo uses the online training and supervision programs for handouts and to troubleshoot when she and Janelle hit a hard spot. One hard spot comes in the beginning: Janelle initially finds the coping skills hokey and skips a few sessions, in part because she is stressed with school and in part because she feels anxious about the trauma narrative and exposure parts. Dr. Soo anticipates these concerns and talks about them with Janelle, validating the teen's worries and admitting that the coping skills can feel forced at first. She encourages Janelle to stick with the program. Janelle eventually finds that music and baking (something she used to do with her mother) help her relax, and that grounding techniques such as a cold shower or holding an ice cube can jolt her out of the moment when things get really bad. Janelle and Dr. Soo share some of this information with Mr. Charles. That way, when Janelle has acute symptoms at school, Mr. Charles can help her use some of her coping skills (especially music or ice) rather than standing by helplessly or calling EMS. The three of them also discuss how Janelle can ground herself in advance of a trigger she knows is coming (e.g., the chaos of changing classes, going to certain parts of her neighborhood) by consciously trying to be mindful of where she is, taking deep breaths, and reminding herself that she's safe.

Knowing that the hallucinations don't mean she's crazy makes them bother Janelle less, so she and Dr. Soo focus the treatment on the flashbacks related to being raped. Janelle creates a trauma narrative about the rape, but remains hesitant to share it with her father. She does give the okay for Dr. Soo to meet alone with her dad, to talk about how best to support her without yet sharing the details of the sexual assault. Dr. Soo is impressed that Janelle's dad wants to help, although he's not a very emotionally demonstrative guy, and she gives him a few tips to show how much he cares when Janelle seems distant or shut down, which he finds helpful. After a few months of treatment, Janelle starts feeling empowered by the gradual exposure to trauma reminders, like she's showing she can face anything. She finds as she does these exposures that the flashbacks begin to lessen and it's easier for her to focus and feel safe at school. After some time the psychiatrist gently encourages Janelle to think about processing her mother's death. But Janelle is hesitant as she feels she is doing much better. Besides, she has been talking about her mother's death with her father and grandparents, which has helped a lot. Janelle and Dr. Soo agree that because she has been doing so well, they'll start to meet every other week, and Janelle keeps checking in with Mr. Charles every month. As the year goes on, Janelle is proud to be able to show him her improving grades, and Mr. Charles smiles when he sees her chatting in the hallway with her new friends.

Family involvement is key for youth experiencing these severe symptoms, both to enhance the effectiveness of the treatment and to ensure that family is supporting the youth and monitoring the progression of symptoms. In many cases, such as Janelle's, as youth start to feel that their family "gets it," there is an increase in openness, trust, and involvement. Families can also benefit from parenting support (as learned in TF-CBT or, for families with significant stress or multiple systems involvement, Trauma Systems Therapy; see Chapter 3, "Aggression"), which can reduce stress in the home by contributing to symptom remission and reducing the youth's risk of developing schizophrenia or other serious illnesses.

Medications can be used in youth with flashbacks, dissociation, or hallucinations, but their use is complicated and should be driven by an understanding of underlying diagnosis. Medication should not be given as an isolated treatment, because medication will have little effect in the absence of therapy.

Antipsychotics can be prescribed for teens with schizophrenia and PTSD, but trauma-related hallucinations don't respond as well to antipsychotics as do hallucinations that are not related to trauma. For youth with PTSD-related hallucinations but not schizophrenia, antipsychotics can be used for acute treatment of hallucinations that are disruptive or distressing to the youth, but antipsychotics will not be effective unless combined with trauma-focused therapy.[14] Antipsychotics also have not been shown to decrease risk of schizophrenia in prodromal or at-risk youth. Clinicians may wish to prescribe antipsychotics to address anxiety or mood dysregulation in PTSD, but this treatment has not been shown to be effective and the serious side effects likely outweigh the potential benefits. Clinicians may be tempted to prescribe benzodiazepines to address anxiety or flashbacks, but benzodiazepines are not recommended because they are addictive and can often make symptoms worse. Antiadrenergic medications such as clonidine, prazosin, or guanfacine may be safer and more effective. Prazosin is especially effective for nightmares. Antidepressants are also not recommended for treatment of PTSD or trauma-related hallucinations, unless the hallucinations are stemming from underlying depression.

Trauma-informed, family-oriented treatments such as those described above do not work immediately, but they can provide significant relief and have the potential to be a cure, even for youth with severe symptoms like Janelle's. For youth with more long-term or complex trauma than Janelle experienced (e.g., long-standing abuse by family members or multiple traumatic experiences in foster care), long-term trauma therapy may be needed. Long-term treatment can also be helpful to provide support as youth move through stressful transitions such as finishing school, leaving home, and starting to become more independent. Symptoms may flare up again during these times of stress, but talking to youth about this in advance and planning for how to cope can keep symptoms from derailing the teen in the future.

Online Resources

Medical University of South Carolina, CTGWeb, a web-based learning course for Using TF-CBT With Childhood Traumatic Grief: ctg.musc.edu

Medical University of South Carolina, TF-CBTWeb2.0, a web-based course for Trauma-Focused Cognitive Behavioral Therapy: https://tfcbt2.musc.edu

National Child Traumatic Stress Network treatment finder: http://www.nctsn.org/trauma-types

References

1. Maijer K, Begemann MJH, Palmen SJMC, et al: Auditory hallucinations across the lifespan: a systematic review and meta-analysis. Psychol Med September 28, 2017 [Epub ahead of print] 28956518

2. Daalman K, Diederen KM, Derks EM, et al: Childhood trauma and auditory verbal hallucinations. Psychol Med 42(12):2475–2484, 2012 22716897

3. McCarthy-Jones S, Longden E: Auditory verbal hallucinations in schizophrenia and post-traumatic stress disorder: common phenomenology, common cause, common interventions? Front Psychol 6:1071, 2015 26283997

4. Lanius RA, Vermetten E, Loewenstein RJ, et al: Emotion modulation in PTSD: clinical and neurobiological evidence for a dissociative subtype. Am J Psychiatry 167(6):640–647, 2010 20360318

5. Teicher MH, Andersen SL, Polcari A, et al: The neurobiological consequences of early stress and childhood maltreatment. Neurosci Biobehav Rev 27(1–2):33–44, 2003 12732221

6. Ruby E, Polito S, McMahon K, et al: Pathways associating childhood trauma to the neurobiology of schizophrenia. Front Psychol Behav Sci 3(1):1–17, 2014 25419548

7. Thompson JL, Kelly M, Kimhy D, et al: Childhood trauma and prodromal symptoms among individuals at clinical high risk for psychosis. Schizophr Res 108(1–3):176–181, 2009 19174322

8. Copeland WE, Keeler G, Angold A, et al: Traumatic events and posttraumatic stress in childhood. Arch Gen Psychiatry 64(5):577–584, 2007 17485609

9. Kessler RC, Chiu WT, Demler O, et al: Prevalence, severity, and comorbidity of 12-month DSM-IV disorders in the National Comorbidity Survey Replication. Arch Gen Psychiatry 62(6):617–627, 2005 15939839

10. Corcoran C, Malaspina D, Hercher L: Prodromal interventions for schizophrenia vulnerability: the risks of being "at risk." Schizophr Res 73(2–3):173–184, 2005 15653260

11. Cohen JA, Mannarino AP: Trauma-focused cognitive behavior therapy for traumatized children and families. Child Adolesc Psychiatr Clin N Am 24(3):557–570, 2015 26092739

12. Fowler DR, Garety PA, Kuipers L: Cognitive Behaviour Therapy for Psychosis: Theory and Practice. Hoboken, NJ, Wiley, 1995

13. Cloitre M, Cohen LR, Koenen KC: Treating Survivors of Childhood Abuse: Psychotherapy for the Interrupted Life. New York, Guilford, 2006

14. Strawn JR, Keeshin BR, DelBello MP, et al: Psychopharmacologic treatment of posttraumatic stress disorder in children and adolescents: a review. J Clin Psychiatry 71(7):932–941, 2010 20441729

CHAPTER 8

Implications of Trauma for Sexual and Reproductive Health in Adolescence

J. Rebecca Weis, M.D.

Aron Janssen, M.D.

Jeremy A. Wernick, L.M.S.W.

Charlotte is a 16-year-old girl who lives with her mother, father, and younger brother. Her parents immigrated to the United States about a year before Charlotte's birth. They have struggled to build a better life for their children and feel very proud that their children were spared the hardships they themselves faced growing up. Recently, though, tension has escalated between Charlotte and her parents. Charlotte's parents have very traditional expectations for girls, and Charlotte doesn't agree. In fact, recently she started dating a girl, and her parents saw the two of them kissing outside near their school. When her parents confronted Charlotte about this, she told them she is bisexual. Her parents were incredulous and confused. Charlotte's mother tried to talk sense into her while her father sat silent, a dark look on his face. Charlotte had dated boys in the past, her mother said, so how could she be gay? Charlotte tried to explain that she is attracted to people not because of gender but because of personality, but this only confused her parents more. Charlotte and her mother argued for an hour before finally Charlotte's father jumped in, frustrated. He said if she wanted to live under his roof, she had to break up with her girlfriend. So Charlotte packed a small bag and left.

Exploring sexuality is a normal part of adolescence, but for teenagers like Charlotte this process presents unique challenges and risks. To examine these risks, we must first have the language to understand what Charlotte is experiencing. Key terms and definitions used throughout this chapter are clarified in Table 8–1.

Gender and sexual development are complex and different for each individual. The process begins at birth, when the child's *birth sex* is assigned based on physical and biological characteristics (although this seemingly simple assignment can be complicated in situations such as when children are born with ambiguous genitalia). *Gender identity*, the sense of self as male or female, begins to develop during the first years of life. It includes the way a person identifies with the behaviors, attitudes, role expectations, and physical characteristics typically associated with being male or female,[1,2] as well as the way a person feels he or she fits into a certain gender group.[2,3,4] By age 3 years, most children are aware of their own birth sex and the differences between males and females.[4] This is the beginning of gender identity. Most children develop a gender identity consistent with their birth sex[2]; however, *gender-variant children* as young as age 3 or 4 might make statements about wishing to have the genitalia of the other sex and/or may play as the other sex in games with peers. As children reach age 6 or 7, they develop *gender constancy*, the understanding that their birth sex remains the same over time even though their bodies change in other ways (like height and hair length).[4] At this point, gender-variant children may begin to experience *gender dysphoria* (discomfort with their birth sex). As children begin school, they are more aware of gender, and gender-variant children often begin to experiment more with different *gender roles* (societal/cultural expectations for behavior based on one's gender). This can sometimes lead to rejection or isolation from peers. It is important to note here that gender dysphoria and gender role experimentation early on do not necessarily correlate with a complete cross-gender identity later in life. The majority of gender-variant children exhibit more gender-typical behavior by adolescence.[1] As children enter adolescence, there is even greater pressure to conform to distinct gender roles. As cognitive development and physical puberty advance, gender-variant adolescents become increasingly aware of gender discomfort in social contexts, such as team sports, where groups are often separated by gender and organized around typical gender roles.[1,2] Some adolescents will experiment with their gender identity expression. Those who present as gender nonconforming and

TABLE 8–1. **Key terms and definitions related to gender and sexuality[a]**

Birth sex	Sex assigned at birth based on physical and biological characteristics (although assignment can be complicated in situations such as when children are born with ambiguous genitalia).
Cisgender	Describes a person whose gender identity is aligned with the sex they were assigned at birth.
Gender constancy	The understanding, beginning at age 6 or 7, that birth sex remains the same over time even though bodies change in other ways.
Gender dissonance or incongruence	The feeling that one's gender identity is not aligned with the sex assigned at birth and the gender roles and expression typically expected.
Gender dysphoria	Discomfort with one's birth sex.
Gender expression/ presentation	Behavior, clothing, interests, attitudes, and preferred roles in various settings interpreted expected of males or females or typically masculine or feminine.
Gender identity	The sense of self as male or female; includes the way a person identifies with the behaviors, attitudes, role expectations, and physical characteristics typically associated with being male or female as well as the way a person feels he or she fits into a certain gender group.
Gender nonconforming	May be used broadly to describe individuals who experience dissonance between their affirmed gender and assigned sex or to characterize individuals whose gender expression and role preferences are incongruent with their assigned sex. Term may also be used by individuals who feel they are neither male nor female, or identify outside the typical gender binary. Other terms for this include "gender variant," "genderqueer," and "gender fluid."
Gender roles	Societal/cultural expectations for behavior, dress, appearance, and relationships based on one's gender.

TABLE 8–1.	Key terms and definitions related to gender and sexuality[a] *(continued)*
Gender variance	A broad term used to describe individuals whose gender expression or presentation does not conform to the expectations of binary gender norms or roles.
Intersex	Describes a person whose physical sex characteristics do not fit with typically expected male or female bodies.
Queer	May be used to describe several groups of people who defy societal expectations in terms of their sexual or gender identity.
Transgender	Typically used to describe a person who consistently experiences dissonance between affirmed gender and assigned sex. "Transgender male" may refer to a person who identifies as male and was assigned female at birth. "Transgender female" may refer to a person who identifies as female and was assigned male at birth.

[a]Distinction between terms is based solely on how a person chooses to identify and how the person is comfortable being referred to.

reject typically expected behavioral norms may experience scrutiny or hostility from peers, and may feel a greater awareness of gender incongruence as a result.[2]

Gender and sexuality are related but separate. Sexual identity and orientation are defined by how a person thinks, feels, and understands his or her own sexual or romantic attractions and chooses sexual partners. Sexual identity develops along a continuum from homosexual to heterosexual. According to Holden and Holden,[5] within that continuum are five dimensions of sexual identity: 1) sexual orientation, 2) attitudes toward one's own sexual orientation, 3) private sexual behavior and contacts, 4) others' perceptions of one's sexual orientation, and 5) nonsexual behavior and contacts. Individuals can be in different places on the spectrum from homosexual to heterosexual for each dimension, and this can change over time, even into adulthood.[5,6] As mentioned previously, gender and sexuality development begins at an early age, and the Gender Unicorn (Figure 8–1) is a valuable resource to help young people explore the interrelated components of their emerging identities.

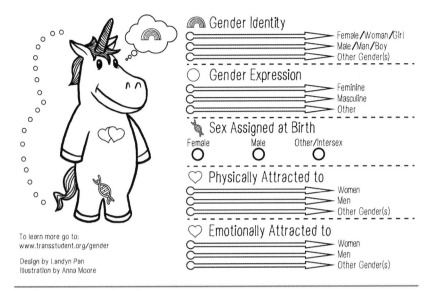

FIGURE 8-1. The Gender Unicorn.

Source. Reprinted from Trans Student Educational Resources. Available at: http://www.transstudent.org/gender.

A child's shifts in gender identity and sexual identity during adolescence can be confusing for parents or other adults, who may perceive identity as fixed. Fluidity over time is actually normal, especially in adolescence, and does not mean a teen is "looking for attention" or "saying she's gay because all her friends are doing it."

Sexual identity generally develops before either sexual desire (interest and motivation to engage in sexual activity) or sexual behavior with others (actual participation in sexual activity). Youth typically begin to experience sexual attraction between ages 7 and 13. However, most 13-year-olds have not had any sexual contacts, and only 7% of teens report sexual intercourse by age 13.[7] Even once a teen begins to engage in sexual activity, the gender of the sexual partners does not necessarily correlate with the teen's sexual orientation.[6,8]

Asking Why: What Puts LGBTQ Youth at Greater Risk for Trauma?

Gender and sexual identity development occurs in the context of race, ethnicity, class, religion, immigration status, and other aspects of identity.[6,9] Lesbian, gay, bisexual, transgender, and queer (LGBTQ) youth all too often experience stigma and discrimination in multiple contexts, including home, school, medical and mental health care, and social services.[10,11,12] This stigma can make it harder for teens to find a positive social support system. Some, like Charlotte, will even choose to leave the social supports they do have because of conflict over sexuality. Without positive supports, LGBTQ teens can be more likely to engage in high-risk health behaviors. This can include early tobacco, alcohol, and other drug use; sexual activity without protection against pregnancy or sexually transmitted infections; unhealthy eating habits; and avoidance of physical activity.[13] These behavioral choices can in turn increase risk for ongoing substance use, mental illness, HIV/AIDS, suicidality, and exposure to traumatic experiences.[12] Even if they do not engage in high-risk behaviors, LGBTQ youth are common targets of verbal harassment, physical threats, or acts of violence and sexual assault.[14,15,16] LGBTQ youth unfortunately are victims of sexual assault, violence, and other trauma more often than their peers. Those youth who have been victimized might not reach out for help because of their prior experiences of stigma and discrimination. If they do reach out, they might still experience discrimination, harassment, blaming, or lack of understanding around their gender or sexuality, even when attending programs designed to help victims.[17]

Finding the Frame: Creating a Therapeutic Space for LGBTQ Teens

Anyone working with LGBTQ teens should take steps to provide a safe and comforting environment for LGBTQ youth, and recognize the high rates of trauma exposure in this population. Assessing for and treating trauma is important, but to do so requires a level of trust between patient and provider. For LGBTQ youth to be able to develop trust, it is vital that those working with them use gender- and sexuality-affirming language throughout the process to avoid inadvertently replicating past experiences of stigmatization. As providers, we can create an environment of safety by being familiar with the specific vulnerabilities and strengths of the LGBTQ population and openly discussing their needs without judgment. Providers hoping to become more comfortable discussing gender and sexuality may find it helpful to practice with a colleague until the language feels more familiar.

After leaving home, Charlotte stayed with her girlfriend for a few days but then realized that she missed her younger brother too much to stay away from home. She tried to explain this to her girlfriend, but they just started arguing, as they did every time Charlotte tried to talk with her girlfriend about the stress of things at home. Frustrated and hurt, Charlotte decided to break up with her girlfriend and return home. Charlotte's parents were thrilled to have her back; her mother thanked God for hearing her prayers, and her father gruffly commented that Charlotte had made the "right choice." When she appeared sad about her girlfriend, they would try to make her feel better by bringing up how she used to date boys and telling her to just "get over it with that girl."

In an attempt to appease her parents, Charlotte starts dating a neighborhood man in his 20s. Although her parents feel worried about his age, they choose to keep the concern to themselves because at least he's a man, not a girl, and Charlotte seems happier. Charlotte goes out with him a few times, but one night she does not come home. Her parents frantically search for her. After a tip from a cousin, they go to the man's apartment and find Charlotte there. They take her to the ER to be "tested in case he took advantage of her."

Parental acceptance or nonacceptance of a child's gender and sexual exploration/identification during the teen years has a huge impact on emotional well-being. How parents react (or even just how teens think their parents will react) can influence whether teens explore their sexuality in safe or unsafe ways. Higher rates of family rejection are associated with much higher rates of suicide, depression, use of illegal drugs, and engagement in unprotected sexual intercourse.[18]

Many families need assistance in learning to support their LGBTQ adolescent children without rejection. The Substance Abuse and Mental Health Services Administration has published a resource guide for practitioners aiming to support these families.[19] Providers should keep in mind that families that are ambivalent or rejecting of their teen's sexual or gender identity are not beyond hope. Even rejecting families become less rejecting over time with education and support. Helping families support their LGBTQ teen starts with a nonjudgmental approach. It is important to meet the family "where they are," recognizing that this is difficult for them and that they love their child. It is also crucial to educate them about the impact of their reactions on their teen's health and well-being.

In the ER, the staff notice how tense things are between Charlotte and her parents. They call the social worker, Maria. Maria interviews Charlotte individually before speaking to her parents. She asks Charlotte about the man she was with. Charlotte denies that he assaulted her and senses that Maria actually believes her, unlike her parents and the ER doctor. She hesitantly shares with Maria that since being intimate with this older man, she has been thinking about something that happened when she was age 6. A friend of her parents, a man in his 20s, had stayed with her family for about a month. Three times, when her parents were sleeping, he came into her room and told her to take off her pajamas so he could look at her. He threatened that if she told anyone she would get in trouble for taking her clothes off for a man and that her family would throw her out, so she had never told anyone until now. She hasn't seen the man in years. Maria starts to ask Charlotte if she would be willing to tell her parents now, but Charlotte tearfully begs her not to make that request.

Maria agrees not to disclose this information to Charlotte's parents but encourages Charlotte to see a therapist to talk about all of this. "But I'm not crazy," Charlotte starts, and Maria reassures the teen that she will be in charge of what she wants to talk about and that the goal will be about helping her feel more comfortable in relationships and with her parents. Charlotte is skeptical but reluctantly agrees. Maria tells Charlotte's parents that she would like to refer Charlotte for therapy because she seems worried about a lot of things. Her parents agree, hoping that the therapy will "fix the problems" Charlotte has been having.

Two weeks later, Charlotte attends her first appointment at the mental health clinic. Charlotte and Linda, the mental health clinician, make small talk for a few minutes before Linda asks how the last 2 weeks have been. Charlotte feels anxious but tells Linda a little about home and school. Then Linda tells Charlotte she'd like to ask some questions to understand the bigger picture of how she's feeling. She asks about a long list of symptoms, and Charlotte says yes to some of them, including nightmares, difficulty concentrating at school, and frequently feeling on edge around men. Linda is fairly direct in asking Charlotte about her sexual and romantic relationships. Charlotte feels weird at first talking about this with an adult, but after a few minutes it becomes sort of a relief to have a place to talk about sex and relationships without feeling judged. Charlotte starts seeing Linda every week. She starts to open up to Linda about the older man she has been dating. She admits that even though he has never forced her to do anything, she feels numb when she is intimate with him. Linda helps Charlotte to see how her numbness, nightmares, trouble concentrating, and jitteriness around men are all related to the sexual abuse she experienced as a child. Eventually, Charlotte decides to stop seeing the older man. She has never felt that strongly for him, and mostly started dating him out of frustration with her parents' pressure to be straight. Also, she doesn't want him to face legal consequences for dating someone underage. Charlotte opens up to Linda about her former girlfriend and how much she misses her. She tells Linda about the day her father gave her the ultimatum, telling her to move out if she did not end the relationship with her girlfriend. Looking back, she can see how it reminded her of when she was a child and the man who abused her said her parents would throw her out. Linda empathizes with how painful this was and reflects on how Charlotte's early traumatic experience still affects her. They talk about how Charlotte might benefit from trauma-focused treatment, and even though it is painful to think about those memories, Charlotte agrees to give it a try.

Charlotte, like many teens who have experienced trauma, has kept her abuse a secret for years. She is initially resistant to disclosing the abuse, to mental health treatment, and to trauma-focused treatment specifically. Individuals who have experienced trauma avoid talking about their trauma because doing so triggers feelings from the past. Victims of childhood sexual abuse may carry additional shame and self-blame that compound emotional distress related to the abuse[20] and make seeking treatment more difficult. As in Charlotte's case, many perpetrators of child sexual abuse shame their victims or tell them it's their fault. Young children are already developmentally predisposed to egocentric thinking (believing they have more control or power than any child really does) and lack the sophistication to be able to question such shaming and blaming (e.g., to reality-test that a young girl could not possibly physically fight off a grown man). As a result, children often have cognitive and emotional distortions about abuse they have suffered, and unless these distorted beliefs are made explicit and questioned, children will carry those damaging beliefs about themselves well into adolescence or adulthood.

Because trauma survivors are psychologically and neurobiologically driven to avoid thinking about their trauma, they often worry that they will be forced to talk about it in therapy. When traumatized youth are referred for therapy or begin trauma-focused treatment, the provider should educate the youth about trauma symptoms and trauma therapy right away to reassure them and assuage their fears. The following are important strategies, with samples of wording that could be used.

- *Naming:* "That thing you experienced was a trauma. Trauma means it's a stressful thing beyond what we're supposed to have to go through, especially when we're young."
- *Normalizing:* "Unfortunately, trauma happens to a lot of us. When we experience a trauma, very often it affects our thinking in certain specific ways. Because thinking about what happened is stressful, we sometimes try to avoid anything that reminds us of what happened, but the thoughts and memories keep coming up anyway, in our thoughts or in our dreams.

After trauma some of us get more sad, irritable, or numb and find that it is harder to think positively about the future. Some people feel on edge a lot of the time. All of these reactions are typical after trauma. They don't mean you're crazy, and they're not your fault—they just mean you went through a really bad experience."

- *Explaining:* "We have learned that we can help people recover from trauma through therapy. Sometimes medication might also be helpful. It's really important for you to know that you will be in charge of deciding when you are ready to talk about your trauma. Our first focus will be to work on strategies you can use to feel better right now. If we think medication will be helpful, we'll tell you and explain why, but it's your decision and we would never force you to take medication if you don't want to. We will work together to decide what is most helpful for you."

When you are working with sexually traumatized LGBTQ youth, it is also important to provide psychoeducation to parents, and if necessary to the teen, about gender and sexual identity development to clarify that sexual identity and orientation can be informed by, but are independent of, exposure to trauma.

Trauma and Reproductive Health

A few months later, Charlotte comes into Linda's office looking anxious. She says she has not had her period in the past 2 months, and although she initially just blamed this on stress, she finally took a pregnancy test and the results were positive. Linda helps Charlotte reflect on what to do next. They set up an appointment at the local family health clinic, where the nurse confirms she is pregnant. Charlotte tells Linda that she wants to continue with the pregnancy, although she has mixed feelings about becoming a mom and is terrified about telling her parents.

Clinicians and parents may forget to counsel LGBTQ youth on safe sex and contraception, thinking that they are not at risk for pregnancy. But LGBTQ youth are actually 2–10 times more likely to get pregnant (or get someone pregnant) compared with their heterosexual peers.[21] This fact underscores the difference between sexual identity and sexual behavior, as discussed above. Youth like Charlotte who have experienced sexual abuse, and those who have experienced physical abuse, are also at greater risk for teen pregnancy, with sexual abuse doubling the risk.[22] Nationally, about 11% of teenage girls will give birth before their twentieth birthday, and the majority of these pregnancies are unplanned.[23] These young mothers are less likely to finish high school, are at higher risk for depression and substance abuse, and are more likely to live in poverty in the future. Their babies are at increased risk of preterm delivery, low birth weight, and neonatal death.[24,25] As they grow, children of teen parents are at higher risk for abuse and neglect, problems with language and learning, mental health issues, and, later on, teen parenthood and dropping out of school.[26]

Obviously the most important aspect of dealing with teen pregnancy is prevention. Teens need good information about sexual health and contraception. Medical and mental health professionals must learn how to engage in open discussion that incorporates understanding of the difference between sexual identity/orientation and sexual behavior. Remember that sexual identity and sexual behavior are not the same thing, so a teen who identifies as lesbian may still have vaginal intercourse with men and need contraceptive counseling. Learning how to ask questions that affirm the teen's experience and identity while also getting an accurate picture of the teen's potential needs is vital. Clinicians and other adults who work with youth should also be prepared to dispel misconceptions about pregnancy and contraception and give guidance about effective contraception methods, including condoms and hormonal methods. Long-acting reversible contraception (LARC) methods such as implants and IUDs are a good option for adolescents, because these methods are much more effective than others in preventing unwanted pregnancies.[27] Because many young women are ambivalent about using contraception, motivational interviewing approaches can help young women (including teens who have already had a baby) decide whether they want to use LARC.[28]

Using Motivational Interviewing Techniques to Discuss Contraception Use

You were referred here to talk about contraception, but it sounds like you have some other concerns that are important to you as well. Where do you think we should start?

What do you want to accomplish before you have another baby?

What needs to happen for you to reach your goals?

What would make it worth your while to use contraception?

> ## Using Motivational Interviewing Techniques to Discuss Contraception Use *(continued)*
>
> You mentioned that you want to wait at least 2 more years before you have another baby, so what options do you think are available to you to help you reach that goal to waiting at least 2 years?
>
> Are you interested in hearing some options that may help you reach your goals?
>
> On a scale from 0 to 10, where 0 is "not important" and 10 is "the most important," how important would you say it is for you to start using contraception?
>
> What concerns you most about using contraception?
>
> If you were to start using contraception, how might things be different in the future?

Linda helps Charlotte think about how to tell her parents about her pregnancy and they practice together what Charlotte could say. Charlotte feels sweaty and shaky when she sits her parents down in the living room to tell them. But to her surprise, they say they will support her in having the baby. Charlotte suspects they are still holding on to an idea that she is "not really bisexual" and hoping that having a baby will guarantee she will not date any more girls. When she shares this worry with Linda, Linda suggests that they invite Charlotte's parents to a therapy session to talk about it.

When Charlotte's parents do join a session, Linda facilitates the dialogue but lets Charlotte take the lead in educating her parents about gender and sexuality. Charlotte uses the Gender Unicorn (see Figure 8–1 earlier in this chapter) to help explain who she is and who she finds attractive. Her parents begin to soften their views, and Charlotte decides to tell them about what had happened long ago with the family friend. She decides it is important because it has influenced some of her thinking about sexuality and might help her parents understand her better. Charlotte's mother begins to cry as Charlotte shares what happened. When Charlotte is done, her mother hugs her while her father tries to hide the tears in his eyes. After a moment, Charlotte's mother discloses that she also had been molested by an uncle when she was young. "I told my parents," she says, her voice breaking, "but they didn't believe me. I would never want you to feel that way." She feels terrible that she had not been able to protect Charlotte. She admits that at the time she had felt worried about having the man stay with them because she saw how anxious Charlotte was around him. But she had doubted her suspicions, thinking her own history of abuse had made her "paranoid." Charlotte and her mother hug for a long time. They decide to meet together with Linda a few more times to work through all of this.

Trauma and Teen Pregnancy: Supporting Moms for Healthy Babies

Once a teen is pregnant and has decided to continue the pregnancy, it's important to focus on how to support the teen. This means both helping the teen stay in school and helping her prepare to become a parent. A number of programs have been designed to prevent the negative outcomes associated with teen pregnancy and parenthood noted in the previous section. Such programs can be implemented through home visiting, schools, and clinics; some examples are below.

Home visiting programs send doulas, nurses, social workers, or other providers to the expecting teen or new mom where it is most convenient: at home. These programs have been extremely successful with high-risk moms of all ages and are increasingly available across the country. The provider meets the new mom at home, sometimes starting even before the baby is born to connect and help the mom prepare both emotionally and practically. Once the baby is born, the provider gives support and parenting advice for the new mom and teaches her about caring for the baby and about normal development. The provider also monitors the baby's development and monitors the mom for postpartum depression and other mental health needs, and refers to other providers and services if needed.

> Home visiting programs for new moms can be found through Nurse-Family Partnership and Healthy Families America (see "Resources and Additional Reading" at the end of this chapter). The Web sites for these programs have information about how to access these services in different parts of the United States.

School-based programs designed for teen parents usually offer on-site prenatal and family planning services, day care, and other supportive services. Unfortunately, these programs fail to reach the mothers who have dropped out of school either before or during pregnancy; those moms are better served in a clinic-based program (as described in the next section). Programs utilizing a multidisciplinary medical home model have proven quite effective. Prenatal care is combined with social services, mental health care, and parenting classes or other group programming to give pregnant teens a chance to connect with one another. After the baby is born, the collaborative approach continues. Each visit, regardless of the "identified patient," is utilized as an opportunity to check in with both mother and baby along with other family members when available.[25]

It is also extremely important to appreciate the role of maternal mental health during and after pregnancy. Pregnant teens are susceptible to perinatal depression at higher rates than older mothers and same-age nonpregnant peers. Trauma is all too frequently present as well. "One study found that on average, teenage mothers had experienced >5 traumatic events."[28] Mothers with a history of childhood sexual abuse, as in Charlotte's case, may carry increased risk for perinatal anxiety.[29] The experience of pregnancy, prenatal care, and childbirth, which are stressful for all women, can be profoundly triggering for women who have experienced trauma, especially sexual trauma. The American College of Obstetrics and Gynecologists has advised that all women be screened for a history of sexual abuse and that their obstetric care be modified to avoid retraumatization.[30] For example, during the first prenatal visits, a woman might be given a choice to undergo a pelvic or breast examination right away or to allow herself a bit of time to adjust after explanation of what will occur. During labor and delivery, the feelings of loss of control over one's own body (felt by most women as a typical part of delivery) may in trauma survivors powerfully replicate the feelings that were present during episodes of abuse. When doctors, nurses, midwives, and doulas understand this connection to past trauma, they are more able to reassure the woman that she is safe and help her stay grounded and feel in control. These strategies can prevent dissociation and flashbacks during labor and delivery.[31]

In both medical and mental health settings, using standardized questionnaires to screen for depression and for history of abuse can be extremely helpful to enable both providers and teens to feel more comfortable addressing these sensitive topics. When presenting a questionnaire, you may find normalizing and explaining to be useful:

> We have learned that many pregnant women and mothers struggle with sadness and many have suffered a lot of stress in their lives. We have also learned that when we help a woman identify these problems, we can offer support that improves outcomes for both mother and baby. We are asking all the women in our clinic this set of questions so we can talk with you about it if you are struggling.

Many teens will feel more comfortable revealing symptoms on self-report questionnaires than in interviews, although teens with low literacy may need help completing questionnaires. Questionnaires should then lead to an in-person discussion with a care provider. When talking with teens about their mental health during or after pregnancy, providers should use a non-judgmental and open-ended approach. For example, they might say, "Sometimes people notice that their mood changes while they're pregnant. How has your mood been recently? Have you been feeling more sad or worried than is usual for you?" When providers are comfortable asking patients these questions, the patient feels reassured. Providers who are not accustomed to asking these types of questions may find it helpful to practice a few times with someone who is not a patient first.

The intergenerational transmission of trauma also deserves mention here. Much new research focuses on this topic, exploring both psychological and biological (epigenetic) mechanisms through which this may occur.[32] As demonstrated in Charlotte's story, she and her mother both experienced childhood sexual abuse. The mother's experience, by her own admission, caused her to doubt her correct maternal observations, making it more difficult for her to protect her child. Unspoken and unaddressed, these types of patterns can extend through generations. Engaging Charlotte and her mother in trauma-focused treatment can break this cycle and create a different course for Charlotte's child.

Treating the Dyad: Supporting Attachment and Healthy Development for Parenting Teens

Linda helps Charlotte find a prenatal clinic with special support services for teen parents. There are groups she can attend for support when she goes to her OB-GYN appointments and a social worker who helps her sort through options for continuing high school and finding daycare options for after the baby comes. She continues to see Linda in the mental health clinic as well. Charlotte's mom starts attending some of her prenatal appointments. The father-to-be also comes occasionally and promises to help with financial support for the baby, although he and Charlotte are not dating. In fact, Charlotte and her previous girlfriend have started dating again. Charlotte's parents are still not entirely comfortable with this or welcoming to the girlfriend, but they accept Charlotte's choices and are relieved to see Charlotte appearing happy and loved in the relationship. Charlotte's delivery proceeds smoothly, as does the initial postpartum period for mother and baby. Charlotte starts receiving support through a home visiting program that provides parenting support. Charlotte's mother changes her shifts at work so she can help with the baby during the day, and she takes care of the baby once Charlotte returns to school. At the baby's 1-year well-child visit, it is clear by observation that Charlotte's baby, Crystal, is strongly attached to her grandmother, perhaps even more so than she is to her actual mother.

Charlotte's process adjusting to pregnancy and parenthood as detailed above demonstrates the inherent complexity of teenage parenting. There are concrete issues such as plans for continuing school, living arrangements, and financial support that must be addressed. In addition, the psychological transition to becoming a parent is complicated by the developmental stage of the teen mother. Personal identity consolidation and individuation from family of origin are two of the most important goals of adolescence. Reaching for these goals requires that the teen be more self-focused and increasingly autonomous. Being self-focused, however, does not jibe well with having a newborn. It is challenging for many teen mothers to be consistently sensitive to their infant's cues and to engage in *reflective functioning* (imagining what the baby wants or needs). Traumatized mothers can struggle with this as well. For example, a woman who experienced physical abuse or domestic violence as a child may be triggered by the baby's crying and thus unable to respond appropriately to the infant's distress. Mothers who have suffered abuse or neglect may also be more likely to misinterpret the baby's crying. The teen might think "the baby hates me, just like my stepfather hated me," and then disengage, missing cues that the baby is hungry, uncomfortable, or simply in need of being held. Mothers who have experienced trauma are also at increased risk for postpartum depression, compounding risk. Therapists, home-visiting nurses, and providers in multidisciplinary medical home clinics can support maternal sensitivity and responsiveness through attention to the special needs of these mothers. Simple empathy ("Being a new mom is so hard"), normalizing ("All babies cry, and it's tough for every new mom—we all feel at first like we're doing everything wrong"), reflective functioning ("When she cries like that, I wonder what she's trying to tell you?"), validation ("When you picked him up, look how he stopped crying—that was just what he needed"), and support can make a huge difference. Sensitive parenting education and guidance can improve child outcomes over time (Table 8–2).

The broader family and social context also plays an important role for teen parents. Many teen mothers are unable to consider leaving home in the near future because they rely on their parents' support. Additionally, the Personal Responsibility and Work Opportunity Act of 1996 required that teen mothers live with a parent or guardian in order to receive public assistance, thereby significantly reinforcing many teen mothers to continue living with their own family. The teen's mother can help the teen transition to parenthood, but this can also be a source of conflict. If the teens have an open, communicative, and flexible relationship with their own mothers, they are more likely to show positive parenting behaviors toward their own chil-

TABLE 8–2. Evidence-based treatments for traumatized moms with young children

Evidence-based treatment	Age range	For more information
Child Parent Psychotherapy	0–5 years	http://childtrauma.ucsf.edu/resources-0
Parent-Child Interaction Therapy (PCIT)	2–7 years	http://www.pcit.org
Triple P	0–16 years	http://www.triplep.net/glo-en/home
The Incredible Years	4–8 years	http://www.incredibleyears.com
Attachment and Biobehavioral Catch-up (ABC)	0–2 years	http://www.infantcaregiverproject.com

dren.[33] The balance of caretaking is important. When the teen's mother provides the majority of direct infant care, the teen may develop less self-efficacy in the parent role and less appreciation of the challenges of child-rearing, which increases risk for repeat teen pregnancy.[33,34] This can be prevented in a few ways. First, providers can help the teen's parents understand the complexity of their dual role and help them find the balance necessary to parent a parent. On a more concrete level, helping teen mothers and their mothers resolve conflict helps the well-being of both baby and caregivers.[35]

When a teen's mother plays a strong attachment role in the grandchild's early childhood, such as is noted for baby Crystal above, this will need to be respected as the child grows older. For instance, if Charlotte and baby Crystal move into their own home in the next few years, frequent ongoing contact between Crystal and her grandmother will likely be important to prevent Crystal from experiencing a serious attachment loss.

Teen mothers are less likely to be married or living with the father of their child compared to women who have children later in life. Although certainly a father does not have to live with a child to be involved, access is often limited when parents are not living together, and studies have suggested that father involvement decreases over time for children born to adolescent mothers, although more research is warranted. Children who have involved fathers do better academically and socially, and fathers of children born to adolescent mothers typically want to be involved but don't know how. There are practical barriers to their involvement as well, including economic and social factors and the need for parenting skills. Providers can engage fathers with support around educational, employment, social, and mental health needs, and also teach parenting skills to help them be more present for their children. Providers can also support both adolescent parents in navigating the difficult task of coparenting, including coping with or putting aside prior conflicts in the relationship to focus on what is best for their child.

Many teens will cycle through numerous romantic relationships on the pathway to adulthood. Given how important relationships can be for the teen's well-being, these relationships should not be discouraged (as long as the relationships are not maladaptive or dangerous). But when a teen has a baby or young child, the teen may need assistance thinking about how best to navigate involvement of the child in these relationships. Attachment is so critical in early childhood that sudden disruption of attachments (e.g., loss of a stepfather, grandmother, or mother's boyfriend who had become an important presence) can itself be traumatic. Young parents should be encouraged to think carefully about how much to involve short-term romantic partners in the lives of their children to prevent a sense of instability that can trigger anxiety and behavior problems in the children. Charlotte may ultimately choose to raise her child in a same-sex parenting household. Although research is somewhat limited, studies looking at parenting stress and child well-being have thus far not found consistent differences for same-sex versus dual-sex parenting households[36,37] From a practical standpoint, because same-sex parenting households are less common, children living in these households may need support when other children or adults have questions or misperceptions. Ultimately, the quality of parenting seems to far outweigh any other factors in child outcomes.

Conclusion

The topics covered in this chapter are complex, and we can by no means do justice to all of this complexity in one brief chapter; however, we have attempted to highlight some important points.

1. Trauma is prevalent among LGBTQ youth, as well as among teen mothers and fathers. Past trauma may influence sexual and reproductive health choices and, because of a variety of factors, may also increase risk for additional trauma exposures.
2. Family acceptance and support are major factors predicting positive or negative outcomes for both LGBTQ and pregnant or parenting teens.

3. Supportive services and treatment interventions for LGBTQ and pregnant or parenting teens need to embrace the complexity of their lives. Often in addition to mental health treatment for trauma-related symptoms, mood symptoms, and substance abuse, they will need options for help with social, economic, and educational disadvantages. Standard medical care may need to be adjusted to align with their specific needs.

Although life can seem challenging for adolescents who fall outside of any social "norm," with support and acceptance most emerge into young adulthood with intact identity, self-esteem, and health. LGBTQ and pregnant or parenting youth deserve no less.

Resources and Additional Reading

Online Resources

Gender and Sexual Development

Gender Spectrum (for information and resources on gender development): https://www.genderspectrum.org

National LGBT Health Education Center, part of The Fenway Institute (a great educational resource for LGBTQ health): http://fenwayhealth.org/the-fenway-institute/education/the-national-lgbt-health-education-center/

Supporting Teen Moms for Healthy Babies (Home Visiting Programs)

Nurse-Family Partnership: http://www.nursefamilypartnership.org

Healthy Families America: http://www.healthyfamiliesamerica.org

Attachment and Parenting Young Children

International Attachment Network resource page: http://www.ian-attachment.org.uk/international-attachment-network-information.html

Zero to Three (great resources about parenting infants and young children, and lots of parent support): https://www.zerotothree.org

Working With Teens Who Have Experienced Trauma

Skills Training in Affective and Interpersonal Regulation (STAIR): http://www.istss.org/education-research/traumatic-stresspoints/2015-march-(1)/clinician-s-corner-skills-training-in-affective-an.aspx

Trauma-Focused Cognitive Behavioral Therapy (TF-CBT) training Web site: https://tfcbt.musc.edu

Additional Reading

Cass VC: Homosexual identity formation: a theoretical model. J Homosex 4(3): 219–235, 1979 264126

Chandra A, Mosher WD, Copen C, et al: Sexual behavior, sexual attraction, and sexual identity in the United States: data from the 2006–2008 National Survey of Family Growth. Natl Health Stat Rep Mar 3(36):1–36, 2011 21560887

Cloitre M, Cohen LR, Koenen KC: Treating Survivors of Childhood Abuse: Psychotherapy for the Interrupted Life. New York, Guilford, 2006

Edwards K, Brooks AK: The development of sexual identity. New Dir Adult Contin Educ 84:49–57, 1999

Espelage DL, Aragon SR, Brikett M: Homophobic teasing, psychological outcomes, and sexual orientation among high school students: what influence do parents and schools have? School Psych Rev 37:202–216, 2008

Faber A, Mazlish E: How to Talk So Kids Will Listen and Listen So Kids Will Talk. New York, Scribner, 1980

Flores A, Herman J, Gates G, et al: How Many Adults Identify as Transgender in the United States? Los Angeles, CA, Williams Institute, 2016

Flores A, Herman J, Brown T, et al: Ages of Individuals Who Identify as Transgender in the United States. Los Angeles, CA, Williams Institute, 2017

Gold CM: Keeping Your Child in Mind: Overcoming Defiance, Tantrums, and Other Everyday Behavior Problems, by Seeing the World Through Your Child's Eyes. Philadelphia, PA, Da Capo Press, 2011

Karen R: Becoming Attached: First Relationships and How They Shape Our Capacity to Love. New York, Oxford University Press, 1994

Russell ST, Ryan C, Toomey RB, et al: Lesbian, gay, bisexual, and transgender adolescent school victimization: implications for young adult health and adjustment. J Sch Health 81(5):223–230, 2011 21517860

Savin-Williams RC: Who's gay? Does it matter? Curr Dir Psychol Sci 15(1):40–44, 2006

References

1. Pleak RR: Formation of transgender identities in adolescence. J Gay Lesbian Ment Health 13(4):282–291, 2009
2. Steensma TD, Kreukels BP, de Vries AL, et al: Gender identity development in adolescence. Horm Behav 64(2):288–297, 2013 23998673
3. Bem SL: Gender schema theory: a cognitive account of sex typing. Psychol Rev 88(4):354–364, 1981
4. Egan SK, Perry DG: Gender identity: a multidimensional analysis with implications for psychosocial adjustment. Dev Psychol 37(4):451–463, 2001 11444482
5. Holden JM, Holden GS: The sexual identity profile: a multidimensional bipolar model. Individ Psychol 51(2):103–113, 1995
6. Levy DL: Gay and lesbian identity development: an overview for social workers. J Hum Behav Soc Environ 19(8):978–993, 2009

7. Saewyc EM: Research on adolescent sexual orientation: development, health disparities, stigma and resilience. J Res Adolesc 21(1):256–272, 2011 27099454

8. Zaza S, Kann L, Barrios LC: Lesbian, gay, and bisexual adolescents population estimate and prevalence of health behaviors. JAMA 316(22):2355–2356, 2016 27532437

9. Meyer IH: Identity, stress, and resilience in lesbians, gay men, and bisexual of color. Couns Psychol 38(3):442–454, 2010 24347674

10. Ard KL, Makadon HJ: Improving the Health Care of Lesbian, Gay, Bisexual, and Transgender (LGBT) People: Understanding and Eliminating Health Disparities. Boston, MA, Fenway Institute, 2012

11. Coker TR, Austin SB, Schuster MA: The health and health care of lesbian, gay, and bisexual adolescents. Annu Rev Public Health 31:457–477, 2010 20070195

12. Kates J, Rnaji U, Beamesderfer A, et al: Health and Access to Care and Coverage for Lesbian, Gay, Bisexual, and Transgender Individuals in the U.S. Washington, DC, Henry J. Kaiser Family Foundation, 2016

13. Kann L, Olsen EO, McManus T, et al: Sexual identity, sex of sexual contacts, and health-related behaviors among students in grades 9–12—United States and selected sites. MMWR Surveill Summ 65(9):1–202, 2016 27513843

14. D'Augelli AR, Grossman AH, Starks MT: Childhood gender atypicality, victimization, and PTSD among lesbian, gay, and bisexual youth. J Interpers Violence 21(11):1462–1482, 2006 17057162

15. Grossman AH, D'Augelli AR, Frank JA: Aspects of psychological resilience among transgender youth. J LGBT Youth 8(2):103–115, 2011

16. Mizock L, Lewis TK: Trauma in transgender populations: risk, resilience, and clinical care. J Emotional Abuse 8(3):335–354, 2008

17. Bauer GR, Hammond R, Travers R, et al: "I don't think this is theoretical; this is our lives": how erasure impacts health care for transgender people. J Assoc Nurses AIDS Care 20(5):348–361, 2009 19732694

18. Ryan C, Huebner D, Diaz RM, et al: Family rejection as a predictor of negative health outcomes in white and Latino lesbian, gay, and bisexual young adults. Pediatrics 123(1):346–352, 2009 19117902

19. Substance Abuse and Mental Health Services Administration: A practitioner's resource guide: helping families to support their LGBT children (HHS Publ No PEP14-LGBTKIDS). 2014. Available at: https://familyproject.sfsu.edu/sites/default/files/FamilySupportForLGBTChildrenGuidance.pdf. Accessed March 3, 2018.

20. Whiffen VE, Macintosh HB: Mediators of the link between childhood sexual abuse and emotional distress: a critical review. Trauma Violence Abuse 6(1):24–39, 2005 15574671

21. Saewyc EM, Poon CS, Homma Y, Skay CL: Stigma management? The links between enacted stigma and teen pregnancy trends among gay, lesbian, and bisexual students in British Columbia. Can J Hum Sex 17(3):123–139, 2008 19293941

22. Madigan S, Wade M, Tarabulsy G, et al: Association between abuse history and adolescent pregnancy: a meta-analysis. J Adolesc Health 55(2):151–159, 2014 25049043

23. U.S. Department of Health and Human Services: Trends in teen pregnancy and childbearing. 2014. Available at: https://www.hhs.gov/ash/oah/adolescent-health-topics/reproductive-health/teen-pregnancy/trends.html. Accessed March 3, 2018.

24. Chen XK, Wen SW, Fleming N, et al: Teenage pregnancy and adverse birth outcomes: a large population based retrospective cohort study. Int J Epidemiol 36(2):368–373, 2007 17213208

25. Ruedinger E, Cox JE: Adolescent childbearing: consequences and interventions. Curr Opin Pediatr 24(4):446–452, 2012 22790098

26. Francis JKR, Gold MA: Long-acting reversible contraception for adolescents: a review. JAMA Pediatr 171(7):694–701, 2017 28558091

27. Tomlin K, Bambulas T, Sutton M, et al: Motivational interviewing to promote long-acting reversible contraception in postpartum teenagers. J Pediatr Adolesc Gynecol 30(3):383–388, 2016 27871919

28. Hodgkinson S, Beers L, Southammakosane C, et al: Addressing the mental health needs of pregnant and parenting adolescents. Pediatrics 133(1):114–122, 2014 24298010

29. Gartland D, Woolhouse H, Giallo R, et al: Vulnerability to intimate partner violence and poor mental health in the first 4-year postpartum among mothers reporting childhood abuse: an Australian pregnancy cohort study. Arch Women Ment Health 29(6):1091–1100, 2016 27565802

30. American College of Obstetricians and Gynecologists: Adult manifestations of childhood sexual abuse, Committee Opinion No 498. 2011. Available at: https://www.acog.org/-/media/Committee-Opinions/Committee-on-Health-Care-for-Underserved-Women/co498.pdf?dmc=1andts=20170220T1135255476. Accessed March 3, 2018.

31. White A: Responding to prenatal disclosure of past sexual abuse. Obstet Gynecol 123(6):1344–1347, 2014 24807334

32. Bowers ME, Yehuda R: Intergenerational transmission of stress in humans. Neuropsychopharmacology 41(1):232–244, 2016 26279078

33. Savio Beers LA, Hollo RE: Approaching the adolescent-headed family: a review of teen parenting. Curr Probl Pediatr Adolesc Health Care 39(9):216–233, 2009 19857857

34. Zeiders KH, Umaña-Taylor AJ, Jahromi LB, et al: Grandmothers' familism values, adolescent mothers' parenting efficacy, and children's well-being. J Fam Psychol 29(4):624–634, 2015 26075734

35. Sellers K, Black MM, Boris NW, et al: Adolescent mothers' relationships with their own mothers: impact on parenting outcomes. J Fam Psychol 25(1):117–126, 2011 21219072

36. Bos HM, Kuyper L, Gartrell NK: A population-based comparison of female and male same-sex parent and different-sex parent households. Fam Process February 15, 2017 [Epub ahead of print] 28197994

37. Schumm WR: A review and critique of research on same-sex parenting and adoption. Psychol Rep 119(3):641–760, 2016 27620690

CHAPTER 9

Trauma and Teens With Developmental and Physical Disabilities

Karen C. Rogers, Ph.D.

Trauma and Teens With Developmental Disabilities

Ava, a 14-year-old girl with intellectual disability, tends to be quiet and shy. She speaks in one- or two-word sentences, and people who don't know her can have difficulty understanding her speech. At the beginning of her freshman year, Ava was happy and excited to be in high school and really liked her new classroom. But recently, she has started crying every morning on the way to school. She tells her parents that another student "pushed" and "touched privates." When her mother talks with the school personnel about it, they say it is impossible that another student could hurt or touch Ava that way because Ava, who is in a special education class, is always directly supervised by adults. But Ava keeps getting upset about school and talking about the "bad girl" there. After a few more weeks, she starts having tantrums in the morning and refusing to go to bed at night.

Teens with developmental disabilities (DDs), like Ava, are particularly vulnerable to trauma and abuse. A DD is a mental and/or physical impairment, diagnosed before age 22, that is expected to be lifelong. The individual with DD has substantial limitations in at least three of the following areas of functioning: self-care, expressive or receptive language, learning, mobility, self-direction, capacity for independent living, and economic self-sufficiency. Youth with DDs are diverse and have different needs, but most live in the community and attend public schools.

One in six American children has a DD such as autism, hearing impairment, or cerebral palsy. Research suggests that the prevalence of DDs among children has increased from 12.84% of the population in 1998 to 15.04% in 2008.[1] Despite how common they are, DDs still carry stigma for children and youth. Teens with DDs are often treated as though they are younger than their age. They are not expected to have the same needs for increasing independence, exploration of sexuality, and identity development that typically developing adolescents have. Youth with DDs may have difficulty accessing informal support systems, such as sports teams and extracurricular activities, and services such as counseling and reproductive health care. They miss out on these experiences less because of their disability and more because people wrongly think they won't be able to participate or benefit from such services or supports. Mistaken beliefs about the ability of a youth with a DD to participate in or benefit from such services can be as much a barrier as the functional limitations of the disability. Missing these supports and services can make youth with disabilities more vulnerable to abuse or maltreatment, and results in greater isolation and having fewer people to turn to if the youth are victimized. This is especially troublesome because children and adolescents with DDs are more likely to be targets of abuse.

Asking Why:
How Youth With Developmental Disabilities Can Be Vulnerable to Trauma and Abuse

Teens with DDs are almost twice as likely as teens without DDs to experience some type of victimization, such as physical abuse, sexual abuse, neglect, and emotional abuse.[2] Teens with DDs are far more likely to experience sexual abuse, especially if the disability is severe or if, like Ava, they have an intellectual disability. The abuse is often more severe and goes on for longer before being stopped. Youth with DDs are also more likely to experience abuse from more than one perpetrator.

> Ava's parents aren't sure what to think. The people at school have worked with lots of kids like Ava and are with their daughter all day. They wonder if maybe the school people are right, and what Ava reported could not have happened. Maybe Ava is having behavior problems and needs consequences. But she has never had behavior problems before, and the sudden change really makes them worry. Her dad quits his job at a factory so he can be around more to help take care of her. Her parents try to talk to the school

again about Ava, but the staff continue to say Ava is "making things up" and doing this "for attention," and nothing changes. Finally, they take Ava to see her pediatrician. Her pediatrician doesn't think Ava has a behavior problem at all. She thinks the school staff must be mistaken, and she believes what Ava has been telling her parents. She is concerned that another student may have harmed Ava at school. The pediatrician asks, "Does Ava have morning tantrums or refuse to go to bed on weekends?" Her parents think about it for a minute before shaking their heads no. The pediatrician explains that Ava's tantrums in the morning could be her way of saying she's afraid to go to school. Her refusal to go to bed on weeknights could be about bad dreams of what happened or anticipatory anxiety about school the next morning. The pediatrician recommends that her parents not send Ava back to that school and insist on a change. The doctor writes a letter to the school and the city's department of education and helps Ava's parents call an educational advocacy agency. After a few months and a lot of meetings, Ava starts at a new high school.

Unfortunately, there are many reasons why youth with DDs are more likely to be abused. The reasons fall into three categories: societal risk factors, family risk factors, and individual risk factors. One of the biggest societal risk factors is misconception about emotional development and needs of youth with DDs. Children with DDs are seen as more innocent and less mature than their typically developing peers. As a result, as they grow they rarely receive any instruction or information about sexual health or development. Many adults assume the youth "won't understand." Other adults simply don't know how to discuss, or don't feel comfortable talking about, sexual health or boundaries with the young person. Adding to the problem, adults may ignore the teens' developmentally appropriate need for socialization and opportunities to explore identity and independence. Although parents and other adults will worry about a typically developing teen who doesn't have any friends, they may brush aside concerns about a young person with DD feeling lonely and isolated. Adults may insist that the teen prefers being alone or that the teen isn't aware of the lack of friendships. Alternatively, adults may encourage the teen to tolerate peer interactions characterized by aggression and poor boundaries, when they would expect better for typically developing youth. Teens with DDs who feel lonely and isolated, who have never been taught about safe or appropriate physical, romantic, or sexual interactions, and who have become accustomed to aggression in peer relationships may not know to ask for help when someone mistreats them.

Another societal risk factor is that parents, schools, doctors, and even therapists for youth with DDs often teach youth to be compliant with adults. Youth with autism or other DDs are often sensitive to bright lights, loud noises, or physical stimulation, or become very anxious in new places or so-cial situations. Well-intentioned adults teach youth with DDs to tolerate these situations even when uncomfortable or even painful, because an adult says to do it. Teens with physical care needs are taught to comply with adults touching their bodies, sometimes in intimate ways. Those who want to victimize a youth with DD can take advantage of this same compliance. A compliant youth may not resist physical or sexual harm, especially if the per-petrator is a caregiver or other adult whom the teen has been taught to co-operate with.

Adding to the vulnerability, adults may not believe that youth with DDs are able to perceive and report others' behavior accurately. Teens like Ava can be seen as "confused" or "mistaken" when they report maltreatment. Even when adults recognize that something traumatic may have happened, they may not recognize trauma symptoms when the adolescent also has a DD. Some people mistakenly believe that the disability somehow buffers the teen from painful feelings associated with trauma. They may misinterpret trauma reactions as being behavior problems or part of the youth's disability. For example, staff at Ava's school may have known other students with dis-abilities who resist going to school, tantrum, misunderstand peers' behav-iors, or repeat phrases over and over without understanding the meaning. Although Ava has never shown any of those symptoms before, the adults still misattributed her tantrums to her DD, rather than wondering what else might be going on.

Adolescents may be more likely to encounter abuse within the service sys-tem (education, disability services) simply because they require help from more people. In addition, a societal failure to provide adequate training and support for service providers doing challenging work increases the risk that caretakers will use inappropriate or harmful interventions (e.g., physical punishments, withholding food) or lash out in frustration. Without a good understanding of an individual's disability and strategies to work effectively with that child, adults may view behaviors as intentionally defiant and be an-gry with the teen. Many adults believe that swift and tangible consequences, such as physical restraint, are the best way to intervene when they see be-havior problems, and they don't take time to think about other potential causes. In addition, some sexual abuse perpetrators may choose to work with youth with DDs in order to have access to potential victims. Schools and dis-ability services systems often lack sufficient oversight and monitoring to formally recognize or track abusers, so even if removed from one program, an abuser may easily find a new position working with vulnerable youth. The legal system also may not respond to victims with disabilities in the same way they do to typically developing youth; when people with disabilities disclose abuse, it is less likely to be reported to police or to be investigated, and perpetrators are less likely to face criminal charges. A child with DD may not be seen as a credible witness by people who lack knowledge and understanding of the disability. People working in the criminal justice system do not systematically receive training to help them understand and work with people with disabilities. Even if a judge, prosecutor, or police officer recognizes that a youth with DD is able to report clearly on an experience, they may choose not to move forward out of recognition that the youth will appear less than credible in court.

Family risk factors can stem both from a lack of understanding of the individual youth's disability and from the stress of caring for a young person with special needs. Family cultural expectations can also be important. Families' misperceptions about their children with DDs can increase the risk of abuse. Caregivers may believe that youth are safe in schools and other programs, or they may believe, as Ava's parents did, that professionals know more than they themselves do about their child. They may not talk to their teens about relationships or sexual health or take steps to make sure their teen has friends and hobbies or opportunities to learn basic sex education. The extra demands of caring for a youth with disabilities are not only stressful but also practically difficult for caregivers and can increase risk for abuse or trauma. It may be difficult to find child care, or families may be forced to choose between subpar child care options. Other parents, like Ava's father, may need to withdraw from paid work in order to care for the child, leading to increased financial stress and social isolation. Families may become isolated from friends and extended family due to the time required for care of their teen or because of stigma associated with the disability in their family. Cultural views of disability can increase a family's stigma and isolation in many ways. In some cultures a child with special needs may be viewed as a punishment for parents' past sins. Parents may be told that if they just spanked the child or used other physical discipline, the problems would go away. Parents of teens with DDs can feel judged harshly in their parenting by family members and friends, and may withdraw or not ask for help as a result. Youth who are seen as too different may also be excluded by extended family or friends, even from cultural celebrations. All of these factors increase loneliness and isolation for the family, so caregivers lack practical and emotional support. A caregiver under stress may be too overwhelmed to recognize signs of trauma in their child, or to know what to do to help. Some parents or other family members may be pushed to their limit and lash out at the child.

Aspects of a teen's disability can also lead directly to greater risk for abuse. A youth with communication difficulties may be unable to report maltreatment to others or to effectively say no. Someone with limited mobility may be unable to escape a perpetrator. A teen with an intellectual disability may have difficulty recognizing or articulating that a boundary has been crossed, or understanding that the situation is not their fault. A youth who doesn't know proper names for private body parts may not be understood when he or she tries to report abuse. A teen who doesn't know about body rights and privacy may not recognize when a line has been crossed. A youth who requires physical assistance with self-care may be socialized to be compliant with adults touching his or her body. A lonely teen who experiences stigma, rejection, and lack of a peer support network may mistake exploitation for friendship.

Medical trauma may be another common source of trauma for youth with DDs. Many youth with DDs have experienced repeated medical intervention, including hospitalization or invasive procedures, from a very young age. These experiences can make a child or teen feel powerless, frightened, and confused, and can cause physical pain, and thus can be traumatic. Youth who experience medical trauma may develop symptoms of posttraumatic stress disorder (PTSD); this becomes more likely when there have been multiple episodes of traumatic stress (e.g., multiple surgeries). Prior exposure to trauma, such as from medical procedures, can increase the likelihood of developing mental health symptoms following a traumatic experience in adolescence or young adulthood.

Behavior in Context: Recognizing Trauma Symptoms in Youth With Developmental Disabilities

> After Ava changes schools, things get a little better. She doesn't have tantrums in the morning or cry anymore, but she doesn't seem like herself either. Her parents notice she still isn't sleeping very well, she almost never speaks, and she seems clingy, wanting to stay right next to them all the time, even when they're at home. They discuss their concerns with Ava's pediatrician, who recommends a therapist. Ava's parents are skeptical, wondering how a talk therapist could work with Ava when she barely talks, but they make an appointment to meet with her.

Just as in typically developing youth, the first sign of abuse or trauma in youth with DDs is often a change in behavior. Adults may not recognize that the behavior change is due to trauma because they assume it is related to the disability or part of adolescence. Emotional outbursts, anxiety, difficulty concentrating, problems with sleep, and insisting that things must be a certain way are all common responses to trauma for teens with and without disabilities. But in youth with DDs, these changes may be misattributed to their disability ("just part of the autism") or to the intersection between their disability and a biological process such as puberty. Teens with DDs can react to trauma in unique ways as well. Many teens with DDs who have been physically or sexually abused become preoccupied with violence or sexuality, or start to copy those behaviors, as a way of trying to come to terms with what happened to them. Another common response to stress is developmental regression, when someone "loses" developmental skills they previously had, such as by reverting to the use of "baby talk" or again having toileting accidents. Ava's decreased use of language and clinginess with her parents are examples of developmental regression.

In youth with DDs, as in typically developing youth, adults might see these changes as "behavioral" (meaning volitional) or as adolescent rebellion. This is even more the case if a teen's DD makes it harder for him or her to verbalize what happened so that adults don't recognize that trauma has occurred, or if the disability makes adults less likely to believe the teen. If adults see the changes as "behavioral" or volitional and respond with behavior-focused interventions, such as increased consequences, this can leave the youth feeling more helpless, inadequate, and ashamed and the adults feeling increasingly frustrated. Not only does the young person not receive appropriate support, but his or her self-image and relationship with caregivers can be negatively impacted by the failure of these well-intentioned but misdirected behavioral approaches.

It can be hard for any adolescents to talk about trauma they have experienced and articulate how it has affected them. Teens with communication difficulties or intellectual disabilities like Ava's struggle even more. Their attempts to express themselves are often misunderstood by adults. Teens generally struggle with identifying the link between their current emotions and prior trauma, and this can be even more challenging for a youth who has an intellectual disability. Youth with disabilities may not have had an opportunity to learn and practice a feelings vocabulary or may have been taught not to talk about unpleasant emotions or distress. Sometimes, play can be a useful communication tool when verbal expression is limited, but this requires that adults recognize that the play is communicating something real. Without ways to express distress, youth with DDs may develop physical symptoms as their bodies struggle with the chronic stress. These also may be misunderstood or misattributed by adults. Gastrointestinal symptoms like constipation, physical pain, changes in sleep or appetite, or weight changes are all common physical manifestations of stress that may be misunderstood by adults.

When teens with DDs are unable to talk about how trauma and painful experiences have affected them, adults may believe (or hope) that the teens are unaffected. They may believe that intellectual disability prevents the teens from "understanding" what happened, or that another aspect of their disability somehow makes them less impacted by painful experiences. For example, adults may believe that an autistic teen with social difficulties is not affected by the traumatic loss of a caregiver or parent because the teen doesn't have an intellectual understanding of death. Or they may surmise that sexual abuse is less harmful because the teen "doesn't understand" about sex and personal boundaries. The opposite is actually true, however: teens with DDs may be more likely to develop mental health symptoms following trauma. Navigating daily life with a disability can be difficult, and many teens carry an added burden of stress as a result. A youth who is isolated doesn't have the opportunity to get support from his or her peers when something traumatic happens. Stressed and isolated family members may not be able to be supportive. Adults may not know how to talk to a teen with DD about traumatic events such as the sudden illness or loss of a loved one, or may exclude the teen from hospital visits or funerals. Also, they may not know how to speak on the teen's level to reassure the youth that the abuse is over and the teen is now safe.

It was difficult for Ava's parents to know if the changes they saw in their daughter were from a behavioral problem, a psychiatric disorder, or trauma. Ava tried to let them know what the problem was, but her limited communication skills made it hard for her to explain. When she didn't get the help she needed, she wasn't able to try new strategies or to find other ways to cope with her pain. Because of the school's misunderstanding of her problem, Ava felt powerless, frightened, and hopeless. Even after her pediatrician intervened and encouraged her parents to change schools, no one communicated to Ava ideas like "we believe you," "we'll protect you," or "you're safe now" in a way that she could understand.

Treating More Than Just Behavior: Providing Support to Traumatized Youth With Developmental Disabilities

Youth with DDs who have experienced trauma or abuse need and deserve good treatment. Unfortunately, because mental health treatment traditionally has relied heavily on talking and abstract thinking, many people have believed that those with DDs cannot benefit from therapy. This is wrong. Trauma-Focused Cognitive Behavioral Therapy (TF-CBT) was developed for children and teens ages 3–21 years who are experiencing trauma symptoms. TF-CBT has been demonstrated to be effective in reducing symptoms associated with different types of trauma in the United States and other countries. It has been adapted for working with youth with DDs, including for working with youth with cognitive or language disabilities (see "Online Resources" at the end of this chapter). Specific TF-CBT interventions can be helpful for other common problems for children and youth with DDs, such as sensory sensitivity, impulsivity, and difficulty with problem solving, while also helping the youth cope with trauma symptoms. TF-CBT has eight "PRACTICE" modules to strengthen coping skills, provide gradual exposure to the trauma, and enhance safety skills. TF-CBT uses graduated exposure to reduce a child's anxiety related to the trauma and help the child process his or her experience. The therapist guides the child through the modules in sequence, but the model has flexibility to allow for them to be implemented in ways that will be most effective for an individual client.

- *Psychoeducation and parenting:* providing basic information about trauma and how trauma affects people, and introducing positive parenting strategies to manage children's behavioral symptoms (often a result of trauma) in a supportive way.

- *Relaxation:* using deep breathing and other relaxation strategies to manage the increased arousal that often results from trauma.

- *Affect Identification and regulation:* using a "feelings vocabulary" and ways to manage difficult feelings.

- *Cognitive coping:* identifying and challenging inaccurate or unhelpful beliefs that contribute to emotional distress.

- *Trauma narrative:* using exposure to traumatic material in order to reduce anxiety and process the experience.

- *In vivo mastery:* identifying trauma reminders and how to cope with them.

- *Conjoint parent-child sessions:* increasing caregiver-child communication by sharing the trauma narrative.

- *Enhancing safety and future development:* reducing the risk of future trauma and preparing for a healthy future.

Jennifer, the therapist, takes time to get to know Ava and her family, and she talks with them about how Ava's intellectual disability affects her everyday experiences. Jennifer tells them that she has known other youth with ID and trauma, and how therapy has helped those teens. Ava's mom asks about medicine, because a lot of parents in her online support group say their child takes medication for mental health reasons. Jennifer explains to Ava's family about trauma and how it affects people, and how it is treated. She suggests trying therapy for a little while before trying medicine, since therapy is the best treatment for trauma symptoms. Jennifer tells them she will meet for 45 minutes every week with Ava and her parents, and what to expect.

Over the next few sessions, Ava's parents notice that every session has the same schedule of "hello time, learning time, and goodbye time." Jennifer mostly talks to Ava, but she always give them ideas for how to help Ava practice what she is learning at home. She makes sure Ava understands that what happened to her at school is called "abuse" and that it wasn't okay. They talk about things like how abuse makes kids feel, and whose fault it is. Jennifer teaches Ava how to blow bubbles and gives her a bottle and wand to take home and practice. This helps Ava learn to take deep, calming breaths. She shows Ava faces with different feelings and teaches her the names for them: happy, sad, mad, and scared. Ava's parents practice with her between therapy sessions, and after a few weeks, Ava starts using those words at home. They talk a lot about private parts and touching rules, and Jennifer tells Ava how smart and brave she was to tell about the kid who touched her. Jennifer gives Ava a coloring book about "ok" and "not ok" touching, and she helps Ava to make a picture book about what had happened to her at the old school. Over the weeks of working with Jennifer, Ava's parents notice that Ava starts to seem a little happier at home, and one day they realize that she hasn't had a bad night in a while.

Ava's therapist uses many adaptations to make TF-CBT work for Ava. She uses visual prompts, like the feelings faces and coloring book, to demonstrate the material she is teaching. She includes Ava's parents in sessions and teaches them how to help Ava practice new skills at home. Jennifer holds shorter sessions, with a predictable structure (including hello time, learning time, and good-bye time), and spends more sessions on each module. She uses verbal and nonverbal strategies (e.g., making a picture book instead of developing a verbal trauma narrative) to help Ava process the trauma she experienced.

> Teens with DDs may need the mental health provider to present information differently than typically developing peers need.
>
> - Provide information in multiple sensory modalities, including both verbally and visually (using diagrams or charts), and encourage the teen to use multiple ways of expressing his or her thoughts and feelings.
>
> - Break information down into coherent chunks, present it at a slower pace, and plan for repeated exposures to new material, regardless of whether the intent is to teach content, build skills, or obtain information from the teen.
>
> - Check regularly for understanding by asking the youth to repeat back what was just said or to say it in a different way.
>
> - Give the teen opportunities to practice new skills across different settings, such as at home, at school, and in the community, to help him or her use those skills in the environments where they are most needed.

For Ava, as for so many youth with (and without) DDs who have experienced trauma, getting the right help was critical to her feeling better. Moving into a school environment that was safer for her helped but did not resolve Ava's distress. Even with her parents' support, she continued to demonstrate trauma symptoms. To heal, she needed the opportunity to engage in exposure therapy and process her trauma. Ava was lucky that her family found a treatment provider who understood how to work with a teen with intellectual disability. Too often, mental health providers think that symptoms are the beginning of a psychotic disorder, or that a youth with DD can't benefit from therapy. This can result in the teen being placed on antipsychotic medication or mood stabilizers, which carry significant side effects and are not the standard of care for trauma symptoms.

Including parents in treatment is key in TF-CBT. Youth with DDs often rely on family members for support, guidance, and physical care. Engaging family members can help the teens practice and reinforce what they are learning in therapy. Increasing social support for caregivers and other family members is equally important. An isolated, overwhelmed caregiver is less able to provide emotional and practical support to a youth experiencing trauma symptoms. A caregiver who feels responsible for the safety and well-being of a child with disabilities may be devastated to learn that the youth has been victimized. Vicarious trauma can lead to PTSD symptoms on the part of caregivers, compounded by feelings of sorrow and guilt for not protecting the teen from harm.

> After Ava makes a book about her experience, she and Jennifer and her parents read it together a few times. Ava's parents get to meet with Jennifer alone so they can talk with her about how upset they were to think about what had happened to their daughter. Ava's dad admits that he is worried that Ava will never be the same because of the abuse. Ava's mom shares that she feels that it was her fault for making Ava go to school when her daughter didn't want to. Although it is hard for them to talk about this, they find it useful to talk about it with Jennifer, who empathizes with, validates, and reassures them. It also helps them to reflect on how strong and brave Ava was to speak up, and how much she seems like her "old self" these days. Jennifer helps them tell Ava how proud they are of her. She teaches Ava more ways to stay safe and helps her practice what to do if someone tries to give her a "not okay" touch in the future. Ava really likes it when they practice saying "NO!" She laughs a lot and tells her parents, "I am brave." The family feels sad when they say good-bye to Jennifer after the last session, but they are proud to celebrate Ava's graduating from therapy.

One of the most important ways to support caregivers of a traumatized youth is to communicate respect and empathy.

- Caregivers may expect to be blamed for the harm their child has experienced, and it is important for professionals to reassure them. Take a strength-based approach that starts with identifying specific parenting strengths as a resource to help the teen and the family recover.

- Linking families to resources to address practical needs and to reduce social isolation can help reduce stress for caregivers.

- When a caregiver's emotional well-being is significantly impacted by distress about a child's difficulties, a referral to therapy for the caregiver may also be required.

Trauma and Teens With Physical Disabilities

Edward is a 17-year-old boy with Duchenne muscular dystrophy (DMD) who uses a power wheelchair. One night, when he is in bed with his breathing machine on, he hears yelling. Edward has difficulty getting out of bed on his own, but he struggles to get up as he hears his mother screaming. After a few minutes that feel like forever, he hears a crash and someone yelling, "Get down. Police!" The man from the apartment next door runs into Edward's room and tells him that he heard the screaming and called 911, and that Edward's father had broken into the apartment and attacked Edward's mother with a knife. The police arrest Edward's dad and rush his mom to the hospital. They take Edward to the hospital too, to get him checked out. Edward has to talk to the police about what had happened, then tell the story again to a social worker who shows up. The cops are cool, but the social worker talks to him like he is a little kid. Plus, Edward has to tell the social worker how to help him get back into his wheelchair from his bed, which is embarrassing. Because Edward doesn't have any other family nearby, the social worker has to find a place for him to stay. He hears the social worker griping about finding a placement for a "crippled kid." Edward isn't surprised that no one wants to be around a freak like him. He feels so worthless. He hates needing help. He knows it was his fault his parents split up, because he heard all the fights about how hard it was to take care of him. And he had known his dad had started drinking again but hadn't told anyone. He feels like he should have been the one who got stabbed, and he is so mad that he hadn't done anything to help his mom.

At the hospital, Edward asks what's happening to his mom, but the social worker just says "don't worry" in a way that makes Edward feel stupid. Edward has to wait all night and most of the next day before finding out he has to go to a group home because there are no foster families that would take him. The group home turns out to be kind of weird. There are other kids there who use wheelchairs and braces and stuff. The staff there talk to Edward like he deserves respect. They act more interested in his sense of humor and his love of Star Wars than his physical limitations. Even though they seem to be accustomed to helping kids like him, Edward is still careful not to ask for help. He won't talk about what happened either, because he is ashamed that they might find out the truth about how he let his mom get hurt.

Edward's daily functioning is significantly impacted by his DMD. He uses a wheelchair, has to have treatments at home daily, and has a number of ongoing medical appointments. As a result of his illness, Edward had already experienced a great deal of hardship in his life, even before his parents' separation and then this acute trauma. Edward's disability also changes his experience of trauma. He was unable to help his mother or to try to stop his father from hurting her. The first responders he encountered didn't understand his medical needs, and his social worker's prejudice against Edward because of his disability impacted Edward psychologically and practically.

In other ways, Edward's response to acute trauma—his drive to be independent, his unrealistic expectation that he should protect his mother, and his hesitance to open up to others due to shame and fear of embarrassment—is typical of normal adolescent development.

> Edward's mom ends up needing surgery, but no one tells Edward what is happening because they think he can't handle it, emotionally and cognitively. Eventually his mom gets out of the hospital, and after a few months of rehabilitation she and Edward get to go home. Edward is so glad to get out of the group home and be with his mom again. Edward's dad goes to jail. Even though he knows his father can't come back again, Edward has trouble sleeping and keeps his phone right by his pillow. He feels jumpy all night and all day. He can't concentrate at school, and his grades have fallen. Whenever he hears loud voices, memories of his mom screaming pop back into his head and bring back those feelings of helplessness and shame that he couldn't do anything to help her. It makes him so mad, and a bunch of times he gets in trouble for yelling at kids or teachers at school. Edward doesn't tell anyone at school what happened; he just can't stand the thought of talking about it. He knows it would upset his mom too much if he said anything to her about what he's thinking and feeling. He just keeps to himself more and tries to make it through another day without thinking about it.

Edward's emotional response to the trauma is no different from that of any other teen. He doesn't want to think or talk about what happened, he worries about his mother's response to reminders, and he feels responsible for not stopping his father. But adults keep seeing him through the lens of his physical disability, and in seeing him as a "disabled kid," they miss opportunities to explain his mother's condition, help him process what happened, or try to understand his thoughts and emotions.

Providers should try to see teens as more than just their diagnosis or their disability. One way to demonstrate this awareness is through person-first language (e.g., saying "a youth with disabilities" rather than "a disabled youth").

- Talk directly to teens, rather than talking to the adults who accompany them.

- Do not assume that youth with physical disabilities have intellectual impairments. Give the youth information about what to expect, or about why you are working with them. Giving teens choices demonstrates respect for their independence and competence.

Prevention: Reducing the Risk of Victimization for Youth With Developmental or Physical Disabilities

Although there are many reasons why youth with developmental or physical disabilities face increased risk of trauma, providing youth and caregivers with information and skills can reduce this risk. One program that does this is Making Friends and Staying Safe (MFSS), which has been offered for over 10 years to children, youth, and their caregivers through Children's Hospital Los Angeles. In MFSS, a group of youth meets weekly for a psychoeducational and skill building program. For many of the teens, participating in MFSS is the first time in their lives they have had a group in which they felt like they belonged, the others liked them, and they had friends.

> Andres, a 13-year-old middle school student with autism spectrum disorder, starts going to a program on Tuesday evenings with his mom. Andres and six other kids his age meet together with group leaders Caitlin and Laura, while his mom goes to another room with the rest of the adults. Andres isn't sure about the program at first, but after a few weeks, he starts really liking it. The other kids seem happy to see him when he gets there. He finds out a couple of the other boys like the same video game that he does, and one of the girls is really pretty. They are learning about interesting stuff, too: feelings, and who likes which sports, but also about private parts and how boys' and girls' bodies change when they became teenagers. Andres is really interested in biology, and nobody acts like he's weird when he explains what he has learned about hormones and puberty. Plus, at home his mom tells him she is learning about some of those same things in her group. She tells him she wants him to understand about bodies changing and sex and all of that kind of stuff, and she thinks it's normal for him to be curious and have different feelings about it. Andres is relieved that his mom isn't mad and that the things he is feeling and thinking are normal. He thinks it's really great to have friends who aren't mean to him and don't call him weird. He thinks about that a lot on the Tuesday when a kid at school punches him about a million times in the ribs. He decides that wasn't okay, and when he gets to the program he tells his friends and the group leaders what had happened and they help him to tell his mom too.

MFSS covers four main topic areas, based on individual risk factors for abuse: social skills, body rights and privacy, age-appropriate sexual education, and risk reduction skills. Basic social skills include identifying and expressing feelings, self-esteem and identity development, how to tell if someone is your friend, and how to make new friends. Like Andres, teens who know the difference between friends and "frenemies" and who can identify and express their feelings are better able to disclose mistreatment and are less vulnerable to exploitation.

> Even though he knows a lot about biology, sexual reproduction, and the medical names for most body parts, Andres has never heard his mom say "penis" or "vagina" and he's pretty sure those are bad words you're not supposed to say. He feels a little nervous when they talk about it in group, even though Caitlin and Laura said everybody's parents knew they were going to be saying it, and wanted them to practice. But later that week, his mom talks to him about how it is okay to use those words if you need to, and they even practice saying them!

Youth with disabilities may not have access to the same age-appropriate information about sexual development as their typically developing peers. Family members' natural reticence to discuss sexual matters openly, coupled with a view of these teens as more childlike than their chronological age, can make it difficult for caregivers to bridge the gap. Youth who are comfortable using "doctor names" for private body parts can disclose sexual abuse in a way that adults are more likely to understand and respond to. If a teen does not learn about sexual development from a trustworthy source, he or she may seek this information in ways that increase risk, including from online sources or from others who will take advantage of them. Understanding private parts and learning to differentiate "okay" versus "not okay" touch can be especially important for youth who are accustomed to intimate physical care due to their disability.

Abuse resistance skills include learning what people should do if someone tries to abuse them: say "no," get away if possible, tell a "helper," and keep telling until somebody helps. In MFSS, this is shortened to make it easy to memorize: "no, go, tell." Participants practice saying "NO" assertively and identifying multiple specific helpers they know. This is important because the first person a child tells may not respond in a protective way. Teens may also learn basic self-defense skills, which will increase their ability to "go" or get away from a perpetrator.

The MFSS content can alternatively be provided to teens and caregivers in an individual setting. One-on-one sessions can be helpful when a teen or caregiver is especially anxious about the content, or if the youth is struggling with the impact of previous sexual abuse. Private sessions also allow for individualized pacing of the material to fit the specific learning needs of both teen and caregiver.

> Carmen, Andres's mom, is used to taking care of her son by herself. Andres's father left when Andres was first diagnosed with autism spectrum

disorder. Her family thinks the teen's problem is that she "spoiled him" and they no longer invite Carmen and Andres to family events because Andres makes them "uncomfortable." When Carmen learned that a boy had beaten Andres up at school, she didn't want to believe it. The other parents in the group really helped her. Nobody asked "What did Andres do this time?" or implied that it was Andres's fault that it happened, like Carmen's family usually did. After talking with the other parents and the group leaders, Carmen decides to go to Andres's school the next day to report what had happened and make sure they keep Andres safe. When she gets there, they tell her the principal is busy and can't talk to her. Before, Carmen would have felt helpless and afraid to make the school mad. But this time, with the support of the group in her mind, she decides to wait for the principal. She would wait all day if she had to. Before long, the principal comes to talk to her and assures her that the school will keep Andres safe. Carmen knows from her friends at the group that she will have to keep speaking up and watching out for Andres, but she feels proud of herself for making a start.

Caregivers are an important component of MFSS, and the curriculum for the caregivers' group is designed to address some of the family risk factors for a teen's maltreatment. There are unique benefits to offering this program in a group format to a population that often experiences rejection and social isolation. Caregivers have the opportunity to learn from each other and, like Carmen, can feel more confident and stronger with the support of other group members. Many caregivers report that nobody has ever explained their child's disability to them and they are not sure what to expect as their child moves through adolescence. They often feel frightened to think about these children reaching adulthood and worry whether their children will be able to live independently, marry, or become parents themselves. One of the first topics for the caregivers' group is helping the parents to understand their children's disability diagnosis and talk with each other about their hopes and fears.

To increase family communication about sensitive topics, the caregivers learn the same material as the teens, as well as ways they can support their children's practice at home. Group leaders take care to explain why the sexual information is important for the youth, and invite the caregivers to talk about the values they want to teach their teens about sexual behavior and relationships. Often, families' cultural values are an important part of this discussion. In addition, caregivers learn specific parenting strategies to support their children through puberty.

The caregivers' group provides a valuable peer support network, as Andres's mother experienced. Getting to know other parents who understand what it's like to care for a child with DDs reduces the isolation many families experience. Parents learn from one another and develop skills to navigate the service systems their children need. Finally, the discomfort of talking with their own children about sexual matters can be greatly reduced when they have an opportunity to review and practice with other parents facing the same challenges.

Carmen was able to be a good advocate for her son when he faced abuse in school. Advocacy is often an essential component of helping a youth with disabilities and their caregivers recover from trauma. The common misconceptions about teens with disabilities, underrecognition of the relationship between trauma and symptoms, and systemic barriers such as a lack of integration between mental health and DD service systems can all present substantial challenges to addressing the needs of traumatized youth with DDs. Individualized advocacy can involve providing information to professionals about trauma and DDs to increase understanding of a teen's needs. By attending service planning meetings such as Individualized Education Plan (IEP) meetings along with caregivers, providers can facilitate trauma-informed plans being implemented. Families may need to link with local advocacy (e.g., disability rights) organizations. Often, families need more than a phone number to call for help; providers can place the call while meeting with the family, give additional information to the advocate about the youth's needs, or join in the meetings between the advocacy organization and the family.

A teen and family who are worried about basic survival will have more difficulty engaging in treatment. Link them to support and advocacy services to address crucial barriers that families face. Consider the need for the following:

- Educational advocacy

- Disability rights advocacy

- Victim's rights or victim/witness programs

- Access to benefits such as Supplemental Security Income (SSI)

- Housing, food, and medical resources

Youth with disabilities, who face increased risk of trauma relative to typically developing peers, deserve to have access to treatment services and supports to help them recover from trauma. Caring for youth with DDs is not a specialized area for which only a select few are prepared. All providers with skill in working with youth are well prepared to meet the needs of trauma-exposed teens with DDs. By tailoring interventions to an individualized understanding of a child's developmental level, learning style, and preferences, providers can address trauma for all teens in need of support.

Resources and Additional Reading

Online Resources

Trauma-Focused Therapy for Youth With Developmental Disabilities

National Child Traumatic Stress Network: Facts on traumatic stress and children with developmental disabilities. Available at: http://www.nctsn.org/sites/default/files/assets/pdfs/traumatic_stress_developmental_disabilities_final.pdf. Accessed March 4, 2018.

National Child Traumatic Stress Network: The road to recovery: supporting children with intellectual and developmental disabilities who have experienced trauma. Available at: https://www.nctsn.org/resources/road-recovery-supporting-children-intellectual-and-developmental-disabilities-who-have. Accessed July 2, 2018.

Advocacy

ACLU Disability Rights: https://www.aclu.org/issues/disability-rights#current
National Disability Rights Network: http://ndrn.org/index.php

Parents of Children With Developmental Disabilities

Center for Parent Information and Resources (also information on sex education and developmental disabilities): http://www.parentcenterhub.org/#

Additional Reading

Brown LK, Brown M: What's the Big Secret? Talking About Sex With Girls and Boys. Boston, MA, Little, Brown, 1997

Grosso CA: Children with developmental disabilities, in Trauma-Focused CBT for Children and Adolescents: Treatment Applications. Edited by Cohen JA, Mannarino AP, Deblinger E. New York, Guilford, 2012, pp 149–174

Holmes MM, Mudlaff SJ, Pillo C: A Terrible Thing Happened. Washington, DC, Dalmatian Press, 2000 (useful in psychoeducation about trauma and trauma reactions)

McIntyre LL: Promoting well-being in families with children with intellectual and developmental disabilities. Available at: http://www.apa.org/pi/disability/resources/publications/newsletter/2016/09/family-developmental-disabilities.aspx. Accessed March 4, 2018.

References

1. Boyle CA, Boulet S, Schieve LA, et al: Trends in the prevalence of developmental disabilities in U.S. children, 1997–2008. Pediatrics 127(6):1034–1042, 2011 21606152
2. Crosse SB, Kaye E, Ratnofsky AC: A Report on the Maltreatment of Children With Disabilities (Contract No 105-89-1630). Washington, DC, National Center on Child Abuse and Neglect, 1993

PART 2

Working With Systems and Traumatic Stress

CHAPTER 10
Acute Psychiatric Services

Schuyler W. Henderson, M.D., M.P.H.

Blake Phillips, M.D.

Fifteen-year-old Taylor is hospitalized following a Tylenol overdose that fortunately spares her liver serious damage. This is not her first suicide attempt; nor is it her second or third. An honors student through middle school and a perfectionist to her core, Taylor has spent the past 2 years battling a profound and persistent sadness. Her feelings of worthlessness, hopelessness, and shame and her recurrent suicidal thoughts seem unshakeable despite the best efforts of her caring family and a rotating cast of social workers, psychologists, and psychiatrists.

Taylor had been a bright, cheerful A student throughout grade school. She spent her days playing soccer with friends; painting her nails with her mom; roughhousing with her adoring younger brothers, Timothy and Thomas; listening to old Beatles records with her dad; and writing and sketching in the yard. She lived in a safe neighborhood and went to a well-regarded public school.

As middle school started, Taylor had her typical teenage moments, rolling her eyes at her parents and taking too long in the shower. But in the middle of eighth grade, after she broke up with her first boyfriend, everything seemed to change. Taylor's parents had been hesitant to let Taylor date, but her first "puppy love" was with a sweet boy from down the street, whose parents they knew well. Taylor had nursed a crush on the boy forever, so her parents were surprised when, after only a few months of dating, she abruptly announced that she didn't want to see him anymore. They were even more surprised when she started withdrawing from friends and seemed anxious and irritable around family friends and neighbors. She no longer wanted to roughhouse with her younger brothers, shrieking if they surprised her from behind or barged into her room without knocking. She stopped playing soc-

cer and sketching, and only wanted to listen to the music on her headphones, never the oldies on her dad's record player. But she continued to be
a stellar student, so her parents told themselves it must just be adolescent
moodiness. Besides, whenever they asked, Taylor vehemently denied that
anything was wrong. Taylor had always been close with her parents and open
with them whenever she had problems, so they believed her when she said
"everything's fine." Imagine their shock, then, when she attempted suicide
for the first time. On a crisp September day during Taylor's freshman year
of high school, Taylor's mother came home to find a note on the kitchen
counter that read, "I love you all so much, but I'm sorry, I just can't do it anymore." She tore around the house before finding Taylor lying unconscious in
a pool of blood on the bathroom floor, arms covered in cuts. Nine-year-old
Timothy called 911 because his mother couldn't speak, while 11-year-old
Thomas ran to get a neighbor. Taylor's mother rode with Taylor in the ambulance to the hospital that first time, clutching Taylor's hand, holding on
for dear life.

Teens are brought into emergency departments (EDs), inpatient psychiatric units, crisis stabilization units, and other acute psychiatric treatment programs for treatment of a variety of symptoms and behaviors, such
as aggression, school refusal, running away from home, mood dysregulation, suicidal thoughts, self-injury and suicide attempts, psychosis, and
risky behaviors. The adults bringing them for evaluation, and often even
the teens themselves, typically lack any awareness of the role that recent or
distant trauma might play in the teens' current behavior or symptoms. The
clinical staff in acute psychiatric treatment settings should know better, because studies have shown between 46% and 96% of youth on inpatient psychiatric units have experienced trauma, with 21%–29% meeting full criteria
for posttraumatic stress disorder (PTSD).[1] Many clinicians, however, are
unaware of how common and how devastating childhood trauma can be for
teens. Clinicians in EDs and inpatient units are also in a difficult position,
expected to make a rapid diagnosis and treatment plan with little time and
often little concrete information. Many clinicians look narrowly for PTSD
but forget that in children and teens, PTSD can look and sound like so many
other disorders and that many mental health issues can stem from trauma.
Until proven otherwise, trauma should be assumed to be part of the story
for every teen presenting to the ED or inpatient unit. This is even true for
teens like Taylor, who come from a "good" home and a "good" community
and may not seem to be at risk. Understanding this role of trauma in youth
presenting for acute psychiatric treatment is critical because it ensures that
the care provided is therapeutic and that treatment is effective rather than
retraumatizing.

Trauma needs to be a consideration in the assessment of any adolescent brought into an acute psychiatric care setting. This question needs to be considered: Is this behavior, which has reached such an extreme that this teen has been brought in for an emergent psychiatric evaluation or hospitalization, related to recent or past trauma? A traumatic event, however distant, can have long-standing psychological and developmental repercussions that affect multiple domains of a child's life. These include social functioning, such as engaging in bullying or being bullied, friendships, dating, sexuality, and conflicts with family and authority figures; academic performance, such as issues with focus in the classroom or responses to a teacher; and psychological well-being, including mood regulation and self-esteem.

After Taylor is medically stabilized following the Tylenol overdose that is her fourth suicide attempt, she is scheduled for transfer to an inpatient psychiatric unit. Seeing her name on the planned admissions board, many of the hospital staff roll their eyes. During the previous three hospitalizations, they experienced a different Taylor than the one her parents know. The Taylor the hospital has seen is an angry, jaded, willful, and defiant teen who is confrontational and disrespectful, a "troublemaker." Taylor's first three hospitalizations followed a typical pattern. She would be willful and irritable with nursing staff and guarded with the clinical team. She engaged only superficially when asked about her own symptoms and history, seeming bored or overintellectualizing in a way that frustrated the clinicians. But her passion would flare when she advocated for her peers, especially those too lost in the storm of their own emotional turmoil to speak up for themselves. Her righteous, accusatory tone irritated the staff. Labels like "borderline traits" were added to her long list of diagnoses and problems. Now some hospital staff have even started suggesting that Taylor keeps returning to the hospital because she wants attention, noting how comfortable she always seems on the inpatient unit.

Over the course of her past three hospitalizations, Taylor has become more aware of the team's frustration with her. Well-intentioned comments from staff make her feel invalidated and rejected. "You know what, Taylor, you really gotta cut it out with this stuff. Nobody's impressed. Besides, you can't spend your whole life in the hospitals; you're better than that," one of Taylor's favorite nurses said last time she was admitted. This and other similar comments made Taylor feel like the staff didn't want her there. The first time she felt this way, Taylor tried to relieve her distress by cutting herself with a broken plastic fork. The unit staff demanded that she relinquish the "contraband." When she refused, they physically held her to take away the fork. Being touched in this way set something off in her, and she began screaming and biting until multiple male staff carried her across the length of the unit, arms and legs flailing, to restrain her on her bed. This made her feel even angrier, and some other feeling she couldn't really name, a desperate sensation of being out of control and outside her own body. After that, when the feelings of rejection and invalidation would build, she would simply announce that she was better, would promise not to hurt herself, and be discharged back to the same problems. Shortly thereafter, the cycle would begin again, sometimes only weeks later, with Taylor getting rehospitalized after another suicide attempt.

The first goal of acute psychiatric treatment programs is to *provide a safe environment for youth*. This usually means close observation with around-the-clock nursing care and doctors available for urgent issues. But ensuring a safe environment must also include consideration of trauma, because the ED or hospital setting, and even certain aspects of treatment, may be triggering or even traumatizing.[2] The key is to adopt "universal trauma precautions": assume that trauma may be playing a role for every patient *and* be watchful for ways that the hospital setting and treatment itself may be triggering or retraumatizing.

The second goal of an acute care setting is to *diagnose the child correctly*. Many times, diagnoses are seen only as stigmatizing labels. But an accurate and appropriate diagnosis is actually crucially important: it guides treatment planning and informs prognosis, both of which are essential before embarking on any intervention. Why is this so important? *Because a diagnosis is what justifies treatment.* The fact that a diagnosis comes with a prognosis enables us to predict what may happen if the adolescent is not provided with evidence-based treatment. It can also inform what treatment can and cannot do, in terms of improving the long-term course of illness associated with the diagnosis. Before you decide on any treatments, having an understanding of the natural course of illness, and of the predictable outcome of any diagnosis, will guide how you use (or decide not to use) the treatments available. All treatment, including the decision not to provide treatment, comes with a risk: from cost and time to side effects, both physical and emotional. Judging the risks and benefits of an intervention depends primarily on the prognosis, and accurate diagnosis is therefore essential. For example, most of us know that if we get a splinter, we need to take it out. A simple pair of tweezers, some rubbing alcohol, and a bandage are typically all we need to take care of the problem. In more formal terms, we could say that a splinter stuck in a youth's middle finger (diagnosis: "foreign body embedded in third digit") causes pain and could get infected (prognosis: pain and infection requiring intravenous antibiotics), and therefore the usual first-line treatment of splinter removal with tweezers is a justified and appropriate course of action to prevent a poor outcome. Notice here, though, that a more drastic initial intervention, such as amputation, would also prevent a bad outcome and a poor prognosis but wouldn't be our first-choice treatment. Nor would we pick a treatment, such as 10 mg of intramuscular olanzapine, that is unrelated to the problem at hand.

This metaphor can be sustained for a moment longer. After trauma, adolescents often thrust out their middle fingers, and the adults around them think the kids are flipping them the bird. The adults yell at the teens, suspend them from school, and maybe threaten to cut off their fingers. But these kids are giving adults the finger in the hope that one adult will see the giant splinter and do something about it. The misdiagnosis of why the adolescents are holding up their middle fingers leads to the wrong intervention, which does not work to help the real underlying problem in the first place. The prognosis worsens and the cycle continues until the youth ends up in an emergency room somewhere needing an amputation—in the case of trauma, the amputation is the psychiatric admission that separates them from their family, school, and community.

Just as amputating a splintered finger can solve a problem but cause long-term consequences, psychiatric hospitalizations without correct diagnoses can create as many problems as they solve. A psychiatric hospitalization might help with an acute problem (preventing suicide, in Taylor's case), but if the teen is misdiagnosed, there can be negative, long-lasting ill effects (e.g., repeat ER visits with persistent suicidality, as in Taylor's case, or disruptions in school, family, and peer relationships, and in self-concept). Taylor was metaphorically extending her middle finger to the adults around her, thinking the message was clear: *Help me. Someone has hurt me. Don't you see?* But during her multiple hospitalizations, Taylor's history of trauma was never elicited. Trauma was never conceptualized as a core problem, and certainly not as the main underlying problem. Also, Taylor's resiliency factors, strengths, and her family's and community's resources were never factored into her treatment planning. This oversight happens for a multitude of reasons—lack of awareness, short length of stay, insurance reimbursement issues, staff shortages and burnout, lack of resources, and other barriers to holistic treatment planning—but the consequence is ineffective care.

> Following her fourth suicide attempt, Taylor's pattern in the ED appears set to repeat. Having received an EMS report of a Tylenol overdose, the initial ED team caring for Taylor quickly pegs her as needing "medical clear-

ance for psychiatric admission." She has an extensive medical record at this hospital, so they focus on medical stabilization, without asking her or her mother about recent or prior psychosocial stressors or any psychosocial history. Taylor is placed on direct observation by hospital police in the part of the ED that houses the other psychiatric patients. Today that includes an older woman screaming about being mistreated by the staff, a middle-aged homeless man sleeping off an alcohol binge, and an angry-looking young man handcuffed to a stretcher awaiting "psychiatric clearance" for court. The first time Taylor came to the hospital, she was disturbed by the behaviors she saw from the psychotic or intoxicated patients in the ED. Now she has gotten so used to such behaviors that they no longer affect her. She is more upset seeing family members sobbing after a deadly car accident, a dazed-looking assault victim brought in by police with one eye already swelling shut, or EMS wheeling in a child barely breathing, with a terrified mother in tow. Taylor's mother sits next to her. She watches the other patients in silent terror that one day it will be Taylor not breathing or Taylor restrained to a gurney, screaming her lungs out.

After Taylor is medically cleared, she remains in the ED for 2 days, watching the other patients come and go, until a bed opens up at a psychiatric hospital. At this second hospital, Taylor encounters a second ED team. Having received transfer documentation from the initial ED, this team focuses on fast-tracking her admission. The clinicians assume that Taylor knows they are rushing to avoid having Taylor sit endlessly in another ED, but they don't say that to her, and she assumes they just want to get rid of her. She senses that all of these adults view her as no more than another suicide attempt.

When she finally arrives on the inpatient unit late in the evening, staff have been expecting her. While a few who know her from her last hospitalization tsk-tsk to themselves when they see her back, the on-call resident is new to her and tries to engage her. But Taylor remains guarded and terse, and her one-word answers are frankly a relief to this tired doctor on her twenty-first hour of work.

The next morning, now 4 days after the overdose, Taylor is approached by a social worker to complete additional assessments. The social worker greets Taylor briefly before proceeding to read a series of questions off various forms. The social worker is frustrated by these forms, which she experiences as required regulatory busywork, but she has to go through them, and when she tries to engage Taylor after they're done, she gets little more than a nod. With no real rapport with this new social worker and an overall lack of trust, Taylor avoids any meaningful discussion of her suicide attempt.

As Taylor settles into the unit, she resumes her usual bravado. She flaunts an encyclopedic knowledge of DSM diagnostic criteria and a laundry list of coping skills at her disposal, but quickly shifts to irritability and anger any time her competent persona is questioned. If she can't keep others at a distance by providing the answers they want to hear, she uses defiance and anger to drive them away.

Asking Why: Understanding How Trauma Can Underlie Problematic Behaviors

Although acute psychiatric services such as EDs and hospitals provide a safe environment, if such services are not trauma informed, they may not feel truly safe to youth who have experienced trauma. Part of "universal trauma precautions" is recognizing how the environment can be simultaneously safe and triggering to traumatized youth. The frightening environment of the ER, the physical intrusions by multiple strangers doing exams and blood draws, the noise, the lack of privacy, the separation from family, the loss of control, and the sight of others being physically restrained (or being physically restrained oneself) on the inpatient unit are just a few of the ways that acute psychiatric care settings can be triggering. A staff member's loud voice or even a caring hand on the teen's shoulder can trigger memories of abuse. Seeing a bruised patient in the ED or hearing an agitated peer screaming on the inpatient unit might remind a teen of domestic violence.

The structure of EDs and inpatient psychiatric units—the close supervision, sometimes rigid routines, and restrictions on freedom—can often be triggering for teens who have experienced trauma. The terror of traumatic experiences often involves a loss of control, and the structure of an inpatient psychiatric unit also involves significant loss of control for an adolescent. This structure is key to these settings keeping youth safe, and for many traumatized teens in acute distress, it is the only thing that can keep them safe; however, the structure can also be difficult for teens like Taylor, leading to conflicts and misunderstandings with staff. Despite the importance of consistency and predictability in inpatient psychiatric units, every adolescent has unique needs. Both the adolescents and the adults working with them in acute care settings need to adapt to a dynamic between rigidity and flexibility. This is very hard in a situation where structures are formal and codified by regulations; where it is not clear whether the adolescent requires more consistency or more flexibility; and where a multitude of diverse, often atypical needs must be met simultaneously, with kids who are dysregulated and staff who are typically undersupported, undertrained, underrespected, and underpaid. When youth are traumatized but staff either don't know it or don't understand how trauma impacts symptoms and behaviors, it's harder for everyone to know what kind of approach—consistency or flexibility, consequences or accommodation—will be therapeutic.

Professionals working in acute care settings should consider how, when, and why particular teens may be struggling with the environment, and how trauma might be part of their story. Recognizing that the environment may be triggering is the first step. When the adolescent has a history of trauma, talk openly with the teen about how that trauma may influence his or her response to the environment. Consider both what the teen can do (practice communication or coping skills, avoid triggering peers, etc.) to adapt to the structure and how the structure needs to be adapted to the teen. Explain to the teen the rationale for the rules and the expectations, and discuss in advance what the teen's needs are and how they may conflict with the rules and expectations. Staff should work as a team to decide how to use the environment most effectively for the struggling teen. Some youth will need explicit changes to the environment, including the physical surroundings, structure and routine of the unit, and/or usual therapeutic approaches. Others will need to be taught, in a validating and graduated way, to cope with triggers.

Trauma, and complex trauma in particular, can result in behaviors that conflict with the structure in acute care settings. If the trauma and its effects are not recognized, these behaviors can be misinterpreted. Imagine an adolescent identified as an "elopement risk" because he makes a wild dash to the exit, shoving staff and peers out of the way to escape every time the door is unlocked. This behavior could be perceived as oppositional, aggressive, or even sociopathic, but maybe this teen is using a survival skill developed when his stepfather would beat him and lock him in the closet. A child who refuses to change into hospital pajamas may not be doing so to be difficult; maybe being commanded to undress by an adult triggers memories of sexual abuse. An adolescent who seems to hate a certain type of staff (e.g., security officers) may unconsciously be reminded of someone who hurt her in the past (e.g., the police who arrested her father and then took her away from her family). Lashing out, cursing, and resisting staff instructions are all seemingly "bad" behaviors that may stem directly from trauma, or may be survival behaviors that were highly adaptive in previously traumatic situations.

When adults don't recognize the role of trauma, these "bad" behaviors can lead to negative feelings about the youth, misdiagnosis, and potentially inappropriate treatment decisions. Adults working with traumatized youth in acute care settings need to discuss these responses to "bad" behaviors explicitly, because survival coping behaviors can be tremendously wearing on staff and morale. It is not at all uncommon for a staff member to develop a good relationship with a teen, but then the youth lashes out at this trusted confidant. The staff member feels hurt, angry, or confused and withdraws from the patient. This reaction inadvertently creates a repetition of the adolescent's trauma or reinforces the teen's expectation that all adults will eventually let him or her down. This is one of the most underreported causes of burnout in the mental health field: the feeling that we give so much to kids who eventually act out and reject us. This is dispiriting to staff members and contributes to a form of sympathy burnout for traumatized children. At its worst, it leads to a hostile environment where adolescents are in fact in danger. Providing staff with education, support, and relief is essential to help prevent them from becoming overwhelmed by this dynamic. We can be hurt or annoyed by a teen's behavior, but if we understand the behavior and where it comes from, and are given the space (emotional and physical) to step back and reflect, we can continue to be empathic, therapeutic, and caring.

Behaviors in Context: Understanding and Connecting With Traumatized Youth in the Hospital

We know that youth presenting to acute psychiatric care settings have high rates of trauma exposure and PTSD. How do we improve our capacity to recognize and diagnose these teens the first time around?

> Karina, a psychology intern on Taylor's treatment team, finds Taylor's bravado endearing—it reminds Karina of her younger sister. But Karina can't understand why Taylor, who seems so tough and smart and so able to speak up for others, can't find a way to "survive" outside the hospital. Karina asks to be Taylor's primary clinician. Her supervisor warns that Taylor's "borderline character structure" will make treatment difficult, but Karina persists. Karina tries to talk to Taylor about her suicide attempts, her relationships outside the hospital, and the conflicts she has with unit staff. She smiles fondly at Taylor's swagger but challenges Taylor to think about her own conflicting patterns of behavior. This often causes Taylor to curse at Karina, threaten to kill herself, or storm off, but by persisting through these moments of willfulness, Karina gradually earns Taylor's trust by instilling a sense of constancy. Karina just keeps coming back day after day to meet with Taylor no matter how hard Taylor tries to shake her. Karina empathizes with Taylor's desire to appear well, her frustration with others seeing her as "crazy," and her simultaneous and seemingly contradictory frustration with others thinking she is "fine."

After several meetings with Karina, Taylor reveals her most painful memory, a traumatic event that she has vehemently denied many times before. At age 13, she was raped by her first boyfriend. Taylor speaks of how lucky she felt that the boy she had "liked" for so long was finally interested in her, how exhilarating it felt to kiss him for the first time, how she thought it was okay when he put his hand up her shirt, but how not okay it felt when he started unzipping her jeans. Taylor remains expressionless while she notes how surprised she felt when the kissing became painful and how confusing it was when the exhilaration faded and panic crept in. Karina's heart breaks for Taylor when after a long pause, Taylor whispers her deepest, darkest secret: "I know I said 'wait,' but I honestly don't know if I ever told him to stop."

The assessment of trauma starts not with a series of questions but with the overall approach to the adolescent. The phrase *universal precautions* in medicine means that doctors and nurses assume that all patients might have an infection and take certain steps with every patient, such as handwashing and wearing gloves, to prevent the spread of disease. Similarly, *universal trauma precautions* means assuming that the teen in front of us could be a trauma survivor and always taking basic steps, equivalent to handwashing, to help teens to feel safe. There are four components to this: 1) developing rapport with clear and consistent boundaries, 2) explaining privacy and confidentiality, 3) systematically and repeatedly assessing trauma in a sympathetic way, and 4) recognizing that our understanding of every child changes as trust develops and we get more information. The principles of universal trauma precautions hold true during every encounter.

A trauma-informed approach creates a safe milieu, but this approach may not be enough to ensure that each teen's trauma history is recognized and that trauma's impact on current symptoms is understood. Standardized screening for trauma ensures that every child is assessed.[1,3] Trauma screening provides an additional opportunity for and a different approach to asking tough questions about trauma, which may elicit responses that would not have come up during a clinical interview. Screening also reminds providers to take a trauma-informed perspective, which is especially important when a teen's difficult behaviors are dangerous or emotionally triggering for staff.

The use of standardized screening instruments alone is not sufficient to assess for and understand trauma. As demonstrated in Taylor's case, it was not a screening instrument that rooted out her history of rape and sexual abuse. Rather, it was a trusting relationship in an environment of physical and psychological safety that allowed Taylor to feel comfortable sharing her history. Screening is an important, systematized part of evaluations, but it is only one part of a complex, ongoing assessment. A negative or positive finding on a scale is not the final word on diagnosis. In fact, repeated screening may be helpful in drawing out a trauma history, especially in youth with multiple ED presentations or hospitalizations. Teens will sometimes say "no" on screening several times before, like Taylor, they feel comfortable enough to share their most painful, shameful history. Other teens may endorse one trauma in response to screening, when other more "severe" traumas remain unspoken, either because the latter do not feel as pressing to the teen or because they are too difficult to talk about yet.

In addition to formal screening, careful assessment requires collaboration with family and other caregivers, as well as previous providers, including mental health and medical professionals, and any other important, supportive adults in a teen's life—from teachers and school counselors to coaches and work supervisors. Collaboration means getting input and information from these other adults, and also working with them to ensure the teen has the right supports upon return to the home environment. Teens are often resistant to disclosing traumatic experiences to adults in their lives, especially parents. They often worry that their parents will get upset or angry, and sometimes they are right. But for that reason, the safe, supported environment of an inpatient unit is often the best place to make a disclosure of trauma. Helping teens think through how to talk to family or other key adults, and supporting them in doing so, can ensure that when they return home the teens have someone who knows the full picture and can help them when symptoms inevitably flare.

Treating More Than Just Behavior: Trauma-Focused Treatment in Acute Care Settings

Sharing her trauma history with Karina and experiencing Karina's empathy and acceptance prove cathartic for Taylor. She begins to talk more with Karina about the details of what happened with her ex-boyfriend. Karina is grateful that Taylor opened up to her but concerned about the way heart-breaking memories seemed to be suddenly right at the surface. Karina is honest with Taylor about her concerns and teaches her grounding techniques to keep herself in the present moment when the memories get too intense. Karina also has Taylor practice reaching out for support when she starts to feel overwhelmed; Taylor found this idea hokey and stupid but begrudgingly admits that asking for help had been tough in the past. They talk for a while about telling Taylor's parents before Taylor actually has the courage to do it. Karina and Taylor end up telling her parents together, and

Karina has a few meetings with Taylor's parents afterward to talk about how best to support her.

> *Grounding* is a mindfulness technique that can be helpful for teens with trauma-related symptoms. Grounding helps keep youth in the present moment, rather than getting pulled into a flashback of a dissociative moment. Grounding anchors them to their current environment, reminding them that they are safe. Examples of grounding include body scans, noticing and counting the breath, utilizing the five senses, saying the alphabet backward, and mentally orienting oneself to the external environment with who, what, where, when, why, and how questions.

As Taylor's discharge date approaches, Karina worries about Taylor's fragility and advocates for Taylor to be discharged to a partial hospitalization program (PHP). She is grateful when Taylor's insurance approves this 5-day-a-week intensive step-down program, so Taylor can continue with intensive trauma-focused therapy when she returns home. She expects that Taylor will be happy with this plan and will see that Karina gets how important Taylor's trauma history is and feel validated and understood. But Taylor is livid and storms out of session when Karina tries to tell her about the program. Karina is confused, but with the same curiosity and empathy that she brought to their first meetings, she is able to understand Taylor's anger. Taylor wants to continue this work with Karina, the person with whom she entrusted this secret and made herself vulnerable. The prospect of starting anew with anybody else, allowing herself to be vulnerable again and to trust someone else, seems too difficult. Karina validates these fears and sets up a joint meeting with Anik, the therapist from the PHP, before Taylor's discharge. Although their first meeting is rocky, Anik is able to make Taylor laugh at the end, and she begrudgingly agrees to keep working with him.

Taylor is discharged to the PHP. Over the next 8 weeks, Taylor and Anik work on understanding the connections between her trauma and her current feelings of emptiness, shame, and depression, as well as her recurrent suicidality and urges to cut. In group sessions, Taylor learns distress tolerance, self-advocacy, and emotion regulation skills from Dialectical Behavior Therapy (DBT). Her parents come in for group sessions with other parents, learning how to coach Taylor in times of distress and how to accept that sometimes they won't be able to make it all better for their daughter. Anik helps Taylor to articulate the sadness that is underneath her anger and defiance, and the psychiatrist starts her on an antidepressant medication to address her trauma-related depressive symptoms. Taylor finishes the PHP and transitions to outpatient therapy with Jane, a licensed clinical social worker trained in Trauma-Focused Cognitive Behavioral Therapy (TF-CBT). Jane reinforces the coping skills Taylor has learned and helps Taylor write her trauma narrative. Taylor shares the narrative with her parents, who are supportive and caring. Her brothers even come to a few sessions, and though she doesn't share the story of her rape with them, they discuss how scary her suicide attempts have been for them, and she shares with them how hard she has been working to get better. Working with Jane, Taylor feels a contentment and stability she hasn't felt since the trauma first occurred.

Effective treatment requires thoughtful consideration of the interplay between biological and psychological sequelae of trauma. Youth whose symptoms are so severe that they are admitted to locked inpatient facilities are usually those who need the most intensive interventions. Accordingly, psychopharmacology for the treatment of trauma goes hand in hand with psychotherapy, and most youth admitted to psychiatric facilities, especially those who have multiple hospitalizations, will be treated with psychotropic drugs. No medications are curative or fully treat PTSD in adolescents the way that trauma-focused therapy does, but sometimes symptoms are so acute or severe that meaningful engagement in therapy is impossible. Therefore, trauma-focused therapy should be considered as first-line treatment, with medication added for symptomatic relief or as an adjunct to therapy.

Selective serotonin reuptake inhibitors (SSRIs) can be used for adolescents who are experiencing severe anxiety or depression in the aftermath of trauma. Depression in adolescents can look like irritability, not just sadness, especially in teens who, as a result of trauma, have nervous systems that are chronically in fight, flight, or freeze mode. SSRIs can potentially mitigate mood and anxiety symptoms in this context, although SSRIs have not been proven to directly treat PTSD-related anxiety, reexperiencing, avoidance, or hyperarousal.

PTSD symptoms of hyperarousal and reexperiencing may be better treated with α_2-agonist medications, such as guanfacine and clonidine.[4] Prazosin, an α_1-blocker, can be helpful for posttraumatic sleep disturbances including nightmares.[5] Clinicians treating youth with severe mood dysregulation, irritability, or aggression after a traumatic experience sometimes prescribe antipsychotics like quetiapine, risperidone, and aripiprazole. This class of medication carries a high risk for side effects and generally should not be used as an initial treatment. If a teen does have a comorbid disorder, the medications used to treat it (e.g., stimulants for attention-deficit/hyperactivity disorder) may be helpful to reduce impairment from that disorder but will not impact trauma symptoms. Before prescribing any medication, the provider should include the teen and his or her caregiver(s) in the treatment decision and explain why medicine is recommended, what it will and won't do, how long it needs to be taken, what side effects may occur, and when alternatives may need to be considered. Psychiatric medications are highly stigmatized. If teens feel that they are being asked to take medication because people think they're "crazy," they won't take it and may even drop out of treatment.

Psychotherapeutically, the focus on acute care needs to be on stabilization, education, and developing a plan for outpatient treatment. Psychoeducation for the teen and caregivers should be provided, including information about diagnosis and different therapeutic options (including TF-CBT and other evidence-based treatments). There is no specific evidence about which short-term psychotherapeutic options are best in an acute care setting. Most trauma-informed therapies, including TF-CBT, are longer-term treatments designed for use in the outpatient setting, although parts of these treatments (such as psychoeducation and coping skills) could be started on an inpatient unit or even in the ED. Some trauma-focused therapies, such as the adolescent group therapy modification of Skills Training in Affective and Interpersonal Regulation (STAIR-A), have been used on inpatient units.[6] Although trauma group programs are not widely available on inpatient units, a number of goals can be accomplished during even a short inpatient stay and without a formal group therapy program. For example, psychoeducation can help the teen (and family members) to identify the relationship between past and current experiences. Psychoeducation can also help teens better understand their own reactions by appreciating the connection between triggers in the environment, thoughts, feelings, and behaviors. Teens should also be coached to identify or develop coping skills to have more effective and adaptive behaviors in response to negative thoughts and feelings. However, identifying coping skills is not the same as being able to access a coping skill when acutely distressed. The biggest missed opportunity in acute care settings, whatever the length of stay, is the chance to practice these coping skills. Expecting Taylor to remember to ground herself when she sees her ex-boyfriend in the park, if she has never practiced a grounding technique, is a setup for failure. Coping skills must be practiced and paired to appropriate situations. For example, deep breathing or distraction may work for a minor stressor, but the best coping strategy for facing your rapist in person may be to make a police report, get a protection order, or find another park to visit.

There is another therapeutic opportunity that is sometimes missed in acute care settings: explaining unexpected behaviors. Negative behaviors, especially outbursts and aggression, are often described as "coming out of nowhere" or happening "for no reason." Generally speaking, behaviors occur in context and many serve a purpose, even those that are destructive. When a symptom or behavior presents unpredictably, the treatment team should consider why that behavior emerged. Performing a functional chain analysis around that behavior can be useful—first without, and then with, the assistance of the teen.

> Two weeks prior to her sixteenth birthday, Taylor comes to see her therapist, Jane. She sits with eyes downcast, appearing hesitant and uncertain for the first time in months. After a brief period of silence, Taylor begins, "I don't know whether I should ask you this." She goes on to ask about safe sex and birth control, sharing that her relationship with one of her best friends had become romantic and she wants to have sex with him for the first time on her sixteenth birthday. She wants to "be smart about it" and hopes Jane can help her think about "protection." Jane is pleased that Taylor feels comfortable asking her about this and walks Taylor to the adjacent adolescent medicine clinic to schedule an appointment. When Taylor returns the following week, she happily shows Jane the pack of birth control pills and condoms and expresses pride that she has moved past her trauma and can have a healthy sexual relationship. Jane praises this but also tries to manage Taylor's expectations, normalizing how first sexual encounters can be awkward and encouraging Taylor to consider possible negative feelings that might come up. But Taylor is confident that things with her boyfriend won't be "like that." Taylor calls to cancel her next week's appointment, citing a school conflict and saying she is feeling really good.
>
> A week later, Jane gets a telephone call from a local ED, informing her that Taylor is being evaluated following a suicide attempt. The ED physician says that Taylor was brought by her mother earlier that morning following the discovery that Taylor had ingested 80 capsules of valerian root. The circumstances surrounding this suicide attempt are unclear because Taylor is largely refusing to speak. Jane advocates for Taylor's transfer back to the inpatient unit where she had last been hospitalized, as the staff there know her well, and it is the unit with which Jane and the partial hospital program are affiliated. But because a bed on that unit isn't immediately available, Taylor is transferred to a different facility.
>
> On transfer, Taylor remains resistant, refusing to divulge details contributing to her suicide attempt. Instead, she repeatedly and willfully insists that she is "fine." The inpatient team seeks collateral history from her mother, who describes this suicide attempt as completely unexpected. Taylor had been doing very well over the course of the preceding few months, her mom says, and was particularly elated regarding her recent sixteenth birthday. Her mother notes that Taylor has been having a little trouble with sleep, something about bad dreams, but otherwise has been doing well with no known stressors. Taylor's inpatient treatment team never attempts to contact Jane or get any records from the inpatient unit or partial hospital program that had treated Taylor before.

Taylor's inpatient team concludes that this highly impulsive suicide attempt in the setting of being "elated," superimposed on a history of depression, was reflective of bipolar disorder. They stop both the SSRI (escitalopram) and the α_1-blocker (prazosin) that had been prescribed for nightmares following disclosure of her trauma, and instead start an antipsychotic medication (aripiprazole). Taylor remains irritable, oppositional, and stubborn throughout this hospitalization, refusing to engage and consistently denying any psychiatric symptoms or suicidal thoughts. She is discharged quickly with a plan to continue working with Jane, who was not provided with any information prior to Taylor's arrival at their next regularly scheduled session.

The detrimental consequences of misdiagnosis of traumatic stress symptoms have been discussed elsewhere in this book (see Chapter 1, "Teens and Traumatic Stress"), but it bears repeating that misdiagnosis occurs commonly in EDs and on inpatient units. Trauma-exposed teens can be misdiagnosed with bipolar disorder, conduct disorder, oppositional defiant disorder, and even schizophrenia in EDs, inpatient units, and other acute care settings.[7] Misdiagnosis can make teens feel misunderstood, ashamed, and stigmatized. It can lead to inappropriate treatment, like Taylor's being taken off her antidepressant and prescribed an antipsychotic, which exposes youth to the risks and side effects of medications that may not be indicated for their symptoms. It is essential to understand that oppositional or aggressive behavior, severe mood dysregulation, and even psychotic-like symptoms may be a consequence of traumatic experiences.

During her first postdischarge appointment with Jane, Taylor continues to appear irritable, defiant, and agitated. But Jane knows Taylor well enough to validate, empathize with, and thoughtfully interpret Taylor's irritability, and Taylor quickly softens. Gently and without making Taylor feel judged or ashamed, Jane asks if the decision to have sex for the first time since she was raped might have been triggering. Taylor explains that the sex itself was not what drove her to overdose again. Although she acknowledges that sex had proven to be mildly triggering, she has no regrets regarding that decision. But, she says, when her boyfriend unexpectedly broke up with her a few days after, she was overwhelmed with sadness, guilt, and shame, as well as anger. This breach of trust by the individual with whom she had allowed herself to be most vulnerable made her question all other relationships in her life. She began to feel that the progress she had made in recent months wasn't real, and was overcome by worthlessness and thoughts of suicide too strong to resist.

Taylor admits that her most recent hospitalization had done little to alleviate her feelings of hopelessness. The antipsychotic medication makes her feel simultaneously jittery and numb and makes it hard to think clearly. When Jane asked directly, Taylor admits to ongoing suicidal ideation. Jane is honest and transparent with Taylor about how much she fears for Taylor's safety. Taylor eventually agrees to go with Jane to the hospital's emergency room, and Jane is able to arrange for Taylor to be readmitted to the inpatient unit where Taylor first worked with Karina. After calling Taylor's parents, and before she leaves for the night, Jane tells Taylor that she is confident the inpatient team will be able to help Taylor overcome this setback.

Effective treatment of trauma does not end with discharge from an inpatient unit or completion of a partial hospitalization program. Acute care settings are designed for immediate stabilization: they provide a safe space where adolescents can be temporarily removed from stressors and engage with a therapeutic team that will accurately diagnose them and initiate treatment. Discharge from acute care settings requires establishing a safe, reasonable plan that can include a return to home, outpatient follow-up, provision of in-home services, and reentry into school. The team should anticipate trauma-related barriers to adjusting back to the community, such as how to cope with trauma reminders in the home or neighborhood, or how to make friends in a new school after a long history of bullying. Family and other adults can be critically important here. Teens can work on coping skills and safety plans while in the hospital, identifying triggers for distress and ways to respond, but they will also need coaching and reminders to utilize these plans during moments of stress after discharge. Family can also help to identify what is feasible and which skills the teen might need to practice more before discharge. For example, if "calling 911" is on a safety plan, then the hospital staff should help rehearse what the teen would say, what he or she would expect to hear, and how to ask someone else to call if needed. Similarly, developing coping skills to address symptoms and to prevent dangerous behaviors is a key part of many acute psychotherapeutic interventions, but planning in advance how to use them in triggering situations should accompany the learning of these skills. The provider should identify maladaptive avoidant behaviors and situations in which they may arise outside of the acute care setting, and make a plan in advance in order to cope with these effectively.

The capacity of a teen to function better in the community will depend in large part on how effectively the team in the acute care setting has prepared the teen for discharge, and this means directly thinking about, addressing, and preparing for what is going to happen on return to the community. Disposition planning should start early and take into consideration what needs to change in the teen's environment to maintain the gains made in the hospital. Family-based treatment or family involvement in the teen's trauma therapy is often helpful. This can start in the hospital but should continue on discharge. Teens who are discharged from the hospital remain highly vulnerable. Family involvement in treatment can ensure that the teen has support and coaching at home to cope more effectively with triggers and traumatic stress symptoms. Family-based treatment can also decrease triggers by addressing and preventing arguments and disagreements between parents and teens. Trauma-informed family treatment is especially important for already stressed families, families with intergenerational trauma, and homes in which multiple members are suffering from mental illness and PTSD. The teen may also need adaptations at school, such as quieter testing environments, or even an alternative school placement.

Returning to acute care settings is often seen as a failure. However, teens like Taylor have every right to return to safe settings for more intensive treatment when the skills and insights they have learned and developed in acute care settings cannot sustain them in a world that can be viciously and sometimes overtly traumatizing. Unless the world becomes free of trauma, acute care settings need to be available, so that passionate, fiercely driven adolescents like Taylor can be kept safe and get the help they need.

Additional Reading

Azeem MW, Aujla A, Rammerth M, et al: Effectiveness of six core strategies based on trauma informed care in reducing seclusions and restraints at a child and adolescent psychiatric hospital. J Child Adolesc Psychiatr Nurs 24(1):11–15, 2011 21272110

Bloom S: Creating Sanctuary, Destroying Sanctuary, and Restoring Sanctuary. 1997. Excerpt available at: http://sanctuaryweb.com/Portals/0/Bloom%20Pubs/1997%20Bloom%20Intro%20Book%20Creating%20Sanctuary.pdf. Accessed March 5, 2018.

Martin A, Krieg H, Esposito F, et al: Reduction of restraint and seclusion through collaborative problem solving: a five-year prospective inpatient study. Psychiatr Serv 59(12)1406–1412, 2008 19033167

References

1. Havens JF, Gudiño OG, Biggs EA, et al: Identification of trauma exposure and PTSD in adolescent psychiatric inpatients: an exploratory study. J Trauma Stress 25(2):171–178, 2012 22522731
2. Bloom S, Farragher B: Destroying Sanctuary: The Crisis in Human Service Delivery Systems. New York, Oxford University Press, 2010
3. Mueser KT, Taub J: Trauma and PTSD among adolescents with severe emotional disorders involved in multiple service systems. Psychiatr Serv 59(6):627–634, 2008 18511582

4. Keeshin BR, Strawn JR: Psychological and pharmacologic treatment of youth with posttraumatic stress disorder: an evidence-based review. Child Adolesc Psychiatr Clin N Am 23(2):399–411, x, 2014 24656587

5. Keeshin BR, Ding Q, Presson AP, et al: The use of prazosin for pediatric PTSD-associated nightmares and sleep disturbances: a retrospective chart review. Neurol Ther 6(2):247–257, 2017 28755207

6. Gudiño OG, Weiss JR, Havens JF, et al: Group trauma-informed treatment for adolescent psychiatric inpatients: a preliminary uncontrolled trial. J Traumatic Stress 27(4):496–500, 2014 25070927

7. Cohen JA: Practice parameter for the assessment and treatment of children and adolescents with posttraumatic stress disorder. J Am Acad Child Adolesc Psychiatry 49(4):414–430, 2010 20410735

CHAPTER 11

School Systems and Trauma

Patrick Heppell, Psy.D.
Komal Bhasin

"The sixth fight this week, and it's only Wednesday!" exclaims Howard School's recently hired dean of students as he and the school safety officer walk back into the office after breaking up a brawl involving five students. The principal looks up. "I know. What's in the water these past few weeks?" None of them say it, but all three have been silently questioning themselves and feeling that they are losing control over their own school. Ms. Pitts, the tenth-grade English teacher, is requesting a transfer to another school in the district. Mr. Jimenez, the eleventh-grade social science teacher, announced his retirement last week, saying that the school was "out of control and I'm too old for this crap." The school counselor's waiting list has increased threefold this past month. Suspensions and detentions have been handed out left and right, but things are just getting worse. Parents are complaining more than usual, asking why safety cannot be maintained at the school.

At the next all-staff meeting, the principal and dean of students try to lead a conversation with the staff to figure out what is going on. Teachers and security staff have lots to say about the ongoing fighting. They argue that the fights aren't isolated incidents, but rather part of a larger wave of anger, frustration, and reactivity dominating the hallways and classrooms. "The disrespect and the talking back," one teacher shouts. "I've been a teacher for 12 years here and I have never experienced anything like this before." Many others agree. An older teacher pipes up to add, "It's not just anger, though. Lots of students also seem quiet and distant. Even the motivated students aren't engaging in my lessons." This statement generates lots of side conversations and nods of agreement from the others. The school counselor jumps in: "Yeah, the kids aren't talking anymore—they're shutting down. Something is going on." "The new dean just doesn't have it in him," whispers one teacher to another. "I'm losing control," the principal and the dean think to themselves.

Schools are home to separate small communities within the larger whole. Students have cliques and teams and clubs, and even teachers, supporting staff, security staff, and administrators will form their own groups. But the school as a whole forms one community, one culture. The school community reflects the temperature of what is happening in the school and what is happening outside as well. At times, it's one student or one group that dictates the temporary vibe of the school. Other times, it might be an event or series of events. Like a sponge, the student body and school personnel absorb and respond and react to significant events inside and outside the school's walls.

Asking Why: How Trauma Can Disrupt School Communities

When an abrupt change disturbs a system or a community, it is human nature to try to find an explanation for the changes. We do this with the evidence available to us, but often we don't have all the facts, and it is easiest to blame one individual, especially one sitting on top such as the principal or dean of students. Other times we blame the ones who seem most directly involved in the problem, in this case the students. Or we blame ourselves. But when something disrupts an entire community, the problem is rarely one person; it is usually something bigger that is affecting the system or the culture.

Feeling like she's losing control of the meeting, the principal asks with desperation, "What do you guys think might explain all of this?" One senior teacher speaks up: "Maybe I'm just getting old, but these kids nowadays have no respect for authority. When you talk to the parents, they don't want to set any kind of limits. They just want to be the kid's 'friend.'" Several others agree. "They just care about themselves and their selfies and Instagrams," another teacher adds, miming a selfie pose; this prompts a few chuckles and loosens up the group. "No, it's the hip hop that kids listen to these days, garbage…." Several teachers laugh and nod while others roll their eyes.

"The neighborhood has been kind of hot lately," shouts one of the staff from the back who is definitely not laughing. The principal asks him to elaborate. "These two gangs have been battling over this community for years now—we all know that—but the violence had been kept pretty minimal. The last few months, though, it's like the peace treaty has been abolished. Lots of shootings, killings, revenge….The police came in, so you know, lots of arrests and stuff, and then the Drug Enforcement Administration and the Department of Child and Family Services come in, and you know what that means: arrests and removals." The room is silent as everyone considers this. The principal and the dean of students look at each other, both shocked. "I had no idea," the dean thinks with embarrassment.

Systemic traumas affect entire communities. These include obvious or newsworthy traumas, such as natural disasters, terrorism, or school shootings, but systemic traumas don't always make the front page of the paper or blow up the Twittersphere. Community violence, bullying, death of an important member of the community, immigration raids, and other more private traumas can still have broad impact. That impact is felt privately by individuals and families and may be felt strongly by groups of students or adults within a school. Those not directly affected by the trauma may be unaware of it, because often the trauma is not talked about. Just as an individual will avoid the painful memories and unpleasant feelings attached to his or her own traumatic experience, a system or a community will also avoid bringing up a trauma. Adults may feel it is not appropriate to discuss at work, whereas teens believe it is not safe to discuss with adults. Others yearn to talk about the event but think, "If no one else is talking about it, it must not be that bad after all, and I should be able to tolerate it too." Cultural beliefs and expectations may also contribute to the silence, because no one wants to be weak or snitch or "air the family's business." Others wait for "someone else" to say something.

> Watch out for upsetting or stressful events that may happen within the school or in the broader community. Even sociopolitical events, far-away conflicts, or incidents with heavy media coverage may impact the school as a community or subgroups within the school. For example, immigrant families may be affected by international conflicts, whereas others in the community may be shaken by episodes of police brutality, changes in immigration policies, shifts in political leadership, or highly publicized deaths or suicides, even if these occur geographically far away. Teachers, school counselors, parent coordinators, parents, and auxiliary staff often have insight into what is going on in the school's ecosystem.

Specific subgroups might be at elevated risk for experiencing traumatic symptoms. Students who are living in poverty, students from ethnic and racial minorities, and gay, lesbian, bisexual, and transgender students are unfortunately more vulnerable to experiencing traumatic events, as individuals and as a community.

> The staff meeting is silent for a moment before people start to speak again, quieter and more serious now, as if seeing the problems they've been experiencing in a new light. "It's like I've been teaching and talking to a wall," one says. "My classroom was not like this a few months ago." "Last week I tried to talk to a student about how she seemed tired in class, suggested she go to bed earlier. She yelled at me and ran out of the room!" "Half my class bombed the last exam, and I practically gave them the answers in the study guide." "We read about the death of Martin Luther King, Jr., last week, and a bunch of kids cried, but no one was willing to talk about why." "A lot more kids have been showing up late to first period, and lots are leaving early too. It's like the last month of school but it's only October!" "A bunch of 'em are coming to school high, more than before." "Marcos told me he has had to say good-byes to many of his homies this past few weeks."

As discussed in Chapter 1 ("Teens and Traumatic Stress"), individuals have different reactions to trauma. This is especially evident when a system trauma affects many students in a single school. A wide range of trauma responses can be seen in school, such as these:

- Anxiety, fear, and worry about safety of self and others
- Worry about recurrence or consequences of the violence or other trauma
- Changes in behavior, such as
    - Withdrawal from others or activities (e.g., clubs, sports teams)
    - Irritable or oppositional attitude with peers or teachers
    - Hostile or angry reactions to authority, redirection, or criticism
    - Angry outbursts or aggressive behavior
    - Overreacting (or underreacting) to bells, doors slamming, sirens, lighting, sudden movements, or physical contact
    - Worsening academic performance
    - Poor attention and/or concentration
    - Hyperactive behavior or seeming "jumpy" all the time
    - Absenteeism
    - Increased impulsive or risk-taking behavior
    - Writing, drawing, talking, or searching online about morbid topics such as death, dying, or suicide
- Talking repeatedly about the traumatic events, or refusing to talk about them at all
- Discomfort with, and refusal to talk about, feelings (e.g., anger, sadness, thoughts of revenge)

- Feelings of numbness or hopelessness
- Difficulty trusting others (peers or adults)
- Increased drug or alcohol abuse
- Sleep problems, that manifest with kids falling asleep in class, not paying attention, making "stupid" mistakes, or being unusually hyperactive or irritable

Trauma affects caregivers, service providers, and educators as well as students. Sometimes the adults are directly affected by the traumatic events, just as the students are. Other times, just hearing about a trauma and seeing its effects on students day after day can be vicariously traumatizing. Seeing teens who are hurt, scared, or struggling, day in and day out, and not knowing how to help, can be exhausting and overwhelming to the adults.

> The principal is astounded. A part of her is relieved that there is an explanation for the changes at her school, that it's not just that she is losing her touch. But her heart breaks to think about how the kids must be feeling. Looking at her staff, she realizes it's not only the kids who are affected. Shaking her head with the sudden clarity, she asks, "How is everyone doing, I mean you guys? How are you doing?"
>
> The responses come quickly and honestly. "I've been bringing more home with me—I mean not actual grading and stuff, I always bring that home—but like the frustration, the despair…. Even my wife is asking me, what's happening?" "Yeah, me too, I've been talking to my partner about this. He don't want to hear it no more." "I'm just tired, tired of the kids challenging me, but also just tired, like, physically and emotionally." "When I get home, I don't even want to think about school anymore. On the weekend, I used to think about special projects and experiments I can bring to my classroom. Recently, I just want to get away." "Me too. The Sunday blues start Saturday night now—I'm just dreading coming to work." "I've been drinking more," shrugs a younger teacher in the back. This gets a good laugh from the crowd, but it quickly settles into a painful silence.

Responses to secondary traumatic stress can mimic typical symptoms seen in posttraumatic stress disorder (PTSD). Unfortunately, it is not uncommon for teachers, administrators, school counselors, and auxiliary staff to experience secondary traumatic stress from their work with students. In addition to the demanding responsibilities of an educator, direct exposure to traumatic events in the community, hearing about traumatic events directly from students or from other sources, and fights or other acute behaviors among the students can all contribute to secondary traumatic stress. Just as kids have different vulnerabilities and reactions to traumatic stress, so do adults. Empathy, isolation, inexperience, and unresolved personal trauma can worsen risk for secondary traumatic stress. So can working in a system that is disconnected or fragmented, that doesn't allow for support or recovery time, or that is constantly under strain or lacking resources.[1]

> After thanking her staff for sharing, the principal ends the meeting with a vague, "We are in this together. We'll get out of this together," but even as she says it she's not sure how they will. As the staff file out, she looks at the school counselor, who quickly looks away and shakes her head. "I have too many on my caseload already!" The principal politely interrupts her: "I know, I know. But I need your help. We need to do something....Let's meet tomorrow to brainstorm. I'll invite a few more staff."
>
> Later that day, walking past room 354, she sees a disturbing sight. Ms. Miller, a diminutive woman who has been an English teacher for 17 years without a single spot on her record, is fully and loudly arguing with one of the students, Tyrese, in the doorway of her classroom while the other students watch from inside. The principal is shocked and steps between Ms. Miller and the boy, facing the teacher. "Ms. Miller, tell me what's going on," she starts, as Ms. Miller continues to yell over the principal's shoulder at the student standing behind her. "Ms. Miller, please, I've got this." As Ms. Miller continues to berate the boy, the principal raises her voice in frustration: "Ms. Miller, please leave the classroom now!" Ms. Miller and the student both fall silent, seeming in shock. Ms. Miller shakes her head as if coming out of a trance, a horrified look on her face. "I'm sorry," she says, backing out of the classroom and hurrying off. The principal wants to go talk to her (though to yell at her or reassure her, she doesn't know), but the students quickly interrupt her thought: "You hear what she called me?" "That was fucked up." "You gonna fire her, miss?" "Tyrese weren't even rude or threatening or nothin', she just lost it on him for no reason." The students are serious, angry. The principal glances at the teacher's aide who nods uncomfortably, confirming the students' report. "Okay! Okay, quiet down everyone. One at a time, tell me what is going on."

Don't ignore the signs!

Signs that educators may be experiencing secondary traumatic stress[2]:

- Increased irritability or impatience with students

- Difficulty planning classroom activities and lessons

- Decreased concentration

- Denying that traumatic events impact students or feeling numb or detached

Don't ignore the signs! *(continued)*
• Intense feelings and intrusive thoughts, that don't lessen over time, about a student's trauma
• Dreams about students' traumas

What to Do First

When traumatic events impact a school, they demand a whole-school response. Helping the students and staff to cope with and recover from a traumatic event requires systemic changes. But first, the principal has multiple "fires" to put out. In this section we'll discuss fair and immediate steps to promote safety, and in the following section ("What to Do Next") we'll discuss the proactive and preventive measures that can prevent the sparks of trauma from catching fire in the first place.

> After hearing from the students, the principal goes to find Ms. Miller. "There's a first for everything, I guess," she thinks, as she ponders the idea of disciplinary action against the woman who has been one of her best teachers. She finds Ms. Miller already waiting outside her office. "Ms. Miller, the students told me…." "I know, I know," interrupts Ms. Miller. "I don't know what happened. I lost it!" "You called Tyrese a lost cause?" the principal asks. "I think I did," Ms. Miller says, a look of horror and shame on her face. "It's so not like me, I can't believe it. But for some reason, I kind of saw this coming. Two days ago, I asked the aide to take over my class. I just couldn't bear the thought of facing the students. I don't know what's happening. Maybe I need to retire. Or…are you going to take me out of my class? Not yet, please, not before the end of the school year…." Seeing the older woman's distress, the principal stops her. "Ms. Miller, I'm going to be honest with you. I don't know what we're going to do. It looks like you're experiencing what we've all been feeling, and it just came out. How can I support you?" Ms. Miller looks relieved but helpless. "I'll be honest, I'm not sure. I don't know if anything could help," she says.

Disciplinary actions, punishments, and shaming do not alleviate symptoms of secondary traumatic stress. Rather, they are more than likely to worsen the problem. At the same time, the role of administrator is to assure that the educators are safe and ready to teach. Although it can be difficult to simultaneously support a struggling teacher and set appropriate limits and expectations for behavior and performance, this is the same difficult task we ask teachers to do for struggling students every day. We can support a struggling teacher and empathize with why that teacher behaved the way he or she did, while setting up a structure to support the teacher to do better going forward.

Seeing the hopelessness on Ms. Miller's face, the principal shakes her head. "Well, we have to find something. I can't have one of my best teachers freaking out at the students again. We're having a meeting tomorrow to talk about what's going on. Think about it tonight, and I'll expect you at that meeting." "But my class…," Ms. Miller protests, "and I'll be so embarrassed!" The principal persists: "Have your teacher's aide take over your lessons. Join us at the meeting. No need to be embarrassed—we're all struggling here. We'll be generating ideas on how to support the students and the staff." Ms. Miller nods and leaves the room. The principal grabs a handful of M&M's from the bowl on her desk. "Stress eating," she thinks, feeling at a loss. "Should we openly process what happened and include the students?" she wonders. But she can't imagine what she'd say, and isn't even sure if it would be appropriate, so she pushes the thought away.

The next morning, the principal, the dean of students, the school counselor, a few teachers, and a few students from the student government gather in the gym to discuss what has been going on and make a plan for what to do. Ms. Miller joins them, looking sheepish. The principal thanks all of them for coming, then opens up the discussion. A student starts: "It has been a while since we've met like this, with students and teachers together." One of the teachers nods. Another teacher adds, "A lot of us have been feeling that disconnect," he says. "Maybe we should do this more often."

Understanding the students' trauma is the first step in building a trauma-informed school. Seeing the connection between the behaviors and struggles displayed by each student as an individual, and by students as a group, with the traumatic events they have experienced helps the adults find more caring and appropriate responses to those behaviors. The principal's initial all-staff meeting where everyone discussed the community traumas affecting students was a good first step. But it's not enough. Helping the school community recover from both the trauma and its effects on students and staff requires a multimodal approach. This should include 1) holding open and continuous conversations between students and staff; 2) promoting safety and a sense of fairness through clear expectations for both students and adults; 3) providing training, specific skills, and self-care opportunities to all individuals who interact directly with students; and 4) supporting students through positive behavior support and connection to nonstigmatizing, trauma-informed, accessible mental health services when necessary.

Holding Open Conversations Between Students and Staff

Traumatic life events, even shared traumas, tend to alienate us from each other. We turn inward with our pain, distancing ourselves from others and disconnecting from activities and engagements. However, traumatic events have the capacity to meaningfully and powerfully bring people together, although this rarely happens spontaneously. To accomplish this within a school, educators and school administrators must take proactive steps in generating, fostering, and maintaining an engaged and connected school community. Small actions from educators and school leadership—for example, saying hi in the hallway, checking in before or after class with students, or inviting students to come chat in the classroom during breaks—make a big difference. Every student should feel connected to and cared for by at least one adult in the building.

Open and ongoing conversations with staff and students are key to maintaining genuine dialogues within the school system. One helpful way to promote such communication is to create an advisory board where active students and staff (and even parents) meet and discuss the traumatic event(s) and its effects. Such meetings strengthen relationships between and among students and staff, enhance trust, and empower the student body and staff to propose and implement solutions. They create buy-in for change and help students and adults see each other as collaborators rather than combatants. An advisory board also provides an opportunity for leadership and educators to hear firsthand about students' and families' experiences.

Homeroom can also provide a setting for students and teachers to talk openly in a safe setting. Openness and transparency are deeply therapeutic for trauma. Speaking sensitively about systemic traumas can have a powerful impact. Talking about trauma shows students that these events are not secret or shameful. Teachers and staff show that they care how youth are affected by the trauma and empathize with the teens' experiences. We as adults can also model for students the difficult behaviors we ask of them but rarely do ourselves: talking openly about our own experiences, feelings, and reactions, and taking responsibility for our own behavior and for change. The school may rely on school counselors, school social workers, and/or school psychologists, as well as conversations in the advisory board, to draft key points on what information should be shared with students and in which format, before the larger student body is addressed.

Promoting Safety and a Sense of Fairness Through Clear Expectations and Restorative Justice

The planning meeting continues. "What are we going to do about all these fights?" one teacher exclaims. "We've been giving out more suspensions and expulsions in the last few months than ever, and nothing has changed!" "No offense, miss, but did you ever think to look at why kids are fighting?" a student asks in response. The teacher replies, "Well, we hear it's all about claiming your hood inside the school, right?" "That might be true sometimes," the student says. "Sh—t, I mean, stuff has to get resolved sometimes. Even the tough kids will tell you though, it's scary out there," as he gestures out of the school. "In the school, at least there ain't no guns. So yeah, when you gotta step up or represent, without maybe dying, stuff will go down in school."

According to the Civil Rights Project at the University of California, Los Angeles, an alarming 3.5 million students were suspended in 2011–2012, resulting in an estimated 18 million instruction days lost and contributing significantly to the high student dropout rates in this country.[3] Zero-tolerance policies may seem like an attempt to take care of the problem and to regulate and regain power and control. However, there is no evidence that zero-tolerance policies lead to any improvement in safety or students' behavior. In fact, schools that rely heavily on punishments, suspensions, and expulsions are less safe, are less academically successful, and are seen as less just by students.[4] Also, when a school has been struck by a systemic trauma that is affecting student behavior, zero-tolerance policies can backfire badly. Educators and administrators in trauma-informed schools structure disciplinary policies in a way that sets clear and consistent expectations and consequences and examines why students are acting up to understand and address the issues at the root of problematic behaviors.

> Safety needs to be promoted from within the school. That does not mean everyone must get searched when entering. If searches are necessary, it is important to remind students about the purpose of the metal detectors: "We care about you, and it is our role to provide you with a safe environment so you can learn as much as you can today." Searches without context make students feel afraid, alienated, or judged.

Consequences for behaviors are necessary; every action has a consequence, positive or negative, and facing the consequence is part of the process of learning and changing behavior. Every action also has a cause: the individual's choice, of course, but also the contextual factors that led the person to make that choice. Trauma-informed disciplinary practices look at consequences but also at causes. If students are acting up, it is important to ask why. Sometimes it is because they are not clear what is expected of them or what constitutes acting "right." Particularly when teens' lives are disrupted by trauma, they need clarity and consistency in school to know how to act to be successful. If expectations and consequences are clear but teens are still acting up, trauma-informed educators and administrators should ask, "Why?" "What's going on?" and "What factors are getting in the way of students doing what they should?" Rather than adopt a "fixed mindset" toward behavior and assume that students act out because they are "bad," a school should consider, as Ross Greene[5] says, that kids do well if they can. If students are not doing well despite clear expectations, opportunities, and incentives to do so, something is getting in the way. Kids act out, fight, yell, and miss school because they are trying to communicate something and do not have the words or the appropriate channel to express themselves.

Trying to understand the "why" behind problematic behaviors does not mean getting rid of appropriate consequences for those behaviors; rather, understanding the root of a behavior helps in finding more effective consequences and in supporting kids to do better in the future. For example, if a student is fighting more in school in part because he is being beaten at home, an out-of-school suspension will not be an effective consequence—it will only expose him more to the traumatizing environment that is triggering the behavior in the first place. How do educators and administrators identify the triggers or the "why" behind behaviors? Engaging students in the process of setting expectations and determining consequences can give students a platform to express themselves and problem solve. Restorative justice practices are one approach to this (Figure 11–1). Restorative justice looks at problematic behaviors in the context of relationships, examining how problematic behaviors affect relationships and using relationships to address them.

Restorative justice gives educators and administrators interventions to pair with consequences to address root causes in a way that prevents recidivism. Restorative justice methods include conflict resolution circles and conferences that bring victims, offenders, and their supporters together in the process of reflecting on the harm that was done, taking responsibility for actions, and coming up with a plan to address the wrongdoing and repair the harm done.[6] By engaging students in this process, the adults can model for them a philosophy of restoration and fairness rather than simple punishment. Restorative justice also gives students an opportunity to build empathy and learn from their mistakes, rather than retreating into defensiveness and shame. Restorative justice practices have been implemented in various school districts around the United States and around the world and have shown impressive results: violence, suspensions, and expulsions decrease, and students feel safer.[7]

Traditional Justice Approach to Discipline	Restorative Justice Approach to Discipline
What rule was broken?	Who has been harmed?
Who broke it?	Who is responsible for what?
What is the punishment?	How can we fix it?

As she listens to the students and teachers talk, the principal thinks back to Ms. Miller's outburst and how to address it. She can't shake the feeling that she wants to address the situation with the students. She decides to take a restorative justice approach. She thinks, "In my old school we had mediations between students after a conflict. There's no reason that wouldn't work between a student and a teacher. Maybe I'll sit down with Ms. Miller and Tyrese this afternoon, and call Tyrese's parents to tell them what happened and what we're going to do to fix it. Then maybe Ms. Miller and I can talk to her class together, tomorrow. She can apologize, and we can discuss with the students about how everyone was affected. Maybe if we, as adults with power, can show the kids we're taking responsibility for something, it'll make it easier for them to take responsibility for their behavior."

Supporting Staff Through Training, Resources, and Opportunities for Self-Care

Everyone who works in education does so out of a commitment to teach, support, and foster students to grow into healthy and successful adults. It can be hard for anyone to honor that commitment, however, when school systems are underfunded and underresourced, when teachers struggle to bridge the gap between ever-growing demands and underprepared students, and when administrations are so distracted by paperwork that they fail to provide opportunities for communication and feedback and staff development. Vicarious traumatization can be the straw that breaks the camel's back for a system already under so much chronic stress.

Fixing this requires building a school culture that supports individuals with necessary resources, communication and connection, opportunities for training and development, and a meaningful commitment to caring for individual students and staff. Staff can only support students if they are

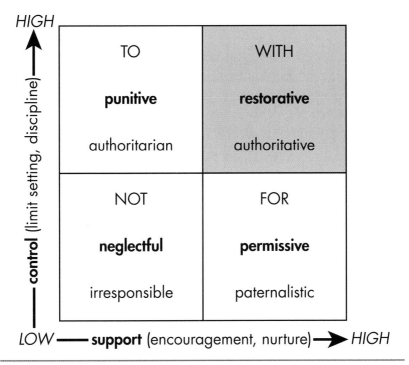

FIGURE 11–1. Approaches to discipline.

There are different types of approaches to disciplines. It is important to consider a balance between the right amount of support given to the students and the right amount of control given to students and educators to be effective. In restorative justice, clear expectations/limits plus support/nurturance help teens make better decisions by having educators and students working together.

Source. Reprinted from Wachtel T: *Defining Restorative.* Bethlehem, PA, International Institute for Restorative Practices. 2013.

equipped with the appropriate skills and if they feel supported themselves. This is true for all staff who interact with students, including administrators, educators, school counselors, auxiliary staff, parent coordinators, bus drivers, school security officers, and anyone else who sets foot inside the school building.

> Back at the planning meeting, "Everyone's so beat, miss," a student tells the principal. "Teachers too—everyone's burnt out," one of the teachers interjects. "We oughta do something to fix that." "Remember last year when we had the teacher's potluck to celebrate Ms. Jones's twenty-fifth year as a teacher?" A few other staff nod in agreement. "That was fun!" "Maybe we should do something like that again?"

School leadership must work to ensure that staff feel supported and connected, especially in times of stress. The school culture should never be neglected. Connection can be fostered through large events such as potlucks,
ordering food for the staff, and appreciation days; these events provide a big
boost of energy and help staff feel appreciated. But these cannot be everyday
things; also, more concrete and specific demonstrations of support and recognition are needed. Check-in meetings, public or private recognitions of
accomplishments, verbal praise, and even just simple and genuine thank yous
let school administrators tell staff just how much they value the hard work
being done every day.

Simple (and Free) Strategies for Staff Appreciation

Write five thank-you notes to individual staff members
each week for specific actions they have taken (even
small ones!). Rotate names, so that every staff member
receives one before starting over.

Hold "office hours" once a week for 20 minutes, when
staff can have lunch with the principal and chat about
what's on their mind, with a focus on administration's
effort to understanding the teachers' experience at the
school.

Encourage staff to choose a weekly "MVP" who is
honored at weekly staff meetings.

One week's MVP can choose the next week's MVP and
determine in what format to honor his or her selection
(e.g., by reading a letter written by a student about the
teacher, with a short video).

Like the saying "show, don't tell," school leadership should also show
appreciation for staff's work and the emotional toll it takes, by fostering a
school culture that allows staff to take care of each other and themselves.
Peer support, both practical and emotional, can help staff solve problems in
the classroom or vent their emotional responses to approach the issue with
more clarity. Ideally the school will have both space and time for such peer
support, which can include team meetings, peer feedback on lessons or in
the classroom, and social events. Self-care is also crucial to reduce the impact of secondary or vicarious traumatic stress and to prevent burnout. Ad-

ministration should acknowledge that self-care is important and ensure that staff members are encouraged to engage in self-care activities. Self-care activities should be individualized for everyone. Some activities can be incorporated during the school day, although some staff will prefer to care for themselves after work. Similarly, some educators may choose to engage in social activities (e.g., walking with a group during lunch time), whereas others may prefer to care for themselves on their own (e.g., going to the gym). Building flexibility and opportunities for self-care into the school culture will be more effective than mandating or scheduling a single activity for everyone.

Strategies to Promote Self-Care

Form a "Sunshine" committee that organizes staff events.

- Based on staff interest, host group exercise classes in the school gym.

- Once a year bring in a masseuse for staff.

Model self-care and be transparent about leaving on time to engage in family activities (rather than visibly staying late).

Rearrange duties to allow people a monthly "appointment afternoon," so they can leave a little early to take care of personal commitments without taking time off.

Professional development is a big part of self-care, because growth is an antidote to burnout. Teaching teens who have experienced trauma requires a high degree of skill, including tolerance, patience, and understanding. We tend not to think of these as skills, but they require practice and reinforcement, just as other skills do. It can be easier to be tolerant, patient, and understanding with traumatized adolescents if we understand the impact of trauma and its manifestations in behavior. Educators also need training in trauma-informed strategies to listen empathically, provide validation, and coach students through challenging situations or trauma reminders. One intervention that supports both students and teachers alike is introducing mindfulness meditation techniques into the classroom. Two minutes of calm time before class can help students relax and focus while setting the tone for learning.

> Do you want to try mindfulness meditation in your classroom? For examples and to hear about students' and teachers' experiences of these practices, please visit the Calm Classroom Web site (see "Resources and Additional Reading" at the end of this chapter).

Another area for professional development is in classroom management in the aftermath of trauma. One of the most difficult aspects of responding to trauma in schools is dealing with the wide range of responses students show. When students are exposed to traumatic events, their presentation in the classroom varies greatly, from zoning out to wilding out. A TF-CBT clinician implementation guide[8] is available to provide guidelines for educators to manage challenging behaviors in the classroom, using LOW and SLOW as reminders:

LOW

- Lower the volume and pitch of your voice.
- Keep a matter-of-fact tone regardless of the situation.
- Speak in short sentences without a lot of questions.
- Don't preach—this is about talking with the student, not at the student.

SLOW

- Slow yourself down by slowing down your heart rate.
- Take slow, deep breaths.
- Slow down your rate of speech and make sure to pause between sentences.
- Slow down your body movements.
- Slow down your agenda and take your time.

These instructions seem simple enough, but actually using them is more difficult. Imagine staying LOW and SLOW in an actual high-conflict situation in the classroom with a+n agitated, disrespectful, challenging, in-your-face (traumatized) student. Practice and rehearsal help to ensure these techniques are second-nature in a crisis.

Supporting Students Through Positive Behavioral Reinforcement and Connection to Nonstigmatizing, Trauma-Informed, Accessible Mental Health Services

Trauma makes people feel isolated and ashamed. Repairing the effects of trauma requires repairing the damage trauma wreaks on school culture. Positive behavioral reinforcement helps teachers and teens feel more connected and cared for, and improves student behavior. Verbal praises, rewards, and catching students "acting good" work not only for little kids. Teenagers (and adults) enjoy being praised and being noticed for doing well. Such recognition reinforces positive behaviors, increases connectedness and confidence, and creates a more pleasant school atmosphere, both for the receiver and giver of the praise.

> Don't wait for students to act up to give them your attention with comments like "Hey, stop that," "Come on man, are you serious," or "I told you not to do that." Instead, catch them when they are doing what you want with an observation like "Thanks for keeping your voice down guys," "I saw how you stepped up for that kid who was getting bullied—that takes guts man," or "You're making your case in a really respectful way, and you're right on point too." This can be done on an individual level for various behaviors, or teachers or administrators can select three or four positive behaviors to promote. Teachers can be supplied with "Caught Being Good" tickets to administer to students with guidelines on how to use them. Tickets should be tied to incentives. These can be known and expected, such as weekly access to the school store or monthly raffles. There can also be unexpected events to keep students on their toes and promote a sense of joyful anticipation. For example, weekly or monthly, the principal could announce over the intercom during lunch that ice cream sandwiches are available in the cafeteria for anyone who earned a ticket that day.

Schoolwide events can also build a sense of community and positivity among students and staff. Regular schoolwide events, such as family potlucks, open-gym hours after school (potentially supervised by parent volunteers), and sporting events, enable students and staff to enjoy each other.

Even students who are having difficulty earning praise or rewards in class due to skills gaps may be able to enjoy themselves and earn praise in these less demanding settings. Students and staff can also come together in support of others or an important cause. For example, a "jeans day" fundraiser (wear jeans and bring a suggested donation of 50 cents, but pay if/what you can) for a cause important to the community (e.g., disaster relief or a local park) can help students and staff feel a sense of community and feel good about helping others.

> At the end of the meeting, the school counselor appears a bit more enthusiastic than she did the day before and is eager to speak. "I chatted online with some other school counselors and school psychologists last night. They had some helpful suggestions. They think a lot of our students will need some kind of counseling or therapy. I'm stretched pretty thin, but we can refer them to some local mental health clinics—I got names of some that offer trauma-informed care. We can also start doing trauma-informed therapy groups here at school." The counselor hands around a quick reference sheet about a group and individual evidence-based therapy called Cognitive Behavioral Intervention for Trauma in Schools (CBITS). She says, "This is a school-based intervention that addresses symptoms of PTSD and also helps students do better with their grades and attendance. I registered through the Web site and now have access to free resources to start implementing CBITS at our school, after some training. I'm excited because so many students have been flooding my office that I can't see them all. I'm exhausted, but also there just aren't enough hours in the day. This will give me a chance to meet with several students at once." The principal, heartened by the counselor's enthusiasm, adds, "I applied for a city program that would give us another social worker, too," she says. "If we get it, he or she could help you with running the groups." "A friend of mine runs groups like that at a mental health clinic down the street. We should see if we can make referrals to that clinic directly," the dean of students suggests. "Also, some mental health agencies can provide school-based services." The counselor nods and agrees to work on building those connections.

> Cognitive Behavioral Intervention for Trauma in Schools (CBITS) is designed for students in grades 5–12 who have experienced one or more traumatic experiences. It is implemented in a school setting, typically by a clinician or mental health provider. It includes 10 group sessions, 1–3 individual sessions, 2 parent psychoeducational sessions, and 1 teacher educational session.

> For more information and to learn how to implement CBITS in your school, see the program's Web site (see "Resources and Additional Reading" at the end of this chapter). CBITS has also been adapted to be led by teachers instead of clinicians. This adaptation is called Support for Students Exposed to Trauma (SSET). Free online trainings in SSET are available at the program's Web site (see "Resources and Additional Reading").

Like most trauma-focused therapies, CBITS follows a phase-based approach. Sessions include exercises related to the following six cognitive behavioral techniques: education about reactions to trauma, relaxation training, cognitive therapy, real-life exposure, stress or trauma exposure, and social problem solving. CBITS is typically provided to students who have a shared traumatic experience, such as the loss of a peer through suicide, the accidental death of a teacher, or community violence. Even when the student body experiences the same trauma, each individual's reaction will be unique. For that reason, the normalization of traumatic reactions and teaching of skills occurs during group sessions, whereas the exposure to the trauma (or trauma narrative) happens during individual sessions.

In-school counseling may not be right for all students. Even though confidentiality remains of utmost priority in school-based mental health services, some students may prefer to meet with a therapist outside of the school to keep their "stuff" private and confidential. In addition, some students with more acute or intense symptomatology may benefit from visiting a mental health clinic with specialized therapies or a higher level of care. Schools should build relationships with outside agencies, including mental health centers, police departments, youth services, and perhaps social services agencies that provide trauma-informed care.

> The National Child Traumatic Stress Network (NCTSN) provides a webinar on how schools and mental health providers can collaborate to provide trauma-informed mental health services and Individualized Education Plans (IEPs) in schools, and methods for integrating these services with school, state, and federal initiatives. The presentation is available at the NCTSN Web site (see "Resources and Additional Reading" at the end of this chapter).

What to Do Next

"Alright everyone, we got plenty to work on in the next few months. I want a few of you to continue meeting to talk about how to be proactive for next year. Who wants to take the lead on this? Ms. Miller?" the principal asks. Ms. Miller nods enthusiastically.

Rather than waiting for negative behaviors to flare up, what if at-risk youth or potential problems could be identified earlier on? Ways to integrate Positive Behavioral Interventions and Supports (PBIS) and Response to Intervention (RTI) to a school system are discussed below.

Implementing Positive Behavior Systems and Response to Intervention

Proactively targeting and reinforcing desired behaviors is much more powerful than simply waiting to provide consequences for undesired behaviors. There is a wide body of research supporting systemwide positive behavior interventions programs in schools. Positive behavioral reinforcement is about catching and reinforcing students doing good things. One version of this, Positive Behavioral Interventions and Supports, is a well-established systemic and data-driven approach that has shown positive results in many schools and school districts.[9,10] Adopting PBIS requires a culture shift across the entire school. This is a difficult task, so professional help or outside consultation may be helpful to implement such programs.

> Positive Behavioral Interventions and Supports (PBIS) assist the school as a whole to create and sustain systems that support every student, targeted groups, and individuals who need more interventions.[11] For more information, see the PBIS Web site (see "Resources and Additional Reading" at end of this chapter).

Using Response to Intervention to Address Emotional and Behavioral Concerns

Several months later, the planning committee is well underway, talking about ways to make the school stronger in the face of the next systemic trauma. In their sessions, the committee members keep coming back to whether they should focus on helping all students or on identifying and aiding those who are really struggling. The dean of student asks, "What if we do it like we do for academics, having interventions at different levels: some for everyone and some for those students who are at risk or struggling?"

Educators are well aware of the Response to Intervention approach to students' academic functioning. In RTI, educators assess all students for their academic functioning and then use evidence-based and individualized interventions for specific groups and individuals. RTI is a layered approach that provides general interventions to all students (Tier 1), more intensive interventions for specific groups who are identified as being at risk (Tier 2), and specifically designed interventions to target those who are identified with skills deficits (Tier 3). Applying this approach to emotional and behavioral issues also makes sense, especially in a school already using this approach for academics.

An example of an RTI approach for emotional/behavioral issues is summarized below. More recently, such an approach utilized for emotional/behavioral issues has been referred to as MTSS (Multi-Tiered System of Support).

Tier 1: Interventions for all students

- Universal screeners for each student to identify students with socioemotional concerns. Such screeners can be used to identify students at risk at the beginning of the year. This establishes a baseline, and then if screening is repeated throughout the year, results can be used to identify changes and prioritize individual students and specific groups for targeted interventions (e.g., groups [Tier 2], counseling [Tier 3]). Examples of screeners widely used in schools include the Strengths and Difficulties Questionnaire (SDQ) for general behavioral issues. For trauma exposure and symptoms screeners, consider the Child and Adolescent Needs and Strengths Trauma Comprehensive (CANS-Trauma), or for more options visit the National Center for PTSD Web site or the Guidance for Trauma Screening in Schools report completed by the Defending Childhood State Policy Initiative (see "Resources and Additional Reading" at the end of this chapter).
- Helpful interventions for all students. These interventions may include use of the positive behavioral system, classroom management skills learned by teachers, and the introduction of meditation practices in the classroom. Another Tier 1 intervention that impacts all students is converting homeroom into an advisory program, in which every staff member participates in leading a 5- to 10-minute advisory group. Activities can focus on get-to-know-you team builders, study skills building, or

conversations to help students feel connection with adults and peers at school.

Tier 2: Additional interventions provided to targeted groups

- Participation in a CBITS or SSET group for teens affected by trauma
- Individual counseling or an extra meditation/relaxation/coping skills group after school
- Creation of an individualized behavior management support
- Involvement of parents and outside community sources (e.g., assisting family with signing up youth for prosocial activities after school)

Tier 3: Individualized intervention for students who continue to have documented struggles despite Tier 1 and Tier 2 interventions

- Referral for individualized counseling and family psychotherapy at school and/or outpatient mental health services
- Consider referrals to trauma-informed evidence-based practices as described in Chapter 2 (see Tables 2–1 and 2–2)

Just as progress is measured throughout the year for academic performances, the impact of each intervention should also be recorded for behavioral issues, using the screeners repeatedly throughout the year.

> NCTSN provides clear guidelines on how to build a trauma-informed school, including an MTSS (see "Additional Reading" at end of this chapter).

Teaching teens who have experienced trauma requires schoolwide efforts. Early identification, prevention, general, and specific interventions comprise an all-inclusive package to target the needs of all students, including traumatized teens. Moreover, trainings, systemwide support programs, self-care, and opportunities for engagement and empowerment for educators and auxiliary staff create the cultural shift required for a school to become truly trauma sensitive. By building trauma-sensitive schools, we can teach our students, educators, and school administrators to weather stress, adversity, and systemic trauma with strength and resilience.

Resources and Additional Reading
Online Resources

Calm Classroom: http://www.calmclassroom.com
Cognitive Behavioral Intervention for Trauma in Schools: https://cbitsprogram.org/

Helping Traumatized Children Learn: https://traumasensitiveschools.org/
National Child Traumatic Stress Network, Schools and Trauma (presentations): https://learn.nctsn.org/enrol/index.php?id=226
Positive Behavioral Interventions and Supports: https://www.pbis.org/school
Support for Students Exposed to Trauma: https://ssetprogram.org/

Screening Tools

Child and Adolescent Needs and Strengths Trauma Comprehensive (CANS-Trauma): http://cctasp.northwestern.edu/pdfs/CANS-Trauma-Comprehensive-Manual-3–22–13.pdf
National Center for PTSD: https://www.ptsd.va.gov/PTSD/professional/assessment/child/index.asp
Strengths and Difficulties Questionnaires: http://www.sdqinfo.com/

Additional Reading

Bloom S: Restoring Sanctuary: A New Operating System for Trauma-Informed Systems of Care. New York, Oxford University Press, 2013
Minahan J, Rappaport N: The Behavior Code: A Practical Guide to Understanding and Teaching the Most Challenging Students. Cambridge, MA, Harvard Education Press, 2012
National Child Traumatic Stress Network, Schools Committee: Creating, Supporting, and Sustaining Trauma-Informed Schools: A System Framework. Los Angeles, CA, and Durham, NC, National Center for Child Traumatic Stress, 2017. Available at: https://www.nctsn.org/sites/default/files/resources//creating_supporting_sustaining_trauma_informed_schools_a_systems_framework.pdf. Accessed July 2, 2018.

References

1. Perry B: The cost of caring: secondary traumatic stress and the impact of working with high-risk children and families. 2014. Available at: https://childtrauma.org/wp-content/uploads/2014/01/Cost_of_Caring_Secondary_Traumatic_Stress_Perry_s.pdf. Accessed March 6, 2018.
2. National Child Traumatic Stress Network: Child trauma toolkit for educators. October 2008. Available at: https://wmich.edu/sites/default/files/attachments/u57/2013/child-trauma-toolkit.pdf. Accessed March 6, 2018.
3. Lösen D, Hodson C, Keit MA, et al: Are we closing the school discipline gap? Civil rights project at UCLA. 2015. Available at: https://civilrightsproject.ucla.edu/resources/projects/center-for-civil-rights-remedies/school-to-prison-folder/federal-reports/are-we-closing-the-school-discipline-gap. Accessed March 6, 2018.
4. Lösen D, Martinez T: Out of school and off track: the overuse of suspensions in American middle and high schools. The Center for Civil Rights Remedies, April 8, 2013. Available at: https://files.eric.ed.gov/fulltext/ED541735.pdf. Accessed March 6, 2018.

5. Greene RW: The Explosive Child: A New Approach for Understanding and Parenting Easily Frustrated, "Chronically Inflexible" Children. New York, HarperCollins, 1998

6. Porter A: Restorative practices in schools: research reveals power of restorative approach, Part I. International Institute of Restorative Practices, March 21, 2007. Available at: https://www.iirp.edu/eforum-archive/4363-restorative-practices-in-schools-research-reveals-power-of-restorative-approach-part-i. Accessed March 6, 2018.

7. Schiff M, Bazemore G: "Whose kids are these?" Juvenile justice and education partnerships using restorative justice to end the "school-to-prison pipeline." Keeping Kids in School and Out of Court, 2012. Available at: http://www.probation.saccounty.net/Documents/Miscellaneous/Other%20-%20Data/Juvenile_Justice_Education_Partnerships.pdf. Accessed March 6, 2018.

8. Community Counseling Center: TF-CBT Implementation Guide. 2018

9. Horner RH, Sugai G, Smolkowski K, et al: A randomized, wait-list controlled effectiveness trial assessing school-wide positive behavior support in elementary schools. Journal of Positive Behavior 11(3):133–144, 2009

10. Metzler CW, Biglan A, Rusby JC, et al: Evaluation of a comprehensive behavior management program to improve school-wide positive behavior support. Education and Treatment of Children 24(4):448–479, 2001

11. Sugai G, Horner RH: The evolution of discipline practices: School-wide positive behavior supports. Child Fam Behav Ther 24:23–50, 2002

CHAPTER 12

Child Welfare and Juvenile Justice

Patrick Heppell, Psy.D.

When Jose and Eva's mother and her latest boyfriend come home one evening, they find Jose, age 16 and visibly intoxicated, with his 15-year-old sister Eva pushed up against the wall, one hand around her throat and the other up her shirt. The boyfriend, horrified, tries to separate them. Jose is fall-down drunk, but he lunges at the older man and the situation escalates into a violent fight. When Jose pulls a knife, his mother calls 911. Jose is arrested and charged with both assault and sexual assault. He is convicted of both, registered as a sex offender, and placed in a juvenile justice facility. Eva is also removed from the home, after a child protective services (CPS) investigation determines that her mother failed to protect her. This is the third time Eva and Jose have been removed from their mother's home but the first time they have been separated from each other.

Ms. Brown, a social worker from the state's CPS, is assigned to Eva and Jose's case. She reviews their lengthy CPS charts. Previous to their most recent removal, Jose and his sister reportedly defied, challenged, and terrorized several foster parents, leading to multiple failed placements and psychiatric hospitals visits. Ms. Brown is shocked to read how young Jose was when he started to fight, gangbang, steal, and carry a weapon. The case notes scream that he is loud, provocative, and aggressive, while at the same time marking him with a string of psychiatric diagnoses. On her first visit to Jose at the juvenile hall, Ms. Brown cannot fail to notice the large tattoos on his back, proudly representing his barrio.

Eva, in contrast, is described as distant, quiet, and detached, though her records list a similar string of failed placements and psychiatric diagnoses. Reports from foster parents and CPS workers note that she is hard to reach, cold, and seems not to care about anyone, not even friends or her biological mother. Some reports say she is sexually promiscuous but seems to have no real relationships. Even with this background, when Ms. Brown meets Eva, she is struck by how disengaged she is, sitting silently for most of the interview and answering questions only with an occasional shrug, as if to say, "I don't care. Leave me alone."

One in 25 youth will interact with the child welfare system each year.[1] That means out of a typical classroom of children, at least one will have his or her family investigated by child protective services or receive support services from a child welfare agency to prevent the child from being removed from the home, or will be placed into foster care. Many abused or neglected youth go into foster care; on any given day, 1 in 184 youth in the United States are living in foster care,[2] and 5.9% of youth will spend time in foster care at some point during childhood.[3] Foster care can mean a private home with a foster parent or family, or an institution (e.g., a residential or group home) supervised (and paid for) by a governmental or social services agency. Adolescents make up over 30% of all youth in foster care.[4]

Children and adolescents enter foster care, broadly speaking, because their caretaker (a biological or adoptive parent, or another relative who has been raising them) is deemed unable to care for them. This can occur after the death or illness of a parent, but typically the child is taken from the caregiver because abuse and/or neglect was reported to a state protective agency and the report was substantiated, meaning determined to be true or likely true. Therefore, by the very nature of foster care, almost all youth in care have experienced trauma. Half of youth in the child welfare system also have mental health issues, some that preceded their abuse or neglect and others that are a direct consequence of the trauma they experienced.

> Keep in mind that the abuse for which an adolescent is removed was a trauma, of course, but the removal (which often occurs in the middle of the night, frequently with police present) and the transitions, uncertainty, change in schools, and separation from family that follow can be traumatizing as well. Further removals often bring up feelings of rejection and sadness that kids often have difficulty putting into words.

The foster care system and the juvenile justice system have significant overlap, unfortunately. The same risk factors that lead to youth being placed in foster care—abuse, neglect, family poverty, poor parent-child relationship, broken home/separation from caregivers, and harsh, lax, or inconsistent discipline—also predispose youth to ending up in juvenile detention. Child abuse or maltreatment specifically increases the child's risk of engaging in criminal activity. Risk of imprisonment is disproportionately high for minority boys like Jose; one in three black and one in six Latino boys will be jailed during their lifetime.[5]

Many youth will be involved in both the child welfare system and the juvenile justice system. Two-thirds of youth referred to juvenile justice systems for an offense have had some involvement in the child welfare system, and of repeat offenders, 9 in 10 youth have been involved with child welfare in the past. Youth with a long history of child welfare involvement were three times as likely to end up in the juvenile justice system compared to youth with no child welfare involvement, and they are also more likely to commit a second offense within 2 years. Similarly, more than 80% of juvenile justice–involved youth report experiencing at least one past traumatic event in their lives, and many of them report multiple forms of past victimization. Youth in juvenile justice also have high rates of mental illness and trauma. Almost 70% of youth who are imprisoned have a diagnosed psychiatric illness and 92% have experienced at least one trauma[6]; between 24% and 32% of youth in detention have posttraumatic stress disorder (PTSD).[7,8] Many youth are revictimized in juvenile detention; as many as 1 in 10 experiences sexual victimization while in juvenile detention, and rates of other types of trauma (which are likely more common) are often not reported.[9,10,11]

Sadly, despite how common they are, mental illness and trauma symptoms in youth in both foster care and juvenile justice are misunderstood, misdiagnosed, underrecognized, and undertreated.

Still shaken from her first encounters with Jose and Eva, Ms. Brown takes steps to better understand each youth. She starts digging around, reading between the lines of the documentation in their charts, getting hold of past mental health evaluations, speaking with a teacher in a class Eva did well in last year, and meeting with a juvenile justice officer who appears to have some rapport with Jose. These conversations help Ms. Brown better understand the kids' prior experiences and why they were so hostile and difficult to engage in their first interactions.

Ms. Brown learns some of the details of Jose's and Eva's prior experiences in foster care. They were first removed from their mother when Eva was age 4 and Jose was 5 after a neighbor found them home alone for several hours; when their mother arrived home visibly intoxicated, the neighbor called the authorities. After being placed in a few foster homes, they moved in with their aunt. She had good intentions and loved the kids, but after a few years of escalating bickering and defiant behavior, she began to resort to frequent corporal punishment. When a teacher noticed a bruise on Jose's leg, the child welfare agency stepped in again. Eva and Jose were sad to leave their aunt, who had been kind and loving to them. They blamed themselves for the times she was violent with them, and (since no one explained otherwise to them) thought it must have been her choice to give them up.

> Try to talk to a variety of sources to best understand each youth and his or her unique needs. Become familiar with the adolescent's likes, strengths, resources, and connections (specific people, activities, groups, sports, school, and religious affiliation). Similarly, learn about the adolescent's triggers (what upsets him or her), warning signs (what he or she looks like before getting upset), and what works for the teen to "cool off."

> Kids are often not given much information about the reasons for removal, upcoming transitions, and their future placement, and in the absence of real information, youth make erroneous assumptions and blame themselves, feel lost and confused, and start to mistrust the "system."

For a while after being taken from their aunt, Jose and Eva, at the time just entering their young teen years, returned to live with their mother, who had completed a parenting class and passed a series of drug tests. But their mother quickly relapsed on drugs and alcohol and once again began inviting many men back to the apartment. When their mother was intoxicated or passed out, Jose was left in charge of the home and his younger sister. One of the men regularly took advantage of the mother's neglect and sexually forced himself on both Jose and Eva. The abuse occurred for several months, but Jose was ashamed and made Eva swear they would never discuss it. The helplessness he felt when being abused, the fear that it might make him gay, the anger at his mother's failure to protect them, his shame at not protecting his sister, and his intrusive thoughts and flashbacks of the abuse stayed with him long after the abuser disappeared. Eva was equally affected by the abuse, although rather than flashbacks or intrusive thoughts, she mostly felt numb. Even though the child welfare agency worker continued to monitor them, neither child disclosed the abuse or their mom's relapse. It was not until their mother failed a drug test and then refused to attend treatment that the court removed Jose and Eva again, this time with police officers bursting in and arresting their mother in front of them.

Over the next year, 14- and 15-year-old Eva and Jose bounced from foster home to foster home, with frequent psychiatric hospitalizations for aggressive behavior (Jose) or for running away and alcohol and marijuana use (Eva). Eva and Jose returned home around the time they turned 15 and 16. Jose spent most of his time on the street, which despite the violence and gang conflicts felt more predictable than home. Eva mostly stayed in her room. It was only a few days later that Jose got blackout drunk, assaulted Eva, and was arrested.

After reviewing all of this background, Ms. Brown chats for a few minutes with Mr. Fields, the juvenile justice officer she had observed playing basketball with Jose. Mr. Fields reflects that youth like Jose "go through a lot of bad stuff before coming in here, and they continue to experience the trauma once they get in here." He adds, "Jose won't tell you or show you, but you can see he is scared as hell inside. I don't blame him; I'm scared too in here sometimes, and I wear a badge and go home at night." Ms. Brown imagines the constant humiliating searches, roll calls, yelling, fighting, isolation, lack of privacy, and guilt that Jose endures in the hall.

Asking Why: How Trauma Affects Youth in Child Welfare and Juvenile Justice

Traumatized youth who enter foster care or juvenile justice are often mistreated by the very systems that are established to help them. When youth are placed in foster care, removal from home often involves child protection (and possibly police) surprising the family in the middle of the night and taking children from their beds. Children are given little understanding of why or where they are going, so foster care can be confusing and frightening to children even if foster parents are kind and understanding. Rates of abuse in foster care are high—studies suggest that there is 3 times more physical abuse and 2–4 times more sexual abuse in foster homes than in the general population.[12] Group homes have more than 10 times the rate of physical abuse and more than 28 times the rate of sexual abuse compared with the general population. Sometimes youth in care abuse each other, but often adults are the perpetrators; in some studies nearly one-third of foster children reported being abused by a foster parent or other adult while in foster care.[12] Equally damaging is the way in which youth in foster care and juvenile justice systems are often judged and stigmatized based on their behaviors and symptoms. The staff, social workers, and therapists working with them often forget that these teens have a history of abuse or trauma, and see only their negative behaviors and "bad attitude." Untreated mental illness further contributes to these behavioral issues; 85% of youth in child welfare who need mental health treatment do not get it,[13] and juvenile justice facilities similarly fail to address the mental health needs of youth. Poor attachment to caregivers can also increase the risk of gang involvement. For many young boys with absent fathers growing up in gang-infested neighborhoods, thugs are their only male role models, and the gang gives an opportunity for connection, safety, money, and status. Once in the gang, it can be difficult to leave these connections (and the pain of being jumped out and removing tattoos is an additional deterrent). When Mr. Fields, the juvenile justice guard, asks Jose why he joined a gang, the teen is quick to reply, "I don't need no one to take care of me. I gots 40 of my boys with me, and I get quick cash moneys."

Even if mental health treatment is available, foster parents, social workers, corrections officers, and judges may not connect a youth's problem behaviors or criminal offenses to mental illness. If a youth is referred for treatment, the information about his or her experiences of abuse and trauma may not be provided to the treatment provider, who therefore hears only about the youth's scary behaviors. The more *intense* the behavior, the more it becomes adults' main point of reference when forming an opinion about the adolescent. The older the adolescent and the scarier the behavior, the more likely it is that adults will fail to see the connection between the behavior and the past traumas and current stressors that contribute to it. These maladaptive behaviors lead the adolescents to being labeled, stigmatized, misdiagnosed, and at times overmedicated. As youth like Jose and Eva age, they are viewed as "failing" foster care. Adults begin to look to the psychiatric hospital or juvenile detention to "fix" them, or for residential programs (within the foster care or mental health system) to "put them somewhere safe." This leads to costly services such as residential facilities and overutilization of psychotropic medications and psychiatric emergency services. It is not only adults who see them as "unplaceable" or ungovernable; this view is also shared by Eva and Jose. Each independently says to Ms. Brown, "No offense, miss, but you can't take care of me. I'm crazy."

> Considering the teens' complex history, Ms. Brown is careful in how she approaches Eva and Jose. She understands that the rejection, abandonment, and neglect they experienced must have been confusing and painful and that the fear of future rejection and disappointment drives their hostile exteriors. She also knows that they have opened up to rare adults in the past, so she is strategic and persistent in approaching them. She opens up the conversation by explaining her role. She casually drops to each youth that she has heard about his or her strengths, letting Eva know she heard from a teacher about her excellent creative writing, while relaying to Jose that the guard she spoke to, Mr. Fields, bragged about Jose's maturity and respectful manners. Both kids shrug off this information, but Ms. Brown notices minute shifts: a drop of the shoulders for Eva, a softening of the jaw for Jose. She is not forceful and respects Eva's and Jose's silence and distance. She is

honest about her limitations, but informs them of what steps she has taken, such as keeping each sibling updated on how the other is doing, finding a creative seminar for Eva, and talking to the guard about getting Jose extra access to the basketball gym. She asks about their goals and needs, although it takes a few more meetings before Eva and Jose open up.

> Youth in child welfare and juvenile justice often feel lost in the system. Make the adolescents feel welcome and safe with you. Orient them to your role and explain what's going to happen, what you know and what you don't know, and what you can control and what you can't. Be reassuring without making promises you can't keep or providing false hope.

"I don't have any friends. People don't get me," states Eva. On the other hand, Jose's approach to relationships is that of an abused alpha dog, more about asserting an "on-top" position than any real closeness. Both of them bring up independently that they don't know anything about their father, other than that he has never made any efforts to love them or locate them. When Ms. Brown asks about visits with their mom, Eva shrugs while Jose murmurs a desire to see her, saying, "She'll always be my moms, no matter what, I guess…." Ms. Brown is surprised that Jose continues to idealize his mom after she has missed countless scheduled visitations that she promised to attend and repeatedly failed to protect them (or even believe them when Eva disclosed the sexual abuse she experienced). Both kids express a sense of regret at having "messed up" their placement with their aunt, with whom they felt safe and cared for.

> Recognize the adolescent's courage for speaking up about the abuse or neglect. There are many reasons why children and adolescents keep silent about abuse: not being sure if what they were experiencing is indeed abuse; fear of retaliation if they disclose the abuse; fear of breaking up the family or upsetting other family members; believing that the abuser is still loving; believing things will change over time; fear that adults won't believe them; and fear of going into foster care. Even after speaking up, even if they are now safe, adolescents often still feel guilt and ambivalence about speaking up. Remind the adolescent that speaking up was the right decision and it took courage to do so. Remind them why they spoke up: to protect themselves and their siblings, and to stand up against something wrong.

With the case records and records from various hospitalizations, Ms. Brown is able to piece together that the kids' behavior in their aunt's home worsened after their mom was granted visitation. Reading about their tantrums and destructive behaviors after these visits, and the lack of support or services at the time, Ms. Brown can empathize with how their aunt lost it and resorted to corporal punishment. Talking to Eva and Jose, she is struck by how being removed from their aunt left them with a sense of being damaged and unparentable. Eva tells Ms. Brown about a moment years ago when, in the back seat of the social worker's car en route to another foster home, she turned to her brother and asked, "Is this our fault?" Jose didn't answer, but Eva says she saw tears slowly falling down his cheeks, the first time she'd ever seen him cry. Hearing this story, Ms. Brown listens quietly and replies, "No, it was not your fault."

> "It's not your fault." Say it. Explain it. Mean it. Adolescents do not enter the child welfare system by choice, but self-blame and guilt can permeate youths' thoughts after the removal or rejection, especially when they are unsure or uncertain about the reason for the removal and unclear about the next steps. Not only is this self-blame inaccurate and unfair, but it also undermines future relationships and placements.

In foster care Eva and Jose felt like "no one could handle us" and spent each placement waiting for the inevitable rejection. With each new placement they both desperately tried not to get kicked out once again, but the pressure was so great that it made them crack. Finally they began to "sabotage" their placements, acting up early on, consciously or unconsciously, forcing foster parents to reject them rather than risk becoming too comfortable or attached.

Behaviors in Context: Understanding and Connecting With Traumatized Youth

Eva is now living with a new foster family but she feels alone. She misses her mother's home, particularly the smell of her mother cooking tortas and tamales. Yet she despises her mother, who, when Eva mustered the courage to disclose her earlier sexual abuse by her mother's "man friend," said Eva must be making it up. Similarly, she is upset with Jose but misses him dearly and is confused about what happened, repeatedly telling Ms. Brown, "He is the only one who has my back and really gets me." Jose also misses his sister, though he never talks about it. He presents a callous attitude, to hide the intense shame and guilt he feels about assaulting Eva; admitting his real feelings would make him too vulnerable in front of the correctional officers and his peers. But slowly and in small ways, he starts to open up to Ms. Brown and Mr. Fields, the guard who spoke well of Jose before, though he still blows off his therapist and grandstands in front of the judge. Ms. Brown struggles to understand why Jose seems to purposefully sabotage these key moments that could help him get out of detention. What she doesn't realize is how the demanding tone of the judge and the forced empathy of the therapist both make Jose feel like everything is his fault. Blowing off these meetings makes Jose feel in control and powerful, at least for a moment.

Posttraumatic symptoms and stress reactions can make it difficult for teens (or adults) to participate effectively in the court processes of both the foster care and juvenile justice systems. Youth may be asked to confront their abuser in court, to speak in front of their family about their abuse, or to take responsibility for crimes they committed. Recognize how avoidance, trauma triggers, flashbacks, anger, and other symptoms can get in the way of youth participating in the legal process, and help youth prepare and plan in advance for how they can regroup if they are triggered or upset in court. Talk to their lawyers and judges to help them understand how trauma can impact the youth's symptoms and behavior in the courtroom.

Youth in foster care and juvenile justice frequently struggle with unspoken and unbearable feelings of guilt, shame, and self-blame. Both Jose and Eva use defiance and avoidance to defend against these feelings, not to mention the flashbacks, trauma reminders, and ongoing stress and helplessness of life in foster care. When internal avoidance fails, Eva turns to marijuana or thinks about running away or suicide as an escape. Jose takes control of every situation, posturing that he is ready to "throw down" in any situation (be it at school or in front of the judge), nonchalantly walking out of the mall with the new red sneakers his foster mother kept promising but never bought for him, letting it be known that he ain't no sucker, and taking what he wants from women (even his sister) to demonstrate dominance. Maladaptive behaviors in youth in foster care and juvenile justice are often best understood as a child's best learned attempts to cope with painful feelings and survive in an unpredictable, chaotic environment while being flooded by memories of prior traumas and triggered by new abuses.

Understand the traumatized adolescent's disruptive, defiant, avoidant, and/or criminal acts in the context of his or her past traumatic experiences. Ask yourself, "Why might this kid be angry, upset, distrustful of adults, or resistant to authority?" or "Where does this behavior come from?" Current behaviors have been learned over time and are influenced by past and current events. Rather than asking, "What's wrong with this kid?" ask yourself, "Why would this teen engage in such risky behavior, defiant behavior, or unsafe behavior?" Adolescents use adaptive and maladaptive coping strategies as they learned them and because they helped them survive past hard times, current trauma reminders, unpleasant feelings, and unwanted thoughts. These strategies, even if problematic in the long term, served them well in the moments of fear, rejection, abuse, and chaos that happen when being abused. Asking a young person to give up what worked and try something new is asking a lot. Teach, model, and have the youth rehearse new adaptive coping skills. Expect that it will take much practice before the new skills stick, and that the youth will go back to tried-and-true strategies when faced with significant stress.

(For more on identifying trauma triggers and trauma reminders, understanding the role of maladaptive coping skills, and replacing those with the use of adaptive coping skills, see the discussion of Trauma-Focused Cognitive Behavioral Therapy [TF-CBT] and Skills Training in Affective and Interpersonal Regulation [STAIR] in Chapter 7, "Trauma and Psychosis," and Tables 2-1 and 2-2 in Chapter 2, "Recognition and Treatment.")

Jose, for example, learned while growing up that he had to remain continuously on guard at all times to protect himself and his sister. He did so without the influence of positive role models, educational support, and appropriate mental health services. He frequently shares with Ms. Brown that he can't trust anyone else to protect them, and that the largely disengaged, burned-out adults he has interacted with in "the system" have made him feel more alone and unwanted. What he doesn't share with Ms. Brown is how ashamed he feels that he failed to protect himself and his sister from the man who abused them, and that he himself hurt his sister. Ms. Brown wonders about this but avoids talking to him about what happened with his sister, wondering how he could do such a thing to the one person who has been on his side all along. Experts have reached different conclusions to explain how victimized youth may in turn victimize others. Probably different victimized youth can become perpetrators in different ways; the behaviors may be about reenacting past abuse, asserting control, preferring to be the offender rather than the victim, not knowing how to connect emotionally due to poor emotional and physical boundaries, or seeing abuse as a normative way of interacting or getting their needs met.

It can be difficult for therapists, case workers, and others to find the time and emotional bandwidth to understand deeply traumatized youth as more than their behaviors. Such work is made more difficult because youth are often resistant to connecting with new adults; this is a form of the PTSD symptom of avoidance—avoiding closeness, avoiding feelings of weakness or vulnerability, and avoiding dependency because the fear of disappointment or abandonment is too great. But it is critical that adults working with traumatized teens persist past this resistance to find a way to connect, because engagement is fundamental to assessment and treatment.[14] Faced with a large caseload, Ms. Brown struggles to find the time to put together all these details about Jose and Eva, but she knows if she doesn't try to understand them, she'll never be able to help them. Understanding the context for their behaviors does not excuse them—particularly Jose's sexual aggression and violence—but it places those behaviors in a larger context of atrocities and unmet needs. When one considers the teens' multiple traumatic experiences (including but not limited to having no father figure, living with their substance-abusing mother, experiencing both domestic violence and physical and sexual abuse, multiple removals from home, and rejections from mother and foster parents), ongoing stress (failing school, living in a juvenile justice facility, separation from each other and from their mother), and underdeveloped self-control and emotion regulation skills, it is more understandable that Eva and Jose continue to behave in ways that jeopardize their placements and chances to move on. Ms. Brown makes the point of holding in mind and sharing this fuller picture (leaving sensitive information out) when speaking to Jose and Eva and with the adults who are making decisions for them (teachers, guards, therapists, judges, foster parents). Slowly, Jose and Eva start to realize that Ms. Brown might see them differently and that she might be fighting for them.

> When working with juveniles who have offended, attempt to view the adolescent as a whole person rather than just the offense. That is, rather than thinking, "Oh yeah, that's the teen who robbed the store," consider, "This kid lost his father at age 2; because his mom was an addict, he took care of his three younger sisters; he writes pretty good slam poetry; and he got arrested last week for robbery." Humanize each youth. Find good to see in each youth.

Treating More Than Just Behavior: Finding Trauma-Informed Treatment Within Child Welfare and Juvenile Justice

As Eva starts to open up more and more, Ms. Brown starts to realize that Eva's ongoing flashbacks, poor self-esteem, and substance abuse are more than Ms. Brown can address on her own. She starts to talk to Eva about participating in therapy, specifically trauma-informed therapy. Eva is at first resistant, but Ms. Brown is patient and understands Eva's hesitation to open up to another stranger. Thinking back to the motivational interviewing training she attended the previous year, Ms. Brown tries to tap into Eva's intrinsic motivation toward change while using a nonconfrontational or directive approach. She reassures Eva that therapy is not for "crazy people" and is not focused only on talking about the past, but rather is about finding ways to move on and build a better future. She assures Eva that she can assume the driver seat and set her own goals of therapy. Eva is hesitant, but when Ms. Brown helps her reflect on how their own conversations have been helpful, Eva agrees to try (especially when Ms. Brown promises to attend the first session with her).

> Become familiar with mental health agencies that provide trauma-informed and evidence-based treatments for adolescents (and their caregivers). Be clear with teens about why you think therapy would be helpful, and how. Include messages such as "Therapy is temporary"; "If you are in therapy, it doesn't mean you are 'psycho' or 'crazy'"; and "You get to choose what you want to work on." Help the teen understand that treatment should be on his or her terms, so if the teen doesn't like the therapist or approach, he or she can ask for something different rather than just dropping out.

Ms. Brown finds a therapist who treats adolescents and is trained in TF-CBT. With Eva's permission, Ms. Brown speaks to the therapist in advance to share some of Eva's history and, more importantly, the strengths Ms. Brown has come to see in Eva. In the initial meeting, the therapist shares some of the good things she has heard from Ms. Brown and says that she is looking forward to working with Eva, even though she gets nothing more than a shrug from Eva in return. Next, the therapist normalizes typical responses to traumatic experiences and how such experiences and responses can make trusting others in relationships tough. Some of what she hears seems to resonate with Eva, though she still shrugs when the therapist asks what Eva hopes to get out of treatment. The therapist describes the usual plan for treatment, and assures Eva that discussing difficult events from the past will only happen after they have built trust and practiced skills to reduce Eva's painful symptoms, and only when Eva feels ready to do so. Later, in the car driving back to Eva's foster home, Ms. Brown asks Eva what she thought. Eva shrugs, then after a long silence expresses surprise that the therapist did not judge her or push her about drug use or risky sex. Eva also adds, "It makes it easier that she already knows some of my story."

> Treatment is important, but it's also very valuable to help teens stay connected to anything positive that they have going on, whether it's a specific person (e.g., a teacher, a counselor, an older brother, a caseworker, an uncle, a former employer, a friend), a group of people, or an activity (e.g., sports, academics, after school, clubs, arts, religious group). Encourage them and help them with concrete steps (consent forms or permission slips) to stay connected. These positive things can serve as distraction, motivation, and connection, and make kids more resilient when things get hard.

Meanwhile, Ms. Brown struggles with how to refer Jose for mental health treatment when he is released from detention. She remembers from talking with Mr. Fields that the staff at the facility were trained with Think Trauma, and how that helped Mr. Fields understand how trauma can lead to maladaptive or criminal behaviors and why understanding and treating the trauma is important, and the training helped him connect with Jose.

> Think Trauma is a train-the-trainer full-day curriculum provided through the National Child Traumatic Stress Network (NCTSN) aimed at creating a trauma-informed setting through increasing staff's knowledge and behavioral modification, in addition to making cultural and organizational paradigm shifts in juvenile justice residential facilities (see "Resources and Additional Reading" at the end of this chapter).

It's a hard sell to get Jose on board with treatment. Ms. Brown starts by talking to him about Mr. Fields. "Mr. Fields, he's my boy," Jose replies right away. Ms. Brown allows a silent moment to pass before Jose adds, "He never judged the things I've done. It's like he knows what I been through. Like without knowing all the fuck'd-up things that has happen to me, he helped me see that's part of why I keep getting in trouble, but like, not excusing my fuck'd-up behavior and not making me feel bad about it either, you know?" "Yes," Ms. Brown replies, "and what if I find you a therapist who can do just that—get you without judging you, help you without telling you what to do, connect you with things you like to do that will also help you get out of trouble, and might get the judge off your back—would you consider therapy then? Or even try it for a little while?" Jose shrugs but doesn't say no.

> Recognize and accept the adolescent's ambivalence about change or treatment by remaining warm, patient, accepting, and empathic. Use a nonjudgmental, non-confrontational, and nonadversarial approach to try to tap into the teen's intrinsic motivations for change.[15,16] If talking about substance abuse treatment, for example, you might say, "I hear you, man. The weed really relaxes you and gives you a break from thinking about what scary thing is going to happen next. At the same time, you are noticing that it's affecting your stamina on the basketball court. I wonder if there is anything else out there that could relax you and keep you fresh and keep your ball skills tight?"

Although Ms. Brown believes she has some momentum in getting Jose involved in therapy after his discharge, actually finding evidence-based treatment has been harder. She believes that Jose would benefit from a treatment similar to the one Eva is engaged in, but many outpatient programs that treat traumatized youth won't take juvenile offenders. Ms. Brown also feels pressure from the court to set up treatment, and knows that when her prior cases haven't had treatment, the teens have often ended up re-offending.

Mental health treatments for youth involved in the juvenile justice systems vary in many ways, including delivery method (individual, group, family, and/or systemic approaches), goal (increasing youth's remorse, responsibility taking, and prosocial future intentions; punishing the youth; restorative justice; and/or rehabilitative objectives), and the setting in which they are delivered (locked juvenile justice facility, nonsecure detention facility, group home, foster home, and/or the youth's family home).

Effective treatment for youth involved in juvenile justice should follow a few basic tenets. Often, youth who get involved in criminal behavior are those who are somehow vulnerable (youth who are impulsive or angry, have problems connecting with others, or are disconnected from their family due to abuse or from their school due to learning problems) and get pulled into criminal behavior as a way to engage socially or find money or safety. The criminal behavior then distances them even more from positive influences in their community and reinforces negative ways of solving problems or connecting with others. Treatment, then, should address all these areas and should be trauma informed and evidence based. It should focus on restoring healthy development, social functioning, and safety (both personal safety and safety of others), by engaging family and community supports and teaching the youth skills to use for managing anger and other painful emotions, navigating social conflicts or disagreements safely, managing anxiety and other posttraumatic symptoms, and making safer choices.

Most evidence-based treatments for juvenile offenders, such as Multisystemic Therapy (MST) and Functional Family Therapy (FFT), aim to "wrap around" the youth with intensive therapy, family treatment (which can occur either in the youth's family of origin or in a foster family, in the case of Multidimensional Treatment Foster Care), and outreach (see Chapter 3, "Aggression"). MST and FFT take a three-pronged approach[17]: First, the therapy team coordinates between families, probation officers, and the court to set clear expectations and contingencies around behavior (including curfews, substance use, contact with criminally involved or otherwise negative peer influences, and other behavioral targets) and thus create a safer environment for the teen. Second, the team works to get the youth more connected to school, prosocial activities, and family; the goal is to help youth gain positive self-esteem from healthy engagement in their community, be it repairing relationships with family members, reengaging with school or a new job, volunteering, or getting involved with sports or arts programs. Finally, intensive individual treatment provides a safe space to break down the teen's denial (because shame and fear of consequences often prevent youth from sincerely engaging) and to promote skill building. The therapist teaches, models, and supports the practice of specific skills for the teen to manage the emotional and behavioral problems caused by posttraumatic stress and to engage more safely and effectively in the world. Youth are taught how snap judgments and erroneous assumptions can lead to unhelpful beliefs and actions. The therapist then introduces skills for identifying and managing emotions, improving interpersonal communication and social problem solving, and, just as in evidence-based trauma treatments, recognizing and dealing with trauma reminders in the environment. The goal of skill building is to prevent becoming triggered, dysregulated, and/or re-offending. The therapist also engages youth in processing and understanding traumatic experiences and sharing those with trusted others, be it family members or a coach from their sports team.

> Check out the NCTSN Web site for a list of questions to take into account when considering what kind of treatment would be the best fit for youth involved in juvenile justice, and which treatments have been shown to be most effective, so you can see what is available in your area (see "Resources and Additional Reading" at the end of this chapter).

In thinking about treatment for Jose, Ms. Brown is also thinking about the upcoming transitions he faces: reentering the community, saying good-bye to Mr. Fields, and aging out of foster care when he turns 18. Although Jose insists he has mastered "rolling with the flow," and although youth like Jose can be eligible for ongoing support from child protective services after age 18 (if they agree to it, which Ms. Brown doubts Jose will), she knows what happens to most youth when they turn 18. Of the 20,000-plus youth who age out of foster care each year, 20% will be homeless, only 50% will be employed by age 24, and 70% of the females will be pregnant by age 21.[18,19,20] Ms. Brown believes that in addition to mental health treatment, Jose needs support through these transitions as well as positive connections to meaningful activity (e.g., a basketball team) to keep him from slipping back into gang life as a way to support himself when he ages out of care. It's the repetitive talks about connection and transition that finally have Jose agree to meet with a MST team. Ms. Brown thus speaks with Jose's MST therapy team about promoting connections to sports and other activities, and about helping Jose work toward his GED or vocational training so he has some work options outside of the gang.

Living in foster care can be painful and complicated, but transitions out of care are also difficult. Most families continue to provide some emotional (or even financial) support to their children after age 18, but for youth who have been living in foster care, turning 18 can mean a complete withdrawal of all of the support, structure, and resources. Youth may outwardly express excitement for their "freedom," but they often don't realize how difficult the transition will be, and many have little sense of how to support themselves financially or manage basic tasks such as budgeting or getting to work on time. Different states have different cutoffs in terms of how long adolescents or young adults can remain in foster care. On paper, a printed number states that a youth enters adulthood at age 18, 20, or 21, but in reality, most young adults may not possess the necessary maturity, resourcefulness, or know-how to access what they need. Therefore, therapists, psychiatrists, case workers, and the child welfare agencies need to take a more active role in preparing the youth for their future out of care.

It is the responsibility of service systems to prepare youth for their transitions out of the system, whether the youth are aging out of foster care, stepping down to a lower level of care, completing probation, or being reintegrated into society from a juvenile justice facility. These transitions are significant, create anxiety and confusion, and require preparation. Start the conversation early with the youth, agency, and caseworker. Consider job training, employment, and independent living. Consider transition to adult mental and medical services. Assist youth in securing identification, such as birth certificates, Social Security cards, and medical insurance cards, and finding strategies to keep these documents safe and organized. It can be helpful to ask the teen to practice navigating on his or her own (in small ways, with you there for support)—for example, by holding his or her own insurance card to show at a medical clinic appointment.

> Adolescents in both foster care and juvenile justice systems will experience multiple transitions and have to say good-byes. A tough teen is unlikely to admit to any anxiety about saying good-bye, but you can share your own sadness about saying good-bye to him or her, or normalize the anxiety by stating, "Saying good-bye can be hard, no matter how much you're used to it." The more you model appropriate goodbyes, the more likely the teen is to eventually open up about his or her feelings. Acknowledge that good-byes create mixed emotions—excitement and sadness, confusion and anxiety. You can offer to stay in touch if you're allowed to, or you can let the teen know that you're not allowed to maintain contact but that you'll be thinking of him or her.

Another resource for older youth in care, or those transitioning out of the system, is advocacy groups. Encourage adolescents to get involved in advocacy groups to help them find connection and purpose. Many youth who have been in the system feel a lot of anger, but they also have learned things that could help other youth going through these experiences. Getting involved in advocacy groups can help them to find a connection and a sense of purpose, and also can keep them involved with prosocial peers and supports. There are local, state, and national advocacy groups for youth and young adults who have been involved in both foster care and juvenile justice.

Resources and Additional Reading

Online Resources

American Academy of Pediatrics handouts for providers and families about working with youth in foster care: https://www.aap.org/en-us/advocacy-and-policy/aap-health-initiatives/healthy-foster-care-america/Pages/ResourceLibrary.aspx

National Child Traumatic Stress Network, Child Welfare Trauma Training Toolkit (2013): http://www.nctsn.org/products/child-welfare-trauma-training-toolkit-2008

National Child Traumatic Stress Network, Juvenile Justice: http://www.nctsn.org/resources/topics/juvenile-justice-system

National Child Traumatic Stress Network, Think Trauma: A Training for Staff in Juvenile Justice Systems: https://www.nctsn.org/resources/think-trauma-training-staff-juvenile-justice-residential-settings

Videos

Matanick N (producer): ReMoved Part 1 (2013): https://www.youtube.com/watch?v=lOeQUwdAjE0andt=6s

Matanick N (producer): Remember My Story—ReMoved Part 2 (2015): https://www.youtube.com/watch?v=I1fGmEa6WnYandt=496s

Matanick N, Kisiel C, Fehrenbach T: Remembering trauma, part 1 and 2: http://www.rememberingtrauma.org

Additional Reading

Beam C: To the End of June: The Intimate Life of American Foster Care, New York, Houghton Mifflin Harcourt, 2013

Lankford SM: Born, Not Raised: Voices From Juvenile Hall, San Diego, CA, Human Exposures Publishing, 2012

References

1. Friedersdorf C: In a year, child-protective services checked up on 3.2 million children. The Atlantic, July 22, 2014. Available at: https://www.theatlantic.com/national/archive/2014/07/in-a-year-child-protective-services-conducted-32-million-investigations/374809/. Accessed March 7, 2018.

2. U.S. Department of Health and Human Services, Administration for Children and Families, Administration on Children, Youth and Families, Children's Bureau: The AFCARS Report: preliminary FY 2011 estimates as of July 2012. No 19, 2012. Available at: http://www.acf.hhs.gov/sites/default/files/cb/afcarsreport19.pdf. Accessed March 7, 2018.

3. Wildeman C, Emanuel N: Cumulative risks of foster care placement by age 18 for U.S. Children, 2000–2011. PLos One 9(3):e92785, 2014, 24671254

4. U.S. Department of Health and Human Services, Administration for Children and Families, Administration on Children, Youth and Families, Children's Bureau: The AFCARS Report: preliminary FY1 2016 estimates as of October 20, 2017. No 24, 2017. Available at: http://www.acf.hhs.gov/sites/default/files/cb/afcarsreport24.pdf. Accessed March 7, 2018.

5. Children's Defense Fund: America's cradle to prison pipeline: a report of the Children's Defense Fund. October 2007. Available at: http://www.childrensdefense.org/library/data/cradle-prison-pipeline-report-2007-full-lowres.pdf. Accessed March 7, 2018.

6. Teplin LA, Abram KM, Washburn JJ, et al: Northwestern juvenile project. U.S. Department of Justice Office of Justice Programs Office of Juvenile Justice and Delinquency Prevention, February 2013. Available at: https://www.ojjdp.gov/pubs/234522.pdf. Accessed March 7, 2018.

7. Burton D, Foy D, Bwanausi C, et al: The relationship between traumatic exposure, family dysfunction, and post-traumatic stress symptoms in male juvenile offenders. J Trauma Stress 7(1):83–93, 1994 8044445

8. Steiner H, Garcia IG, Matthews Z: Posttraumatic stress disorder in incarcerated juvenile delinquents. J Am Acad Child Adolesc Psychiatry 36(3):357–365, 1997 9055516

9. Beck AJ, Cantor D, Hartge J, Smith T: Sexual victimization in juvenile facilities reported by youth, 2012. National Survey of Youth in Custody 2012. NCJ 241708. Washington, DC, Office of Justice Programs, Bureau of Justice Statistics, U.S. Dept of Justice, June 2013. Available at: https://www.bjs.gov/content/pub/pdf/svjfry12.pdf. Accessed March 7, 2018.

10. Dierkhising CB, Lane A, Natsuaki MN: Victims behind bars: a preliminary study on abuse during juvenile incarceration and post-release social and emotional functioning. Psychology, Public Policy, and Law 20(2):181–190, 2014

11. Mendel RA: No Place for Kids: The Case for Reducing Juvenile Incarceration. Baltimore, MD, Annie E. Casey Foundation, 2011

12. National Coalition for Child Protection Reform: Foster care vs. family prevention: the track record on safety and well being. Issue Paper 1, November 9, 2015. Available at: https://drive.google.com/file/d/0B291mw_hLAJsV1NU-VGRVUmdyb28/view. Accessed March 7, 2018.

13. Burns B, Phillips S, Wagner H, et al: Mental health need and access to mental health services by youths involved with child welfare: a national survey. J Am Acad Child Adolesc Psychiatry 43(8):960–970, 2004

14. Cook JM, Newman E: A consensus statement on trauma mental health: the New Haven Competency Conference process and major findings. Psychological Trauma: Theory, Research, Practice, and Policy 6(4):300–307, 2014

15. Miller WR, Rollnick S: Motivational Interviewing: Helping People Change, 3rd Edition. New York, Guilford, 2013

16. Rogers CR: Client-Centered Therapy: Its Current Practice, Implications, and Theory. Boston, MA, Houghton Mifflin, 1965

17. Borduin CM, Letourneau EJ, Henggeler SW, et al: Treatment Manual for Multisystemic Therapy With Juvenile Sexual Offenders and Their Families. Charleston, SC, Department of Psychiatry and Behavioral Sciences, Medical University of South Carolina, 2005

18. Courtney M, Dworsky A, Cusick G, et al: Midwest Evaluation of the Adult Functioning of Former Foster Youth from Illinois: Outcomes at Age 21. Chicago, IL, Chapin Hall Center for Children, 2007

19. Dworsky A, Courtney ME: The risk of teenage pregnancy among transitioning foster youth: implications for extending state care beyond age 18. Children & Youth Services Review 32(10):1351–1356, 2010

20. Pecora PJ, Kessler RC, O'Brien K, et al: Educational and employment outcomes of adults formerly placed in foster care: results from the Northwest Foster Care Alumni Study. Children & Youth Services Review 28(12):1459–1481, 2006

CHAPTER 13

Medical Providers

Alexis K. Yetwin, Ph.D.

At the end of a long day at her pediatric clinic, Dr. Bradley glances at her schedule and smiles. She feels a sense of relief when she sees the name of her last patient. Gabriela is a 16-year-old girl with a keen fashion sense who loves to compliment the doctor's shoes and educate her on the latest clothing trends and viral videos. She is a good student, behaves well at home (aside from the occasional mother-daughter conflict), and loves to go out with her friends. She is usually accompanied by her mother, a sweet woman who rarely voices concerns about her daughter. Gabriela has a history of asthma, but this has been well controlled, and she does not have any other significant medical concerns or allergies.

Dr. Bradley last saw Gabriela for her physical in June, at which time Gabriela informed her that chokers were making a comeback. She had been her usual vibrant, talkative self, and the physical exam was normal. Since that time, Gabriela's mother has called the office twice to seek consultation from a nurse, once about cold symptoms and once about stomach pain. The family did not schedule an office appointment either time, preferring to monitor the symptoms to see if they would resolve on their own.

Now it's mid-January, and Dr. Bradley feels something is amiss as soon as she enters the room. Gabriela is hunched over, her arms crossed over her stomach. She is quiet and her affect is sad. Her mother explains that for the past 6 months, Gabriela has experienced seemingly random bouts of stomach pain with nausea that can last for several days. Originally, the episodes were sporadic, and Gabriela was able to get through them in a couple of hours with heat packs and rest. Now the episodes last longer and are more frequent, and Gabriela has started to miss school. Gabriela has tried over-the-counter pain medications and changing her diet, but nothing helps. Last week the pain became so strong that they ended up in the ER, but the doctors could not find anything wrong (i.e., abdominal ultrasound was normal, urinalysis was negative).

271

During today's visit, Gabriela's medical exam is normal, and a review of systems is negative for fever, chills, runny nose, constipation, and diarrhea. She has occasional heartburn but does not feel that it's related to the abdominal pain. Gabriela reports a decreased appetite, especially when she is in pain; difficulty sleeping; nightmares; and occasional headaches.

The pain has kept Gabriela home from school seven times in the past 3 months, and she has had to leave school early on several other occasions due to the pain. The pain has also made it hard for her to concentrate on schoolwork. Her mother said that Gabriela seems fatigued at home and depressed. She has noticed that her daughter isn't spending as much time with her friends, which she attributes to the pain, but adds that Gabriela still seems to find time to see her boyfriend. Her mother grimaces as she mentions this, prompting Gabriela to quietly comment that she wishes her mother would be more accepting of him. When Dr. Bradley assesses for any recent changes or traumatic events in the family's life, Gabriela and her mother shake their heads. Dr. Bradley refers Gabriela to see a gastroenterologist and orders lab tests to obtain more information.

Given their intimate knowledge of their patients' lives, pediatricians and other medical providers are uniquely poised to recognize when youth have experienced trauma and to help traumatized teens and families. (Although the term "pediatricians" is used throughout this chapter, teens' medical providers might also be family medicine physicians, nurse practitioners, adolescent medicine specialists, and others.) Pediatricians are trained to scan for signs of concern, such as changes in sleep, eating, and toileting, that might signal that something stressful has occurred. Families turn to pediatricians for guidance on issues big and small and trust their pediatricians' expertise and commitment to their children. As such, pediatricians can play a vital role in helping families to understand how trauma can affect teens and connect them to the right kind of treatment.

It is also important for pediatricians and other medical providers to ask about trauma because traumatic stress can have a major impact on physical health. Evidence that childhood trauma can have long-term negative consequences for medical health came from the Adverse Childhood Experiences (ACE) study in 1998.[1] This landmark investigation was a collaboration between the Centers for Disease Control and Prevention (CDC) and Kaiser Permanente. A questionnaire was mailed to 13,494 adult patients who had completed a standardized medical evaluation at Kaiser Permanente San Diego Health Appraisal Clinic between 1995 and 1997; of these patients, 9,508 responded. The questionnaire asked questions about seven categories of adverse childhood experiences (ACEs): psychological abuse, physical abuse, sexual abuse, violence against a mother or stepmother, living with household members who engaged in substance abuse, living with a household member who had mental illness or was suicidal, and having a household member that has been incarcerated.

The ACE study found a graded relationship between the number of ACE categories a participant endorsed and all of the adult health risk behaviors and medical concerns studied.[1] In other words, the more types of trauma a person had experienced as a child, the higher the adult's risk was of having medical problems and engaging in risky behavior, such as alcoholism, drug abuse, sexually transmitted disease, and physical inactivity. Those participants who endorsed four or more ACE categories had a 12-fold increased risk of attempting suicide, were over 4 times as likely to be depressed, had a 7-fold increased risk of considering themselves to be alcoholics, were 2 times as likely to be smokers, had a 10-fold increased risk of having injected drugs, were 1.6 times as likely to be obese, and were 2.5 times as likely to have a sexually transmitted disease. There was also a dose-response relationship between the number of childhood exposures and ischemic heart disease, cancer, chronic bronchitis or emphysema, history of hepatitis or jaundice, skeletal fractures, and poor self-rated health.

The ACE study was so groundbreaking that most pediatricians and other medical providers now recognize that trauma can affect physical health. The trouble is that few adolescents walk into their annual physical and announce, "Here is the terrible thing that happened to me, and here are all the medical and psychological problems I'm having as a result." To find out which teens have been affected by traumatic experiences, pediatricians have to ask. The ACE study shows that pediatricians should ask not merely a single, general question about trauma but rather direct, closed-ended questions about abuse, trauma, and other specific stressors. For most pediatricians facing busy offices and overpacked clinic schedules, the idea of implementing trauma screening is daunting. Indeed, research shows that most pediatricians and medical providers don't ask patients about traumatic experiences in their past. Kerker et al.[2] examined data collected from the 2013 American Academy of Pediatrics (AAP) Periodic Survey, which contained questions about identifying adverse events in children. The survey asked experienced (nontrainee) pediatricians whether they asked patients about seven ACEs, similar to those in the original ACE study: maternal depression, parental separation/divorce, physical or sexual abuse, hostile/rejecting parenting by mothers, domestic violence exposure, parental alcohol/drug use, and an incarcerated relative. Of the 302 pediatricians surveyed, only 4% tended to ask about all seven ACEs and 32% usually failed to ask about any of them. Those who did screen for ACEs tended to inquire about maternal depression (46%) and parental separation or divorce (42%). Only one in nine of the pediatricians surveyed reported being very or somewhat familiar with the ACE study.

> When Dr. Bradley begins to write her note about Gabriela's appointment that afternoon, she reflects further on their time together. Although she still doesn't have all of the information about possible medical causes for Gabriela's current symptoms, she is bothered by how different Gabriela's presentation was from previous appointments. She seemed like a completely different kid. Dr. Bradley starts to wonder if something else is going on. Should she have asked more questions during the appointment or have been more specific? She makes a mental note to assess further at the next visit.

A similar investigation in Canada asked family medicine residents whether they ask patients about ACEs and why or why not.[3] Only 2 of the 112 residents reported screening for ACEs at the first visit, with a bias toward screening women more than men (6.3% screened women and 0.9% screened men). Although 80% of the residents believed it was their duty to assess for trauma, 65% said they did not feel confident about screening for ACEs and less than half said they had received formal medical training about screening. Many residents in the study felt they didn't have time to effectively evaluate and support patients who reported abuse, and several felt there was little they could do to help patients who had experienced traumatic stress.

Asking patients about current or prior trauma does not take a lot of time or skill. There are many resources, as discussed below, to help physicians and other medical providers screen for trauma, assess its impact, and connect youth to the right kind of help. Even if a pediatrics practice has mental health providers on staff, pediatricians should resist the temptation to fully delegate trauma screening to those providers. Adolescents are much more likely to be honest and open with the pediatrician they have known for years than with a social worker or psychiatrist whom they've never seen before. If the pediatrician can screen for and recognize the impact of traumatic stress on a young patient, and then talk to the family about recommended treatment, the family is much more likely to accept that recommendation because it comes from the physician they know and trust.

Another reason why pediatricians and other medical providers must consider the effects of trauma is that the medical setting itself can be traumatizing to patients. Medical traumatic stress may arise for any patient receiving medical care, whether the stress is caused by remembering a previously difficult medical procedure, the fear of being separated from parents during an x-ray, or anxiety about experiencing pain or other medical symptoms. With a trauma-informed approach, the medical team can have a better understanding of the family's re-

Pediatricians and other medical providers may not know how to ask patients about trauma. The AAP has created a Trauma Toolbox for Primary Care to educate and support clinicians in the primary care setting.[4] In one of the handouts, "Addressing Adverse Childhood Experiences and Other Types of Trauma in the Primary Care Setting," the AAP suggests a four-step process to help practices implement effective trauma screening, support, and resources. For practices that are overwhelmed by the idea of formal screening for childhood trauma, the AAP recommends a staged approach, such as initially asking about only one type of trauma or using a broad screening question (e.g., "Has anything really scary or upsetting happened to you or your family since I last saw you?"), followed by more specific questions as indicated.

action to the medical experience and avoid adding to their discomfort. The Center for Pediatric Traumatic Stress at The Children's Hospital of Philadelphia developed the D-E-F model[5] to help providers prevent and address medical traumatic stress in children and adolescents (https://www.healthcaretoolbox.org). According to the model, once medical providers have assessed for a patient's urgent medical needs (using A-B-C in Table 13–1), they should shift their attention to the patient's and family's emotional needs (D-E-F in Table 13–1). Implementation of the D-E-F model can help medical providers identify pediatric patients and families at risk for medical traumatic stress and then develop a plan with the medical team to provide appropriate psychosocial support and mental health resources.

Medical settings can be triggers for traumatic stress in youth with medical concerns, as well as in youth who have or are currently experiencing other types of traumatic events. The Health Care Toolbox Web site (see "Online Resources" at end of this chapter) has handouts for medical providers and for patients and families on how to cope with a child's illness, injury, and hospitalization. The Health Care Toolbox also provides case vignettes to give providers a better sense of how to apply the D-E-F model.[5] For health care providers who wish to learn more about pediatric medical trauma, the National Child Traumatic Stress Network created the Pediatric Medical Traumatic Stress Toolkit (see "Online Resources" at end of this chapter).

TABLE 13-1. A-B-C and D-E-F: Acronyms for assessing patient's physical and emotional health

A	Airway
B	Breathing
C	Circulation
D	reduce Distress
E	promote Emotional support
F	remember the Faith

Source.   https://www.healthcaretoolbox.org.

Over the next 6 months, Gabriela meets with a gastroenterologist on several occasions. Her blood tests (e.g., complete blood count, metabolic and liver panels, C-reactive protein, immunoglobulin E) are found to be normal, and an upper endoscopy reveals no significant pathological abnormalities. However, Gabriela is found to have a bacterial infection in her small intestine, which her gastroenterologist successfully treats with medication. After following the gastroenterologist's recommendations, including prescribed medications and increasing her fiber and water intake, Gabriela finds that she is having less frequent and less intense pain.

When Gabriela arrives for her physical in June, Dr. Bradley is pleased to hear of this improvement. However, Gabriela and her mother do not seem very happy. Gabriela's mother wonders why Gabriela's abdominal pain has not fully resolved and comments that the episodes continue to interfere with her ability to attend school and spend time with family and friends. Last week, they had to go to the ER again. Gabriela still appears sad and withdrawn, not the girl Dr. Bradley remembers. During a review of systems, Gabriela endorses continued difficulty sleeping, nightmares, headaches, difficulty concentrating in school, anxiety, and sadness. Given this constellation of symptoms and the persistence of chronic pain despite treatment, Dr. Bradley wonders if Gabriela has experienced a recent stress or traumatic experience. She knows that emotional distress can lead to somatic and behavioral complaints. She wonders if her patient has suffered abuse or trauma, even though her physical exam does not reveal any bruising or unexplained marks suggestive of abuse.

> The effects of trauma are not always visible. Be careful not to assume that the absence of physical evidence rules out trauma as an explanation for changes in behavior or functioning.

Asking Why: How Trauma Can Lead to Medical Problems

Because teens rarely start a pediatric office visit with a disclosure of trauma, pediatricians and other medical providers need to be alert for common physical or psychological symptoms. The first signs that a patient may have experienced trauma often emerge during a review of systems. Trauma stimulates the brain's reticular activating system, leading to sleep dysfunction; inhibits the satiety center in the hypothalamus, leading to changes in appetite; and increases sympathetic tone and catecholamines, causing anxiety, constipation, encopresis, and/or enuresis.[6] Gabriela's review of systems was positive for decreased appetite and for sleep problems, including frequent nightmares. Nightmares should be further probed, because they can provide clues about possible trauma. A clinician could explore by asking teens whether they are having the same nightmare repeatedly or different ones, whether the nightmares are related to something that has happened to them or something they have seen (although trauma-related nightmares may not match the traumatic event), and when the nightmares began or became more frequent or intense.

Trauma causes toxic stress. As discussed in Chapter 1 ("Teens and Traumatic Stress"), toxic stress affects the brain, and it similarly affects the body. The stress response is designed to protect people by fueling the fight-or-flight response through physical and chemical changes, but ongoing stress is detrimental to emotional and physical health. When a stressor is too intense or chronic, the brain and body become fatigued, and this can cause a range of physical symptoms, including sleep problems, stomachaches, eating disturbances, and physical pains, as well as anxiety, isolation, and irritability.

The gastrointestinal system in particular is very sensitive to stress. Stress heightens a person's awareness of sensations in his or her stomach and can lead to nausea, "butterflies," pain, or vomiting. Stress also affects appetite and digestion, which can cause constipation, diarrhea, acid reflux, and/or heartburn.[7] Additionally, stress increases contractions in the colon, leading to diarrhea.[8]

The AAP advocates for use of an ecobiodevelopmental model in understanding how toxic stress impacts children and then leads to poor health outcomes in adulthood.[9] This model proposes that early experiences and environmental influences (even prenatal stress) affect the expression and activation of genes. Environmental influences are not exclusively negative; a relationship with a supportive adult can buffer the effects of stress, as the child is provided with guidance and support in navigating the stressors. However, in the absence of a supportive adult relationship in times of stress, it is hard for a child to deactivate his or her stress response. Traumatic stress can lead to hypertrophy (enlargement) of the amygdala, the brain's fear center, and a chronically activated stress response, which can cause chronic anxiety. Persistent or severe stress is also associated with decreased neurons and neuronal connections in the hippocampus and prefrontal cortex, which explains deficits in executive functioning, impulse control, and memory in children who have endured toxic or traumatic stress.

In addition to performing physical exams and reviews of systems, pediatricians and other medical providers should take stock in their behavioral observations of teenage patients, because these may highlight additional clues of trauma or prolonged stress. Females, young children, children with ongoing trauma or pain, and children unable to defend themselves tend to display detachment, numbing, compliance, and fantasy. Males, older children, witnesses to violence, and people able to fight or flee tend to exhibit hypervigilance, aggression, anxiety, and exaggerated responses.[6] Gabriela has already endorsed anxiety, and further screening by Dr. Bradley reveals social withdrawal as well.

Pediatricians typically inquire about a patient's academic functioning, and they should keep in mind that difficulty in school could signal potential trauma. Either recently experienced trauma or chronic, complex, ongoing trauma can impact an adolescent's working memory, inhibitory control, and cognitive flexibility. These problems can be demonstrated as trouble staying organized or on top of schoolwork; difficulty learning a complex task that involves rapid interpretation of information, such as driving; and problems with authority. Gabriela mentioned poor concentration in class and decreased school attendance.

Recalling that the family denied recent traumatic events during their January appointment, Dr. Bradley wonders if she failed to thoroughly assess for emotional distress and possible trauma, abuse, or new stressors. She decides to provide some psychoeducation about the body's response to stress in order to provide a framework for her question about traumatic events.

Dr. Bradley says, "When I saw Gabriela in January, she was also experiencing depressive symptoms, sleep problems, and appetite concerns. She was missing school and not spending much time with friends and family, but it all seemed to be related to her abdominal pain. Since treating her bacterial infection, we have seen some improvement in her pain, but the other symptoms have persisted and it's important for us to consider all possible explanations. Sometimes we see these issues arise when a person is experiencing stress, as the body gears up for 'fight or flight.' If a tiger walked into this room right now, your brain would alert your body to get up and climb on top of the table or run out of the room. And to do this, your heart rate would increase and other bodily rhythms would become activated. The stress response is protective because it alerts us to possible danger. However, too much stress can cause problems with sleep, eating, and other areas of life." Dr. Bradley pauses to let this sink in for a moment and then continues: "Has there been anything stressful or scary that has occurred in Gabriela's or the family's life recently? Any big changes, like a move?" After the family continues to deny recent stressors, Dr. Bradley asks more specific questions about abuse: "Has Gabriela ever experienced any kind of abuse, neglect, or a physical or sexual assault? Has she witnessed domestic violence or violence in the community?" pausing after each question to give Gabriela and her mother time to respond.

> Although time is a precious commodity in the medical field, spending a few extra minutes to ensure that your patient's family understands your questions about possible trauma is critical. Providing an explanation for this sensitive line of questioning can disarm families and help them appreciate your thoroughness instead of becoming defensive and feeling that you are dismissing the teen's medical complaints as "all in the head." It will also make it easier to ask more direct questions about specific types of trauma.

Gabriela's mother is unable to think of any recent stressors but reports that Gabriela witnessed domestic violence when she was young. She says that Gabriela's biological father was emotionally and physically abusive toward her, though she tried to shield Gabriela from it. She tells Dr. Bradley that Gabriela does not currently have a relationship with her father, who was deported to Mexico when she was age 7. Gabriela's mother notes that Gabriela has a great relationship with her stepfather, who has taken on the role of being her father. While her mother speaks, Gabriela shifts uncomfortably in her seat and looks down at the floor.

> Gabriela's mother was forthcoming with information about her previous history of domestic violence. But not all caregivers will be as open about their experiences, especially if they are still involved in an abusive relationship. The AAP has provided a comprehensive report offering guidance to pediatricians on how to effectively assess for intimate partner violence and offer appropriate support to affected families.[10]

Emotional abuse and neglect can be just as devastating as sexual or physical abuse.[11,12] Data analyzed from the Lehigh Longitudinal Study found that child abuse and domestic violence both increase a child's risk for engaging in internalizing behaviors (e.g., anxiety, depression) or externalizing behaviors (e.g., aggression or delinquency) in adolescence.[13] Domestic violence exposure was significantly related to withdrawal behavior, depression, and delinquency and predictive of total internalizing behaviors and symptoms of anxiety and depression. Like all traumatic experiences, intimate partner violence is more common than one might assume. One in four women and one in seven men will experience severe physical violence (e.g., being slammed against something, a suffocation attempt) by an intimate partner during their lifetime.[14]

Symptoms in Context: Recognizing, Understanding, and Connecting With Traumatized Youth

It can be hard to differentiate between a moody teenager and an adolescent in danger. As the National Institute of Mental Health[15] explains, the teenage brain is "still under construction" and does not fully develop until early adulthood. Teenagers feel physically and intellectually fit but lack impulse control. Additionally, functional brain imaging studies have shown that adolescents respond more strongly to emotions than do adults or younger children. (No one who has ever been or met an adolescent will be surprised by this, but it is nonetheless remarkable to see the difference in functional magnetic resonance images of their brains.) Adolescence is also a time of significant hormonal change in the areas of reproduction and response to stress, which adds to teens' complexity.

> Dr. Bradley thanks Gabriela's mother for sharing information about her past, explaining that it helps her to understand what the family has been through and how best to support them. Dr. Bradley then requests to meet privately with Gabriela for the remainder of the appointment, as Dr. Bradley always does with teenagers.[16] After Gabriela's mother has left, Dr. Bradley conducts a brief HEEADSSS 3.0 assessment (see Table 13–2) to further explore possible stressors that could be contributing to Gabriela's symptoms.

The original HEADSS assessment was expanded in 2014 to account for additional issues faced by adolescents from using social media[17,18,19] The new version, HEEADSSS 3.0 (Table 13–2), includes additional questions on eating and safety from injury and violence and advocates for a strength-

---

TABLE 13–2. HEEADSSS 3.0

H	Home environment
E	Education and employment
E	Eating
A	peer-related Activities
D	Drugs
S	Sexuality
S	Suicide/depression
S	Safety from injury and violence

---

based approach, because assessments focused solely on risk factors can worsen shame and disengagement. Tips on using the HEEADSSS, including sample questions and recommendations on how to review the limits of confidentiality, are available online (http://www.modernmedicine.com/tag/heeadsss-30-and-sshadess).

> Even adolescents who report being close with their parents or caregivers should be given the opportunity to meet privately with a health professional, to ensure a more accurate and open level of communication about health concerns. Some teens won't share even benign reports, such as increased caffeine intake, in the presence of a parent. One study found that when meeting with providers in the presence of a caregiver, adolescents reported less panic disorder, posttraumatic stress disorder (PTSD), drug use and disorder, and suicidal behavior.[16]

In her individual meeting with Dr. Bradley, Gabriela denies any substance use, noting that her biological father was an alcoholic and she does not want to be like him. She is sexually active but is knowledgeable about safe sex practices and uses condoms consistently. Gabriela continues to deny current stressors or previous abuse but notes some distress related to a recent fight with her boyfriend, who felt she was not spending enough time with him. This is what is making her feel anxious and sad today, she shares, but she didn't want to say this in her mother's presence because her mother does not approve of her boyfriend and would just say "I told you so." Gabriela endorses passive feelings of suicidal ideation, specifically moments when she feels that "it's all too much," but denies wanting to hurt herself. She confirms that she does get along well with her mother and stepfather. During the interview, she frequently checks her phone and apologizes, explaining that she does not want her boyfriend to think she is ignoring him. Dr. Bradley wonders to herself whether this is a healthy relationship, but is unsure if Gabriela would be able to accurately assess this if asked.

After meeting with Gabriela alone, Dr. Bradley invites her mother to rejoin them and engages both of them in conversation about Gabriela's treatment. Chronic pain can be stressful, Dr. Bradley begins, especially since Gabriela has had to undergo many tests and exams and the pain still hasn't gone away. She further explains that stress makes pain worse, and pain is stressful, creating a "vicious cycle." One of the most helpful ways to combat pain is to learn relaxation skills, she says. She recommends that Gabriela begin psychotherapy to learn tools to manage stress and thereby reduce pain. She also notes that people can find psychotherapy helpful for processing prior or currently challenging and threatening experiences.

As she speaks, Dr. Bradley notices Gabriela's shoulders tighten and her face darken. She pauses to let Gabriela speak. After a moment, Gabriela responds, "I don't need therapy. I'm not crazy. I'm just sick. That's what I keep trying to tell people. It's not 'all in my head' like they said in the ER."

"I'm sorry they made you feel that way. I definitely don't think that and I don't want to make you feel that way," Dr. Bradley offers with a kind smile. "Our brains and bodies are connected, which is why pain and stress can create that vicious cycle." She continues to explain how pain can lead to stress and how extended periods of stress can have effects on one's brain and body. Dr. Bradley points out that although therapy is often stigmatized, in reality anyone can benefit from having someone listen to his or her concerns and suggest tools on how to manage stress and difficult events, including physical illnesses. "I also want to make sure we keep meeting to monitor your physical symptoms and your physical health, and to make sure the therapy is helping."

Gabriela's body language softens as Dr. Bradley speaks. After receiving encouragement from her mother to give it a try, Gabriela agrees to meet with a therapist. She makes a point of telling Dr. Bradley that she's still not sure it's for her but she wants to feel better and will see if it helps. Dr. Bradley then provides Gabriela and her mother with a list of therapists in the area that she trusts.

Two weeks later, Gabriela and her mother are sitting in the waiting room of Dr. Perez, one of the therapists from Dr. Bradley's list. Gabriela is still unsure whether this will really help her feel better, but her mother insisted given how down Gabriela has been feeling lately. Dr. Perez initially meets with Gabriela and her mother together, reviewing the limits of confidentiality and obtaining a brief history. Then Dr. Perez meets with Gabriela alone. They start with lighthearted topics, Dr. Perez admiring Gabriela's bright manicure and asking about the novel she had been reading in the waiting area. Gabriela is open and engaged, but constantly checks her phone. She apologizes to Dr. Perez for having to respond to text messages so as not to worry her boyfriend. As Gabriela becomes more comfortable with Dr. Perez over the next few sessions, she talks more about the boyfriend and confides that although she loves him, the relationship is a source of stress.

There are several forms and handouts that clinicians can access for free online that will help families take the next steps in supporting their children after leaving the medical office. The AAP's Visit Discharge and Referral Summary for Family (see "Online Resources" at the end of this chapter) provides the family with a summary of the child's trauma type, trauma symptoms, medical and developmental concerns, and recommendations for treatment. The form has checkboxes, making it efficient to complete, and it serves as a helpful reminder for the clinician of what to do, such as providing a family with a handout about parenting strategies or making a referral for a psychiatric evaluation. Pediatricians are encouraged to gather a list of resources that can be made readily available to families, thus increasing efficiency in the appointment and facilitating linkage to mental health services.

She says that her boyfriend is the only one who really understands her because, like her, he doesn't have a close relationship with his biological father and knows what this feels like. She explains away his possessiveness as a reaction to a previous relationship in which his ex-girlfriend cheated, and it doesn't help that her closest friends are guys. Her girlfriends don't seem to trust him, but she thinks they are just jealous. Her parents don't like him, but Gabriela thinks they would react this way toward anyone she dated. She and her boyfriend have been fighting more recently, but Gabriela feels it is all her fault, because she did things that she knows upset him. Gabriela tries hard to appear confident in her statements, although her voice wavers and she has trouble maintaining eye contact as she speaks.

When meeting with an adolescent, observe the adolescent's body language, especially when assessing for possible stressors or mental health concerns. Teens may be guarded with their responses, so look for clues in affect, body language, and reaction to caregivers and providers.

In the age of reality TV and social media, teenagers are especially susceptible to misinformation about healthy relationships. Supposed "real-life" depictions of intimate relationships are heavily filtered and edited to produce a desired story line. Abuse and violence by entertainment and sports stars and even politicians are portrayed as normal. When people in high positions have been abusive or make disparaging comments about those reporting abuse, adolescents are left wondering what constitutes abuse and whether they will be believed if they report it. Adolescents in abusive relationships are often scared to tell family and friends. They may feel they are to blame for the abuse, which causes shame, or feel that it was justified. If family or friends express concern about these relationships, adolescents' desire to be independent from their parents and align with their peers may skew their perception of these concerns.

> A month after referring her patient for psychotherapy, Dr. Bradley calls Dr. Perez to see how Gabriela is doing. Because Gabriela's mother had signed a release for the two physicians to talk, Dr. Perez shares her concern that Gabriela, like many teens in her practice, has been dealing with an unhealthy and abusive relationship. Dr. Bradley reflects that an abusive relationship could explain the recent somatic and behavioral changes she has seen in Gabriela, because medical tests have revealed very few answers. Dr. Perez agrees that the stress of the relationship has affected Gabriela's behavior, mood, and physical health. Dr. Bradley is surprised that such a smart, strong, vibrant girl would "let herself" get into a relationship like that. But Dr. Perez reminds her that one in four adolescents experiences verbal, emotional, physical, or sexual dating violence. Dr. Bradley is shocked to hear how common this is and wonders aloud how she can more effectively screen for this in her teenage patients. Dr. Perez recommends that Dr. Bradley check out the CDC's Web site about teen dating violence (https://www.cdc.gov/violenceprevention/ intimatepartnerviolence/teen_dating_violence.html) and display the printable fact sheets in the waiting room of her practice, beside other pamphlets.

Although intimate partner violence and abusive relationships are unfortunately common in adolescence, Gabriela has several risk factors that make her particularly vulnerable. These include anxiety, depression, having a conflictual relationship with her boyfriend, and having witnessed domestic violence as a child. Her earliest model of an intimate relationship was fraught with abuse, and she has been given little information about what occurred or guidance about healthy relationships. Gabriela is currently showing signs of dating violence: she is afraid to be unavailable to her boyfriend when he texts her; feels anxious, depressed, and suicidal; and has been isolating herself from family and friends. She has also experienced a loss of appetite, an indirect sign of possible abuse. Although Gabriela's mother has expressed disdain for her daughter's boyfriend, it's unclear whether she suspects abuse. Studies have found that most parents either do not believe that teen dating abuse is an issue or express uncertainty about whether it is a problem.[20] Additionally, a 2009 report on teen dating abuse found that while most parents appear confident in their ability to detect teen dating violence, less than half were able to correctly identify all the warning signs of abuse.[21]

> Interventions aimed at addressing teen dating violence must help the adolescent learn how to identify signs of a healthy partnership. Loveisrespect.org, a project of the National Domestic Violence Hotline, is a site directed at teens to help them learn how to categorize their relationships, spot abuse, and seek healthier partnerships (http://www.loveisrespect.org). The CDC also launched a prevention initiative, Dating Matters: Strategies to Promote Healthy Teen Relationships (see "Online Resources" at the end of this chapter), which targets 11- to 14-year-old youth in high-risk, urban communities. Parents struggling to talk to teens about healthy dating relationships can also find a video on the CDC site for guidance (see "Online Resources").

Treating More Than Just Somatic Symptoms: Engaging Teens and Families in the Recovery Process

During the course of treatment, Dr. Perez notices that Gabriela struggles to connect her somatic symptoms with stressful events and tends to have an easier time identifying her physiological reactions than her feelings. Dr. Perez notices several occurrences when Gabriela reports a recent episode of abdominal pain that correlates with a fight she had with her boyfriend, but Dr. Perez has to point this out to Gabriela, who doesn't recognize the connection on her own. Gabriela also discloses that she has engaged in cutting a few times.

People with trauma histories often experience a disconnection from their bodies and may engage in self-harm behaviors, such as cutting, to feel alive or to regulate emotions. Exposure to chronic trauma leads to decreased medial prefrontal activation, which means that in an effort to shield themselves from painful feelings associated with terror, these people have lost their sense of purpose and direction.[12] Trauma survivors can also struggle with alexithymia, meaning trouble describing feelings and a sense of disconnection between the mind and the body. When asked about feelings, they tend to substitute actions for feelings and register emotions as physical sensations.[12]

Dr. Perez is trained in Trauma-Focused Cognitive Behavioral Therapy (TF-CBT) and uses the PRACTICE model for her sessions with Gabriela. During the psychoeducation phase of treatment, she talks about how Gabriela's early childhood experiences, including the domestic violence between her parents, have shaped her current experiences. She helps Gabriela to reflect on healthy versus unhealthy relationships, and to recognize some of the abusive patterns in her relationship with her boyfriend. Dr. Perez also provides education about how toxic stress impacts the body and can lead to somatic symptoms. Gabriela is still struggling to understand how her mental and physical symptoms are related, but Dr. Perez knows a therapist who is trained in biofeedback, and she has seen this kind of treatment be a useful mind-body intervention for patients who have difficulty in traditional therapy, who feel uncomfortable sharing their emotions with others, and who lack body awareness. Dr. Perez decides to refer Gabriela for biofeedback to supplement their work in TF-CBT, and Gabriela agrees to give it a try.

Gabriela arrives at her first biofeedback session anxious that she will be poked and prodded or put through rigorous medical tests. The psychologist conducting the biofeedback session immediately puts her at ease by showing her the biofeedback equipment, which consists of a laptop computer, a battery pack, and sensors that sit on top of her skin to measure her breathing, heart rate, and other things happening in her body. When the psychologist hooks her up to the equipment, Gabriela is surprised to see immediately how fast her heart is beating and how fast she is breathing. Gabriela is then guided through various exercises to learn how to have more control over her body. Although the exercises are not like the Xbox games she plays with her friends, she's happy to engage in a treatment in which she can play games and learn about her body, and isn't asked about her prior traumas or feelings on a regular basis. She finds herself eager to return the following week to learn more about how to engage in relaxation and to be more in touch with her body. Gabriela continues to see Dr. Bradley regularly to check on her physical symptoms, which remit significantly after some time in biofeedback therapy.

Several psychological interventions have proven useful for treating adolescents who have experienced trauma, including TF-CBT, Cognitive Behavioral Intervention for Trauma in Schools (CBITS; described in Chapter 11, "School Systems and Trauma"), and Attachment, Self-Regulation, and Competency (ARC; described in Chapter 5, "Risky Behavior and Substance Use"). For youth with complex trauma, such as Gabriela, the following accommodations are recommended for TF-CBT treatment: an extended coping skills phase, addressing trauma themes as opposed to one specific trauma, and a longer treatment consolidation phase to ensure maintenance of trust and safety.

Sometimes adding an adjunctive or supplemental treatment can help to make TF-CBT and other therapies more effective. Yoga, biofeedback, and Eye Movement Desensitization and Reprocessing (EMDR) can help teens exposed to trauma reintegrate their minds and bodies. Yoga trains people to focus on sensations in their body and to learn self-regulation.[12] By holding positions for brief periods of time, people learn to increase their tolerance for discomfort. Likewise, biofeedback increases body awareness and one's sense of control over involuntary bodily functions, such as heart rate and breathing.

Stress can lead to panic and decreases the body's capacity for regulation. For example, a study revealed that abuse history in women was related to decreased vagal regulation of the heart and an inability to reengage vagal regulation after mild exercise to return to a calm state.[22] Biofeedback helps people to feel more empowered in times of distress and to engage in relaxation techniques to calm both the mind and the body. There has also been some evidence in support of neurofeedback, a specific type of biofeedback (also called *electroencephalographic [EEG] biofeedback*) that involves brain-wave readings, for treating adults with PTSD. In a randomized controlled trial of adults with complex PTSD who had failed to respond to at least 6 months of trauma-focused psychotherapy, participants who received neurofeedback training twice a week for 12 weeks demonstrated significantly greater improvement with their PTSD symptoms compared with the control group.[23] By the conclusion of the study, the majority of participants (73%) who received neurofeedback no longer had symptoms that met criteria for PTSD. Although there has been some evidence in support of biofeedback or neurofeedback for PTSD in adults, more research is needed regarding the benefits of biofeedback and neurofeedback for children and adolescents who have PTSD.

Another mind-body intervention, EMDR, can help teens and adults with PTSD process their trauma without becoming retraumatized.[12] In EMDR, the therapist guides the patient through recounting a traumatic memory or emotion while rapidly moving the eyes back and forth, a process that usually occurs during rapid eye movement (REM) sleep. While the World Health Organization has recommended EMDR, along with TF-CBT, as a treatment for PTSD in children and adolescents, they acknowledge a paucity of research in this area and advise that it only be provided by competent clinicians trained in this therapeutic method.[24]

Over the course of the next year, Gabriela continues in therapy and makes significant progress with both her emotional and physical health. Her abdominal pain occurs less often now and she is usually able to identify the trigger for an episode. Additionally, her sleep and appetite have improved and she is able to focus more in school. A few months ago, Gabriela's mother starting joining the therapy sessions with Gabriela and Dr. Perez. This was initially hard for Gabriela's mother, as she expressed disappointment with herself for not setting firmer limits with Gabriela about her boy-friend. She felt that she should have known better, especially given her relationship with her ex-husband. She also wished Gabriela had confided in her more. Gabriela's mother meets a few times alone with Dr. Perez for support and eventually decides to pursue her own therapy to process her previous trauma to be able to better support her daughter in her healing process.

Caregivers will have different reactions upon learning about their children's trauma and need to be adequately supported. Some will express frustration that their teen did not tell them what was going on or what happened. It is important to explain to them that it is common for children to keep traumas to themselves for a variety of reasons and to encourage them not to take it personally. Pediatricians can be an important support for families during this time. As noted before, parents trust pediatricians for advice and parenting support. Pediatricians can remind parents that the most important thing right now is that their adolescent feels supported and doesn't regret sharing their trauma narrative with their parents. Pediatricians can also provide anticipatory guidance, as they do for typical developmental milestones and developmental struggles, about the process of trauma-focused therapy, trauma-related symptoms and ways parents can help, and finding a good balance between supporting their teen and still setting appropriate limits and expectations.

Psychopharmacological Options for Managing PTSD in Youth

Some parents ask pediatricians and other medical providers about pharmacological treatments for teens who have experienced trauma. There is insufficient evidence in support of medication for PTSD in youth, and at times medication may be contraindicated. Psychotropic medication should not act as a standalone treatment for PTSD; instead, medication can be a supplement to trauma-focused therapies and psychosocial interventions, to target specific symptoms that are getting in the way of therapy.

Adolescents who are new to trauma-informed therapy often experience high levels of anxiety and distress, which can manifest with irritability, insomnia, withdrawal, and hyperreactivity to small things. Teens and parents (and even therapists) may feel that the teens need medication to reduce these symptoms before they can "tolerate" the hard work of therapy. β-Blockers and α-adrenergic agonists such as clonidine or guanfacine seem to be the best options for reducing anxiety or hyperarousal.[25] Anxiolytics such as benzodiazepines are often requested to address anxiety, but because they can become addictive and have high abuse potential, they are not recommended for prolonged or frequent use. For youth with PTSD who experience nightmares, prazosin has shown some promise, reducing nightmares related to PTSD (which can include nightmares that seem unrelated to the trauma).[26,27] Two selective serotonin reuptake inhibitors (SSRIs), sertraline and paroxetine, have been approved by the U.S. Food and Drug Administration for PTSD in adults, but none have been approved for PTSD in children or adolescents. If a traumatized adolescent is experiencing a major depressive episode, then SSRI medications may be indicated. Antipsychotic medications such as aripiprazole, risperidone, or quetiapine have sometimes been prescribed to quell painful and distressing sensations in those who have experienced PTSD; however, these medications neither resolve the distressing experiences nor teach patients how to cope with them. Antipsychotics can also further promote numbing and decrease pleasure,[12] and they carry a heavy burden of adverse side effects, including weight gain, diabetes, galactorrhea (for risperidone), movement problems, and tardive dyskinesia with long-term use. It is recommended that people taking an atypical antipsychotic have their weight, glucose levels, and lipid levels regularly monitored by a doctor.[28] Regardless of the type of medication chosen, the medication and dose should be reevaluated as the teen completes a course of therapy, as therapy should hopefully reduce the core symptoms and thus reduce (or eliminate) the need for medication. Although families may seek a quick fix by requesting medication, it is actually psychotherapy that will be the key to facilitating healing for adolescents overcoming trauma. Medication should be viewed as a supportive intervention for trauma, such as when trauma symptoms impact the adolescent's ability to engage in psychotherapy and begin the healing process.

Online Resources

American Academy of Pediatrics: The medical home approach to identifying and responding to exposure to trauma. 2014: https://www.aap.org/en-us/Documents/ttb_medicalhomeapproach.pdf

American Academy of Pediatrics: Trauma toolbox for primary care. 2017: https://www.aap.org/en-us/advocacy-and-policy/aap-health-initiatives/healthy-foster-care-america/Pages/Trauma-Guide.aspx#trauma

American Academy of Pediatrics: Visit Discharge and Referral Summary for Family: http://downloads.aap.org/DOCHW/HFCA/DischargeForm.docx

Centers for Disease Control and Prevention, National Center for Injury Prevention and Control: Break the Silence: Stop the Violence (video): https://www.cdc.gov/cdctv/injuryviolenceandsafety/break-silence-stop-violence.html

Centers for Disease Control and Prevention, National Center for Injury Prevention and Control, Division of Violence Prevention: Dating Matters: Strategies to Promote Healthy Teen Relationships: https://www.cdc.gov/violenceprevention/datingmatters/

Children's Hospital of Philadelphia: Health Care Toolbox: https://www.healthcaretoolbox.org/

Children's Hospital of Philadelphia: Health Care Toolbox, Patient Education Materials: https://www.healthcaretoolbox.org/patient-education-materials.html

National Center for Injury Prevention and Control, Division of Violence Prevention: National Intimate Partner and Sexual Violence Survey infographic. 2016: https://www.cdc.gov/violenceprevention/nisvs/infographic.html

National Center for Injury Prevention and Control, Division of Violence Prevention: Teen Dating Violence. 2017: https://www.cdc.gov/violenceprevention/intimatepartnerviolence/teen_dating_violence.html

National Child Traumatic Stress Network: Pediatric medical traumatic stress toolkit for health care providers. 2014: https://www.nctsn.org/resources/pediatric-medical-traumatic-stress-toolkit-health-care-providers

References

1. Felitti VJ, Anda RF, Nordenberg D, et al: Relationship of childhood abuse and household dysfunction to many of the leading causes of death in adults. The Adverse Childhood Experiences (ACE) study. Am J Prev Med 14(4):245–258, 1998 9635069

2. Kerker BD, Storfer-Isser A, Szilagyi M, et al: Do pediatricians ask about adverse childhood experiences in pediatric primary care? Acad Pediatr 16(2):154–160, 2016 26530850

3. Tink W, Tink JC, Turin TC, et al: Adverse childhood experiences: survey of resident practice, knowledge, and attitude. Fam Med 49(1):7–13, 2017 28166574

4. American Academy of Pediatrics: Trauma toolbox for primary care. 2017. Available at: https://www.aap.org/en-us/advocacy-and-policy/aap-health-initiatives/healthy-foster-care-america/Pages/Trauma-Guide.aspx#trauma. Accessed March 9, 2018.

5. Children's Hospital of Philadelphia: Health Care Toolbox. 2017. Available at: https://www.healthcaretoolbox.org. Accessed March 9, 2018.

6. American Academy of Pediatrics: The medical home approach to identifying and responding to exposure to trauma. 2014. Available at: https://www.aap.org/en-us/Documents/ttb_medicalhomeapproach.pdf. Accessed March 9, 2018.

7. American Psychological Association: Stress effects on the body. 2018. Available at: http://www.apa.org/helpcenter/stress-body.aspx. Accessed March 9, 2018.

8. Sapolsky RM: Why Zebras Don't Get Ulcers: The Acclaimed Guide to Stress, Stress-Related Diseases, and Coping. New York, Henry Holt, 2004

9. Shonkoff JP, Garner AS; Committee on Psychosocial Aspects of Child and Family Health; Committee on Early Childhood, Adoption, and Dependent Care; Section on Developmental and Behavioral Pediatrics: The lifelong effects of early childhood adversity and toxic stress. Pediatrics 129(1):e232–e246, 2012 22201156

10. Thackeray JD, Hibbard R, Dowd MD; Committee on Child Abuse and Neglect; Committee on Injury, Violence, and Poison Prevention: Intimate partner violence: the role of the pediatrician. Pediatrics 125(5):1094–1100, 2010 20421260

11. Spinazzola J, Hodgdon H, Liang LJ, et al: Unseen wounds: the contribution of psychological maltreatment to child and adolescent mental health and risk outcomes. Psychol Trauma 6(S1):S18, 2014

12. van der Kolk B: The Body Keeps the Score: Brain, Mind, and Body in the Healing of Trauma. New York, Viking, 2014

13. Moylan CA, Herrenkohl TI, Sousa C, et al: The effects of child abuse and exposure to domestic violence on adolescent internalizing and externalizing behavior problems. J Fam Violence 25(1):53–63, 2010 20495613

14. National Center for Injury Prevention and Control, Division of Violence Prevention: National Intimate Partner and Sexual Violence Survey infographic. 2016. Available at: https://www.cdc.gov/violenceprevention/nisvs/infographic.html. Accessed March 9, 2018.

15. National Institute of Mental Health: The teen brain: 6 things to know (NIH Publ No OM 16-4307). 2018. Available at: https://www.nimh.nih.gov/health/publications/the-teen-brain-6-things-to-know/teenbrain6thingstoknow-508_153233.pdf. Accessed March 9, 2018.

16. Herrera AV, Benjet C, Méndez E, et al: How mental health interviews conducted alone, in the presence of an adult, a child or both affects adolescents' reporting of psychological symptoms and risky behaviors. J Youth Adolesc 46(2):417–428, 2017 26792265

17. Cohen E, Mackenzie RG, Yates GL: HEADSS, a psychosocial risk assessment instrument: implications for designing effective intervention programs for runaway youth. J Adolesc Health 12(7):539–544, 1991 1772892

18. Goldenring J, Rosen D: Getting into adolescent heads: an essential update. Contemp Pediatr 21:64, 2004

19. Klein DA, Goldenring JM, Adelman WP: HEEADSSS 3.0: The psychosocial interview for adolescents updated for a new century fueled by media. Contemp Pediatr January:16–28, 2014

20. Loveisrespect: Dating abuse statistics. 2011. Available at: http://www.loveisrespect.org/pdf/Dating_Abuse_Statistics.pdf. Accessed March 9, 2018.

21. Picard P, Sarmiento K: Teen dating abuse report 2009: impact of the economy and parent/teen dialogue on dating relationships and abuse. June 2009. Available at: https://www.breakthecycle.org/sites/default/files/pdf/survey-lina-economy-2009.pdf. Accessed March 9, 2018.

22. Dale LP, Carroll LE, Galen G, et al: Abuse history is related to autonomic regulation to mild exercise and psychological wellbeing. Appl Psychophysiol Biofeedback 34(4):299–308, 2009 19707870

23. van der Kolk BA, Hodgdon H, Gapen M, et al: A randomized controlled study of neurofeedback for chronic PTSD. PLoS One 11(12):e0166752, 2016 27992435

24. World Health Organization: Guidelines for the Management of Conditions Specifically Related to Stress. Geneva, World Health Organization, 2013

25. Lubit RH, Giardino ER: Posttraumatic stress disorder in children: treatment and management. Medscape, 2016. Available at: http://emedicine.medscape.com/article/918844-treatment#d9. Accessed March 9, 2018.

26. Akinsanya A, Marwaha R, Tampi RR: Prazosin in children and adolescents with posttraumatic stress disorder who have nightmares: a systematic review. J Clin Psychopharmacol 37(1):84–88, 2017 27930498

27. Kung S, Espinel Z, Lapid MI: Treatment of nightmares with prazosin: a systematic review. Mayo Clin Proc 87(9):890–900, 2012 22883741

28. National Institute of Mental Health: Mental health medications. 2016. Available at: https://www.nimh.nih.gov/health/topics/mental-health-medications/index.shtml. Accessed March 9, 2018.

CHAPTER 14

Families and Caregivers Caring for Teens Exposed to Traumatic Stress

Fadi Haddad, M.D.
Gabrielle Carson, Ph.D.

> A caregiver does not have to be a biological parent to be a key support to an adolescent who has experienced trauma. Parents, grandparents, foster and preadoptive parents, or other adults who care about and make a commitment to a teen, even if for a limited time, can be involved in the teen's recovery from trauma. Whatever your role, showing the teen that you believe in, support, and care about him or her can be profoundly therapeutic.

Hannah, age 14, lives with her biological parents and her two sisters, 10-year-old Alyssa and 12-year-old Tara. Hannah has always been a happy kid and a good student, but recently things have started to change. Her teachers note that she seems tired and disengaged in class. She seems more irritable at home, and Tara has caught her crying alone in her room a few times. Tara mentions the crying to her mom, who tries to talk to Hannah about it, but she just says she's "fine" and puts her headphones back on. Hannah's mom is a little worried but suspects that Hannah is probably just mooning over a boy she likes at school. A few weeks later, on Hannah's midterm report card, Hannah's mother notices that Hannah's grades have dropped. When she talks to her husband about it, he notes that Hannah has been staying up too late and is often up at night; he suspects she is distracted with her phone and computer and has been texting her friends rather than sleeping or studying.

When there are changes in a teen, including changes in sleep or mood, increased tearfulness, feeling tired despite being in bed for sufficient time to sleep, or any deterioration in academic or social functioning without a clear reason, parents often wonder if something is wrong. Parents and caregivers tend to assume the explanation is "typical teenage stuff"—either issues such as laziness, defiance, or negative peer influences, or a minor stress such as a fight with a friend or a romantic disappointment. But sometimes these behavior changes are a sign of a more serious issue, such as being exposed to a traumatic event. Teens who are struggling due to a traumatic event often keep it to themselves, even if they have a close relationship with their parents or caregivers; they may not want to worry their parents or caregivers, or may fear that the adults will be angry or not believe them. Parents or caregivers may be unsure how to ask their teens what is going on, and as discussed in Chapter 1 ("Teens and Traumatic Stress"), those conversations may lead teens to become defensive or shut down. Parents and caregivers may not want to consider or believe the possibility that their child has experienced abuse, assault, or another traumatic event—it is simply too painful to even imagine it. Unfortunately, however, the adults' discomfort might make them blind to something important affecting their teen.

Asking Why: Understanding How Trauma Affects Teens and Families

Over the next few months, Hannah continues to seem withdrawn and disinterested at school. Her teachers are surprised, as she was very bright and engaged last semester. They talk to the school social worker, Ms. Hicks, who approaches Hannah gently to ask how she is doing. Hannah insists everything is "fine," denying any problems at home and saying she has just been "tired" and "bored." She promises to make more effort to keep up with her school work. Something about the conversation feels off to Ms. Hicks, but she can't put her finger on it. She asks Hannah to start checking in with her each week so she can provide support; Hannah seems irritated and sort of tense about this, but she agrees.

At their weekly meetings, Ms. Hicks tries to get to know Hannah and engage her. She asks about the New York Liberty stickers on Hannah's notebook and shares that she was on the basketball team in college; Hannah brightens a little with this and shares that she enjoys playing at the local Y and dreams of playing for the school team. Ms. Hicks asks about the music on Hannah's iPhone, the book she's reading, and eventually about her life at home and her relationships with her parents and her sisters. Hannah rolls her eyes when talking about Tara and Alyssa, who always want to be in her business, and Ms. Hicks laughs and shares that she did the same to her older sister when they were kids. Ms. Hicks notices that Hannah seems more subdued and even a bit tearful when talking about her parents, so she takes this opportunity to try to ask more about Hannah's feelings. Hannah eventually admits that she has been keeping a secret from her parents. A few months ago, a friend of her dad's was visiting and tried to molest her. She managed to shove him off and tried to tell him to leave her alone, but he laughed her off. "Or what," he said, "you're going to tell your parents? I've been your dad's best friend since high school. You think he'll believe you over me? And with what you're wearing, you're asking for it." He hasn't come to the house again, but Hannah feels on edge all the time, worrying she might see him. She didn't know how to tell her parents at first, but then she started to wonder if the man was right that her parents wouldn't believe her, especially since her mom said she was "so disappointed" the time she caught Hannah lying about not having homework. She also worries that if her parents find out, they might be mad at her. She and her parents have had fights before about the crop tops and lipstick she likes to wear, and she's afraid they'll say it's her fault. She also notes, darkly, that they must have noticed how she has been feeling depressed and more withdrawn recently, and that if they cared they would have said or done something.

Trauma creates a sense of terror, disrupting a person's ability to experience the world as safe and secure. But equally as damaging, trauma disrupts one's sense of trust and safety in others.[1] Hannah is struggling with the fear and violation of her father's friend attempting to abuse her. She feels ashamed, like maybe it is partly her fault. That shame also makes her fear being blamed and rebuked by others, even her family. Parents and caregivers tend to think, "Of course my child knows I would never blame her or be angry at her," but the nature of Hannah's abuse was that an adult she thought was trustworthy hurt her in a way she'd never expected. When one trusted adult hurts a child in an unexpected way, it can be hard for the youth to feel secure with anyone else, even parents. The perpetrator reinforced this with his shaming comments, making Hannah feel that her parents, whom she previously trusted to protect her, will instead deny or blame her. Hannah also has the typical egocentric adolescent belief that if others care enough, they will be able to somehow "know" what is going on in the teen's mind. The fact that her parents haven't figured it out (even though her mom asked and Hannah said everything is fine, a fact that Hannah has conveniently forgotten) reinforces Hannah's fear that they would blame her or not care.

In other cases, a teen will not tell his or her parents or caregivers about a traumatic event for fear of worrying them, causing stress, or even putting the parent in danger. Adolescents' developing emotional maturity means that they are able to anticipate the emotional responses of others but are not yet able to fully put themselves in others' "shoes." For example, a teen may be able to recognize that a parent or caregiver will feel angry or sad that the teen has experienced a traumatic event, or will feel guilty that the adult didn't prevent it or know sooner. But the teen is unlikely to be able to reflect that the parent or caregiver would still want to know, even if knowing is painful. Or the teen may worry that knowing will cause too much stress for a parent or caregiver who might already be burdened by work, parenting, financial stress, concerns about immigration status, or medical illness. Teens' typical egocentric thinking makes them feel that they are responsible for protecting the parent or caregiver, but adults know the opposite is true. Perpetrators of abuse may feed into this anxiety by threatening the parent or caregiver directly. Therefore, teens often hide traumatic stress from adults, and parents or caregivers feel at a loss to explain the changes in their child.

> Ms. Hicks encourages Hannah to tell her parents what happened, but Hannah begs not to tell. Finally Hannah agrees to tell them with Ms. Hicks's help. The social worker calls Hannah's mother and asks the parents to come to school for a meeting the following day. Hannah's father has to miss a shift at work to come in and worries that his boss will be mad; there have been layoffs recently, so he has been trying to stay on the boss's good side. But he and Hannah's mom come in and wait in the office for Ms. Hicks. Ms. Hicks is a few minutes late, having been pulled into a crisis with another student. When she gets to them, Hannah's parents seem anxious and a little annoyed. Ms. Hicks apologizes for the delay and asks if they have any concerns about Hannah. The parents say they've noticed that her grades have been dropping, but explain that Hannah wasn't focusing because she was upset about the boy at school who didn't return her affections, and that she has been getting "distracted" with Instagram and texting her friends. They deny any other concerns. Ms. Hicks tells them that there is something Hannah has wanted to tell them but didn't feel comfortable, and suggests they bring Hannah in. "She what?" Hannah's mom replies, a skeptical look on her face. "Hannah and I are so close—what do you mean she told you something that she didn't feel comfortable telling us? If there was something going on, she'd tell me. She knows she can tell me anything. When did you even talk with my child?"

Parents and caregivers are often incredulous that their teen would rather share something important with someone outside the family—a friend, counselor, or someone at school—rather than the parent. Parents and caregivers often fear that they have done something wrong or failed in some way if their teen does not tell them, but that is not necessarily the case. As noted above, teens have many reasons for not disclosing the trauma to the adults who care for them. Also, teens may feel that it is a counselor's or social worker's "job" to talk about feelings and therefore the teens may not worry as much about stressing or burdening a professional as they do about worrying the parent or caregiver. Additionally, if the teen feels that adults might not believe the teen or might react with anger or disappointment, the psychological injury of this happening with a relative stranger is much less than with someone close to them. "If my school social worker blames me or suggests I brought this on myself, fine," the teen thinks (consciously or unconsciously), "but to disappoint my dad that way? Better not to tell him than to risk it."

> Although teens are often hesitant to tell their parents or caregivers about traumatic experiences, there are things adults can do to increase the likelihood that their teen will be open. They should not assume their teen "knows" that he or she can come to them or that they'll support and love the teen no matter what. Trauma makes us question those around us, so parents or caregivers need to make these things explicit. If a teen has a notable change in mood or behavior, parents or caregivers should not ask, "What's wrong with you?" or "What's going on?" These questions can put a teen on the defensive. Instead, parents or caregivers should point out what they've noticed: "You seem sad recently" or "I've noticed you've stopped painting/playing with your brother/going out with friends. Is everything okay?" This can give the teen an opening to share without feeling put on the spot. The teen might say everything's "fine," but parents or caregivers should trust their gut and ask again later.

Ms. Hicks brings Hannah into her office, and together they tell Hannah's parents what happened. Hannah starts to say that this is why she hasn't been doing her schoolwork and has been more irritable at home. Hannah's father's face darkens as she speaks, but he stays silent. Hannah's mother is more vocal: "You're saying this is why you're failing out? If this happened 4 months ago, why are you just saying something now? I don't understand!" "I can't believe Tom would hurt my child," her dad says, shaking his head, eyebrows knit together and a frown creasing his face. "I've known him since high school. This can't be."

Hearing that one's child has experienced a trauma can be very painful to a parent or caregiver. Knowledge of such a painful event can cause a huge amount of anxiety, anger, sadness, and blame/guilt,[2] to such a degree that the adult may even subconsciously avoid thinking about it, acknowledging it, or considering that it even happened. Parents and caregivers want to protect their children, and when they are told that something traumatic happened, they can react with anger, sadness, guilt, and even disbelief.[3] Although these are natural and understandable reactions, they can be very painful for the teen who is sharing what happened. Children and teens exposed to trauma generally look to the adults around them for cues as to how to interpret what happened to them, how to react, and whether or not it is okay to talk about the trauma. Teens often feel confused about what is normal and what is not after trauma and rely heavily on the family's response to put things into context. The family's reaction to a teen's disclosure of abuse is critical.[2] The family's reaction indicates to teens whether the family believes the teen and whether the teen should feel responsible for what happened. The family's response also indicates to the child whether the event is something shameful that the child should hide or is something to be faced together head on. Often, when trauma is disclosed, parents and caregivers have automatic, emotional reactions to the painful news, which can impact their ability to be supportive and avoid potentially negatively impacting responses.[4] These unintentional reactions, however, feed into the shame and fear engendered by the trauma and can make the teen feel rejected or blamed. The shame and anxiety that teens feel after trauma means that they are likely to misinterpret even more supportive reactions from their family. For example, Hannah interprets her father's shaking his head and angry face to mean he is upset at her, when in fact he actually is angry at the perpetrator and the situation. Hannah's mother's reaction is part disbelief and part horror that Hannah has been in danger from this man for 4 months without her or Hannah's father knowing. But Hannah interprets the comments to mean, "If you didn't say something then, it probably didn't really happen."

Abuse perpetrated by someone known to the family can be even more complicated for a teen and family to process. The child might feel guilty and betrayed at the same time: guilty for having "caused" the problem with the family member or family friend, and betrayed by the trusted adult who abused her. She might feel angry at the family for (inadvertently) exposing her to someone who hurt her or for not realizing the abuse was going on. Family members close to the perpetrator are often incredulous at first that this trusted person would abuse their child. If confronted, the perpetrator often denies any wrongdoing, leaving family members feeling caught in the middle. Sometimes some members of a family will believe the child while others will not. Confronting the abuse, pressing charges, or even discussing the issue may divide the family or cause a split between family members or friends. In some cases, family members may believe the teen but feel so overwhelmed by feelings of sadness, worry, guilt, and fear that they unconsciously avoid the teen, or seem distant and cold because they don't know what to say. The result is that the teen and each member of the family feel isolated with their feelings and pain.

Ms. Hicks is aghast that Hannah's parents seem annoyed about being called in to school, that they seem disconnected from what is going on with their daughter, and that they react to her disclosure with anger and disbelief. Therapists, school staff, and other adults often feel disapproval toward parents' reactions in these moments. As discussed in Chapter 1, this is the *fundamental attribution bias* at play. If Hannah's parents' reactions are taken at face value, Ms. Hicks's disapproval seems logical. It is necessary, however, to understand the context from which the parents are coming: their worry at being called for a sudden meeting at Hannah's school without knowing why or what is going on; their stress about having to miss work and then wait anxiously for the meeting; the way they have been silently worrying about Hannah but telling themselves there was nothing important because Hannah herself insisted she was "fine"; the horror and grief they feel to learn that Hannah was abused, particularly by someone they knew and trusted; their concern that their beloved girl felt too scared to tell them and suffered alone for months.... Understanding this context and their perspective enables the professional to see their reaction in a different light. The parents' or caregivers' emotional state, cultural background, and personal history all impact their reaction to their child's trauma. Understanding this context is important for helping parents and caregivers say what they want to say but which is so hard to articulate in the moment: "I believe you. I love you. I'm so sorry this happened. We will get through this together."

> Ms. Hicks quickly asks Hannah to step out of the room and calls the school nurse to sit with her while Ms. Hicks talks to Hannah's parents alone. "I'm sorry for having to bring you in to hear this news in this way," she says, "and I'm so sorry this happened to your daughter. I can only imagine how painful it is for you to hear," she continues, *empathizing* with the parents' experience. Hannah's mother starts to cry quietly while her father stands and starts pacing around the office. Ms. Hicks *normalizes* Hannah's difficulty in telling her parents, explaining how the perpetrator made her feel blamed and shamed, and explaining how and why many children hesitate to tell their parents after a traumatic event. She *validates* their feelings of anger,

sadness, and confusion. She provides *psychoeducation* into the various ways kids exposed to abuse or trauma can react. And she lets them cry, vent, ask questions, and even yell a little. Once they are calmer, she talks about how important it is that they let Hannah know, first and foremost, that they love and care about her regardless of what happened. "She knows that—" Hannah's father interjects, but Ms. Hicks continues: "I know she does, but trauma makes us feel unlovable, broken. Even though she knows you love her, tell her again." She gives them some time to compose themselves; Hannah's father wipes the tears from his eyes, while her mother blows her nose. Then Ms. Hicks brings Hannah back in. Her parents quickly stand and envelop her in a hug, and as Hannah relaxes into them, Ms. Hicks hears Hannah's mother whispering into her hair, "I'm so sorry, baby, I'm so sorry." Ms. Hicks breathes a sigh of relief and tears up a little herself.

Hannah's parents, like many caregivers in this situation, feel overwhelmed when confronted with the idea that their child has been abused, and react with sadness, pain, guilt, and anger. Although initially it is easier not to accept or acknowledge that their child has been hurt, with support and some time to process, they are able to gain control of their own emotions to be present for Hannah. Adults who have experienced trauma and abuse themselves can have a particularly hard time coping when their child experiences trauma; in such a situation of intergenerational trauma, knowledge of the teen's trauma can trigger flashbacks or other posttraumatic stress symptoms in the adult. These symptoms may prevent a caregiver from being emotionally available to help the child in his or her emotional struggle. A parent or caregiver who has been through his or her own trauma might think, "It was horrible when it happened to me. How could I let this happen to my child?" The feelings of shame, guilt, sadness, and embarrassment can be strong and can lead to avoidance, displacement of fault, and a possible inability to empathize with the child or to take appropriate action.

Parents and caregivers might not realize how profoundly their responses can affect their teen. ("She seems to ignore everything else I say or do," a parent might think, consciously or unconsciously.) However, although they don't show it, teens are extremely attuned to their caregivers, even to subtle cues that indicate how the parent or caregiver is feeling or reacting. Helping parents and caregivers to *mentalize* about their teen's experience, and about how what they say and do will be perceived by the teen, assists the caregivers to more effectively support their child in that crucial moment.

Talking to the teen about the trauma should be done in a gentle, supportive way. Parents and other caregivers should help the child feel that he or she is loved unconditionally and that they are there for their child to talk, or even just to hold and express love and sympathy. Parents and caregivers can be honest about their own emotional reactions, while making sure that the teen doesn't feel blamed or shamed. For example, parents should make it clear that they are angry at the perpetrator or the situation, not the teen.

> After the initial disclosure and processing of the trauma, families still need support to understand and talk about what happened. Families may feel ashamed of what happened to the child due to guilt, cultural beliefs, or fear that they will be viewed by others as neglectful parents. This shame can lead them to avoid talking about the trauma, and to tell the teen implicitly or explicitly to "get over it." But teens will interpret this to mean that what happened isn't important or that their family is ashamed of them. Help families acknowledge these feelings and understand how important it is for them to process what happened, in order to help and support their teen.[3,4]

Finding the Frame: Understanding and Connecting With Traumatized Youth and Families

When confronted with news that their child has been exposed to trauma, parents' and caregivers' initial instinct is often to jump into action. They may want to learn all the details to find out what happened, who is to blame, and how to make sure it never happens again. They may question why the teen was in a certain place or with certain peers, or whether the teen did anything that put him or her at risk (e.g., using drugs or alcohol, skipping school, lying to parents about where she was going or whom she was with). In their drive to discover the true story, however, parents can make the teen feel blamed and shamed for what happened. Remember that the child never intended to expose himself or herself to any unsafe situation.

> Even when teens did something that put themselves in harm's way, they are still not to blame for the terrible thing that happened. If a teenager feels blamed by parents or other family members, this can lead the teen to:
>
> - Feel guilt and shame.
>
> - Shut down.

- Feel resentment toward the parents.

- Feel that parents misunderstand him or don't care about him.

- Become more vulnerable to depression, risk-taking behaviors, and even self-harm.

Parents and caregivers may alternatively want to jump to blame someone else. In some traumas, such as accidents, natural disasters, and random acts, there may be no one to blame; however, when the trauma or abuse has a perpetrator, parents often direct their anger toward that person and want to press charges, fight the person, or in some way exact retribution. But this may not be what the teen wants or needs in the moment. Supporting the child should be the primary concern. Hannah may fear that the perpetrator might harm her parents if they confront him, or that neighbors or others will hear about what happened and look at her differently. She may not feel ready to press charges, talk to police, or testify about what happened. In some cases in which the teen already has a relationship with the perpetrator (who is perhaps a family member, friend, or romantic partner), the teen may have ambivalent feelings about the person, and may need time and support to decide to press charges or take other actions.

Parents and caregivers who themselves experienced trauma in the past may be particularly anxious to "do something," especially if they never had treatment to resolve the emotions surrounding their own trauma. When these adults blame themselves for their teen being abused, they need to be reminded that they *can* do something about it: they can support their teen in the way they themselves were likely never supported when they experienced abuse.

In other cases, the parents or caregivers want to "put it behind us" and pretend everything is okay. Or they move to protect the teen, such as by keeping him at home, restricting him from spending time with peers or other family members, taking away his phone, or calling and texting constantly to check on him. This can make the teen feel blamed, or the teen can feel that his parents are worrying too much and thus try harder not to show symptoms or feelings, which can make the situation much more complicated.

All of these reactions by the adults are well intentioned but can backfire. The most important thing for parents and caregivers to do is support and stand with their child.[3,4] The child should feel understood by her family, and her feelings of pain and sadness should be respected and validated by family members so she can feel connected and protected by them. Without this support the teen might feel lonely and isolated, or overwhelmed with emotions that could lead to the classic trauma reactions such as reexperiencing, hypervigilance, and avoidance/isolation, in addition to a decline in social and academic functioning. Walking this path between overreacting and underreacting can be difficult. Treatment, support, and guidance in dealing with a disclosure of abuse or other trauma are available through consultation with school mental health staff, a primary care physician, or a mental health professional. Resources are also available online or through support groups for parents in health clinics. Anyone working with parents and teens in this moment can help the adults manage their own emotions, empathize with their teen, and understand the teen's fears, emotional reactions, and need for emotional help in this crisis.

Empathy and understanding are important for healing. But even with family support, teens are still at risk for emotional and behavioral difficulties in the aftermath of traumatic stress. After being informed about the trauma, parents should be alert to and aware of all symptoms that could be related to the trauma in a variety of different ways. As discussed in Chapter 1, the reactions of children and teenagers to trauma can be varied. Some children tend to isolate, hide their emotions, and try to pretend that everything is fine, whereas others experience severe mood symptoms that can appear in the form of aggressive behaviors toward others or self-harm such as cutting, defiance, truancy, or using drugs and alcohol to medicate the painful experience. The range of symptoms is variable, and the severity could be from mild or unnoticeable symptoms to severe symptoms. Parents should be aware that any change, even a mild change, in behaviors, social interactions, or academic performance could be an indication of a severe internal response to the trauma. The child might be struggling to cover up all these symptoms. Awareness on the parents' behalf and openness to discussing these difficulties with the child might ease these symptoms, especially if the parents explain to the child that it is normal to feel the way he or she feels and that they are there to try to help with the struggle.

> Hannah's parents hug her for a long time before they finally sit down. Hannah's father asks if she feels okay sharing more about what happened. She is able to tell her parents exactly what happened with the family friend. Her mom holds her hand, and when Hannah seems upset or her voice starts to waver, her dad squeezes her shoulder. Hannah's parents express shock but also tell Hannah how much they love her. They say they had been concerned about the recent changes in her behavior and didn't know what to do. Hannah's mother acknowledges that she may have dismissed Hannah's

difficulties out of a hope that the problem was something minor because she was worried the problem might actually be larger. She apologizes, and both parents tell Hannah they are proud of her for telling them what happened. Ms. Hicks also praises Hannah's courage in speaking up. Hannah seems relieved, then asks hopefully, "You're not mad?" Her parents shake their heads no. Ms. Hicks talks to Hannah and her parents about some therapists she knows who work with teens who have experienced trauma, as well as some support groups at the local clinic. Hannah's dad asks about pressing charges. Ms. Hicks admits that she doesn't know the process well, so they decide to look into it together but to wait to speak to the police until Hannah decides what she wants to do. Hannah and her parents agree that finding a therapist is a good first step, to help with the depression and problems with focusing that Hannah has been experiencing. "I'm not grounded, right Mom?" Hannah asks.

Following trauma, the most important immediate response is to give the adolescent support and love. The next challenge for families is to determine whether the adolescent needs additional help, and if so, where to get that help. If physical or sexual abuse is suspected, the teen should be taken to a medical professional for an evaluation. Families can ask their pediatrician if he or she can do the evaluation or refer them to a provider who specializes in this type of medical evaluation. Some teens who experience trauma, with support from their parents or caregivers, will be able to move forward without any more involved intervention. Others will need more active treatment in order to function and remain healthy and stable.

Parents and caregivers should monitor children carefully to determine whether additional professional help might be necessary. Any changes in normal functioning or impairment should be considered an indication that the child should be evaluated by a professional. Table 14–1 lists warning signs that may indicate trauma in teens. If families notice any of these changes, their child should be evaluated by a clinical social worker, psychologist, or psychiatrist with experience in child trauma. Providers with training and expertise in child trauma can be located through the Therapist Certification Program for Trauma-Focused Cognitive Behavioral Therapy (see https://tfcbt.org). Schools and pediatricians may also be able to recommend clinicians with this expertise.

When an adolescent is struggling, seeking treatment as early as possible is very important. Knowing what kind of treatment and finding the right treatment can be very difficult for parents who have no experience with the mental health system. Looking for the right mental health professional can be overwhelming for parents. There are many approaches to dealing with and

TABLE 14–1. Warning signs of potential trauma in teens

Changes in sleep	Changes in eating or appetite	Changes in mood
Changes in school performance, grades, or attendance	Changes in interest and participation in normal activities	Engagement in intentional self-harm
Poor hygiene	Increased irritability or aggression	Social withdrawal
Risk-taking behaviors		Any other behavior or affect that is not typical of the teen

treating trauma, and parents can become very confused about where to go and how to choose.

The following steps can help parents and caretakers decide about the right treatment for their child:

1. *Get informed.* Chapter 2 ("Recognition and Treatment") discusses various individual, group, and family treatments for adolescents exposed to trauma. School mental health staff and pediatricians can also help with finding the right treatment. Some online resources are listed in the box below.

2. *Ask potential therapists if they provide evidence-based trauma treatments and, if so, what kind and what is involved.* Ask how you as the parent will be involved in the treatment, and be aware that parents and caregivers should be involved in some capacity with all effective trauma therapies.

3. *Interview the therapist and get a feel for his or her approach, attitude, and personality.* It is crucial to feel comfortable with the therapist who is going to treat your child. Building trust is part of the treatment, and if you don't feel you are able to trust that person, regardless of the individual's degree and experience, the treatment is less likely to be successful. It is important to meet the therapist yourself, most likely more than once before you make a decision.

4. *Collaborate with the treatment team and have scheduled appointments with them to check on the progress of the treatment for your child.* Be involved, ask questions, and get advice.

> Looking for information about evidence-based treatments for adolescent trauma? Check out these resources:

- American Academy of Child and Adolescent Psychiatry: Facts for Families on posttraumatic stress disorder (PTSD): http://www.aacap.org/AACAP/Families_and_Youth/Facts_for_Families/FFF-Guide/Posttraumatic-Stress-Disorder-PTSD-070.aspx

- National Alliance on Mental Illness: Treatment guide on PTSD: https://www.nami.org/Learn-More/Mental-Health-Conditions/Posttraumatic-Stress-Disorder/Treatment

- National Child Traumatic Stress Network: Families and Caregivers page with information on trauma treatments: http://www.nctsn.org/resources/audiences/parents-caregivers

Treating More Than Just the Teen: How the Family Can Help in Trauma Treatment

Families often encounter barriers to obtaining good care, which can include difficulty locating a provider who both accepts the family's insurance and has experience addressing trauma. Families should feel empowered to ask potential providers questions about the approach they use in treating children who have experienced trauma, the number and types of cases they have treated in the past, and their comfort in using a trauma-informed approach. Finding the right provider can take some persistence on the part of families but is an important step in supporting children after trauma. Local teaching hospitals and universities with training programs in psychology or social work can be useful resources and may be able to connect families to well-qualified providers.

Families seeking treatment for a teen exposed to trauma should look for an experienced provider who delivers evidence-based treatment for traumatic stress. In the initial meetings and early stages of treatment, families should continually evaluate whether the provider they've chosen is a good fit and able to adequately treat the child. Sometimes a teen and therapist are not a good match, even if the therapist is skilled and experienced. If therapy is not working, talk to the therapist (or help the teen talk to the therapist) about why, or request a transfer to a different therapist or clinic. Therapy won't work if the teen doesn't feel comfortable with and is unable to open up with the therapist.

How Parents and Caretakers Can Know That Their Child Is Getting Good Treatment

Families should look for several indicators that the therapist they've chosen is able to adequately treat the child. A trauma therapist should:

- Meet with both the child and with caregivers initially and on an ongoing basis (in cases where an involved caregiver is available).

- Make the child and family feel that the therapist is listening to them and cares about their well-being.

- Give a clear outline of what the treatment will involve.

- Discuss the typical reactions that children and teens have following trauma.

- Help the child and family identify the ways in which trauma is impacting the child and family members.

Treatment should be active, meaning that it should address the traumatic event(s) directly and thoroughly and should include skill building, monitoring and tracking of symptoms and problematic behaviors, and help for parents in managing disruptive or risky child behaviors.

The provider should be mindful that the teen may have ambivalent feelings about treatment. Child trauma survivors are often inclined to avoid any reminders or discussion regarding the trauma, including in therapy. This avoidance of a painful and difficult experience is a natural instinct, but unfortunately avoidance makes trauma symptoms worse. When a child struggling to deal with a traumatic event tries to pretend the event never happened and avoids reminders of the event, and when family members avoid talking about what happened, the trauma is usually manifested in unhelpful and at times unhealthy ways. These often include nightmares, irritability, flashbacks, and heightened anxiety. High-quality trauma treatment involves sensitively and directly revisiting and talking about what happened and addressing the trauma openly through an approach called exposure therapy. This approach can be anxiety provoking for the teens as well as for their families, who often want children to "just be able to move on" or don't want to make the child continue to revisit what happened. Once the trauma is addressed, however, children typically feel much better. Directly addressing what happened allows providers and families to help children work through feelings of shame, guilt, and embarrassment as well as help the children to feel in control of themselves and their emotions once again. It is an opportunity to return to the children the control and power that was taken from them. A good provider should be able to discuss this approach with families and address their concerns.

Treatment: Letting Family Members Know What to Expect

Good treatment should target not only the patient but also the surroundings and family environment. As seen in Hannah's story, it is clear that the family plays a major role in alleviating the teen's anxiety or potentially even exacerbating symptoms by denying what happened due to their feelings of shame and guilt. Effective trauma treatment involves the family as much as possible, to help them support the teen and to meet the needs of the family as a whole.[3,5]

What Parents and Caregivers Should Expect

Parents and caregivers should be part of almost any trauma treatment. The parent or caregiver will not go to all the child's therapy sessions, but will typically go to some therapy sessions with the therapist but not the child and some sessions with the therapist and child together. Parents should expect the following from the therapist:

- *Help in dealing with feelings:* Because parents can be overwhelmed with many emotions when issues arise about their child's safety, treatment should help parents express and process their own emotions and reactions to the teen's traumatic experiences. The parents' reactions can include sadness, anger, and shame and guilt for not protecting the child or preventing the trauma.
- *Education about trauma and its effects:* Parents often struggle after trauma to know what is normal adolescent limit testing and what is an effect of trauma. For example, if a teen is up much of the night, is it because he's playing video games, or because of nightmares and insomnia related to PTSD? Treatment should help parents learn the common effects of trauma in adolescence and ways to cope with them.

- *Help with communication:* Living with and communicating with a teen is complicated in the best of circumstances, and trauma can make the situation even more difficult. Therapy should help the teen and parents express their feelings and needs effectively, validate and empathize with each others' experiences, and solve problems collaboratively.
- *Help with parenting:* Knowing how to react to teens' behaviors after a traumatic event can be complicated. Parents often wonder when to set limits or consequences, or when to let behaviors slide. Therapy should help parents know which behaviors are related to trauma, how to set limits empathically, and how to find a "middle path" between being too permissive and too protective.
- *Hearing the teen's trauma narrative:* If the teen's therapy includes creating a trauma narrative, this will often be shared with the parent or caregivers as part of the therapy process.

What Teens Should Expect

Although parents and families should be involved in trauma treatment, the teen should have a lot of control and authority over what is shared or discussed with the family. The teen should expect the following from the therapist:

- *Confidentiality:* The therapist will maintain the teen's confidentiality and be honest about the limits of confidentiality.
- *Help with communicating feelings:* Teens often feel worried about parents' reactions or don't know how to talk about complicated emotions. The therapist can help, either individually with the teen or in a family session.
- *Help in deciding whom to tell and when:* Teens often fear that extended family or others will learn about the trauma and judge them. The therapist can help the teen decide with whom to share the trauma narrative, when, and how.

What Siblings Should Expect

Siblings can also play a role in treatment. Siblings are affected when a teen experiences trauma; they might feel worried about the well-being or safety of the trauma-exposed teen, feel scared or angry about what happened, feel guilty for not protecting their sibling, or even feel upset that the trauma-exposed teen is getting more attention. The therapist should help the parents identify and anticipate the ways siblings are affected. The therapist can also help the teen and parents decide when, how, and how much to tell siblings about what happened.

The therapist should also help to find resources in the community to help the teen. This can include support in school, during after-school programs, or in religious or other community programs. Parents and caregivers and teens can consider sharing basic information with school staff to allow the school to be more supportive for the teen and ease his or her return to full functioning.

Additional Reading

American Academy of Pediatrics: Helping foster and adoptive families cope with trauma. 2016. Available at: https://www.aap.org/en-us/Documents/hfca_foster_trauma_guide.pdf. Accessed March 9, 2018.

Faber A, Mazlish E: How to Talk So Teens Will Listen and Listen So Teens Will Talk. New York, Harper Collins, 2006

Gold C: Keeping Your Child in Mind: Overcoming Defiance, Tantrums, and Other Everyday Behavior Problems by Seeing the World Through Your Child's Eyes. New York, Da Capo Lifelong Books, 2011

National Institute of Mental Health: Helping children and adolescents cope with violence and disasters: what parents can do. 2015. Available at: https://www.nimh.nih.gov/health/publications/helping-children-and-adolescents-cope-with-violence-and-disasters-parents/index.shtml. Accessed March 9, 2018.

Neufeld G, Mate G: H0old on to Your Kids: Why Parents Need to Matter More Than Peers. New York, Ballantine Books, 2006

References

1. Herman JL: Trauma and Recovery: The Aftermath of Violence, From Domestic Abuse to Political Terror. New York, Basic Books, 1997

2. Fuller G: Non-offending parents as secondary victims of child sexual assault. Assault Trends and Issues in Crime and Criminal Justice 500:1–7, 2016

3. Foster J: Supporting Child Victims of Sexual Abuse: Implementation of a Trauma Narrative Family Intervention. Fam J (Alex Va) 22:332–338, 2014

4. Aherns C, Campbell R: Assisting rape victims as they recover from rape: the impact on friends. J Interpers Violence 15:959–986, 2000

5. Tjersland OA, Mossige S, Gulbrandsen W, et al: Helping families when child sexual abuse is suspected but not proven. Child Fam Soc Work 11:297–306, 2006

CHAPTER 15

Advocacy and Systems Change

Making Services Work for Youth Exposed to Trauma and Their Families

Jeanette M. Scheid, M.D., Ph.D.
Sin Chu, M.D.

Everyone who works with adolescents who have been exposed to trauma wants those adolescents to have services and supports that work. Ideally, each of these teens will have a system of care that is family centered, youth guided, and respectful of the youth and family's history and culture, with services and supports that are individualized, coordinated, and grounded on evidence-based and promising interventions. But accomplishing this goal can be difficult. Unfortunately, service systems that serve traumatized adolescents are often underfunded, underresourced, and fragmented. Getting the right care for our youth requires that each of us understands our own role, strengths, and limitations, as well as those of others serving our youth. Often, our teens need us to be advocates as well as therapists, teachers, parents, caseworkers, or physicians. Fighting for them individually helps, but we are most effective when we can build strong teams in our communities and get support from state and national leadership. Building and leading such advocacy efforts requires knowledge of and collaboration with system partners. These include families and family advocacy organizations, child welfare (protective services, foster care services, adoption agencies, and juvenile justice systems), state and federal government, health and mental health providers, schools, and faith-based organizations. Coordinating and collaborating across so many disparate systems and organizations is not easy, but doing so effectively can transform the care available for youth exposed to trauma.

Understanding the Systems Surrounding Traumatized Youth

> Mary first got the idea of becoming a foster parent at church. A social services agency was presenting to her church group about the need for foster parents, and it got her thinking how empty the house has felt since her kids left home. She talks with her husband, Steve, and they decide to explore becoming foster parents. She calls the agency that presented at the church meeting to begin the process of becoming licensed foster parents.

Many social services are delivered by or coordinated through *faith communities*. Faith communities range from small or informal congregations of individuals who share a set of beliefs to large organizations with national, regional, and local governance. Faith communities and religious organizations can serve as sources of support to those in need, including traumatized youth, and those who care for them. They can provide outreach, spiritual, emotional, and material support. Many faith communities run shelters, schools, child welfare organizations, and health or mental health treatment facilities. Faith communities and organizations also regularly engage with state health and human services departments in the systems of care for children and families, and may advocate politically for or against certain social policies. The beliefs and practices of each faith community and religious organization are unique, which can create challenges when working with lesbian, gay, bisexual, transgender, and queer or questioning (LGBTQ) youth or those who have been victims of sexual assault. The specific beliefs held by religious organizations and their members will impact their choices when engaging in leadership and partnership on issues related to services and supports for children and families exposed to trauma.

> Mary and Steve complete the steps to become licensed foster parents, including attending an orientation, completing an application, participating in a home study, and attending a series of trainings. The training curriculum includes information about the challenges faced by children in foster care,

common responses to trauma and the ways trauma may affect a child's be-havior, and parenting techniques that can help a child be comfortable and safe in their home. Early in the process, Mary and Steve invite their two young adult children for a family dinner to discuss their plans. After 6 months, they complete the process and prepare to accept a child into their home.

One month after obtaining their license, Mary and Steve get a call say-ing a 12-year-old girl was removed from her home because of alleged phys-ical and sexual abuse. The next day, a protective services worker and a foster care worker bring the girl, Joan, to Mary and Steve's home. The workers tell them Joan had just been "remanded" into foster care that morning at a court hearing. The caseworkers also bring Joan's Medicaid insurance card and a one-page document with some medical and developmental history and the name and address of Joan's pediatrician. Joan doesn't say much, keeping her head down and kicking the driveway with the toe of her sneaker. Mary won-ders what Joan will think of them and their home.

The foster care worker reminds Mary and Steve that Joan is required to have a health evaluation within her first month with them, so they arrange for her to see the pediatrician who saw their own children. Mary and Steve share with the pediatrician their concerns about the impact of Joan's exposure to trauma and the transition into foster care. The pediatrician has limited experience working with children in foster care. He consults the American Academy of Pediatrics (AAP) Web site and finds the Healthy Foster Care America page (https://www.aap.org/en-us/advocacy-and-policy/aap-health-initiatives/healthy-foster-care-america/Pages/Goals.aspx). He prints out some handouts and information booklets for Mary and Steve to take home.

The AAP Web site has a wealth of resources for parents, pediatricians, mental health providers, and others working with youth who have experienced trauma and those in foster care.

- The Fostering Health manual is a great starting point (https://www.aap.org/en-us/advocacy-and-policy/aap-health-initiatives/healthy-foster-care-america/Pages/Fostering-Health.aspx) and includes a great resource library.

- There are also wonderful handouts and resources for families, like "Helping Foster and Adoptive Families Cope With Trauma": https://www.aap.org/en-us/Documents/hfca_foster_trauma_guide.pdf.

Mary and Steve also enroll Joan in school but don't know whether they should tell the guidance counselor the little bit they know about Joan's past. At home, Joan seems tense and jumpy, speaks very little, and often screams

or cries in her sleep. Mary and Steve wonder if this is normal and feel uncertain of what to do. They review some of the materials from their training
and ask the foster care worker if he has more information about Joan's experiences and history, but he too has limited information.

Child Welfare Services

Child welfare services aim to keep children and adolescents safe from abuse
or neglect. Child welfare gets involved after an allegation of abuse or neglect
and is tasked with three goals: safety, permanency (figuring out where the
child can safely live for the long term), and well-being. Child welfare arranges the child's placement in foster care and coordinates with the courts to
achieve a permanency goal, which could be reunification with the child's
family of origin, adoption, or another living arrangement. Child welfare services are organized and governed at state and county levels and supervised by
the federal government, but the structure, rules, and policies of child welfare
services often vary from state to state. The child welfare system conducts investigations of alleged child abuse/neglect and provides prevention, foster care,
and adoption services. These services may be provided by a state's child welfare
department and or by private agencies that contract with the state. Other support services may include community-based psychotherapy and residential
treatment services for children in foster care. Child welfare typically also includes services and supports provided by the juvenile justice system.

Child Protective Services

The goals of child protective services (CPS) are to investigate allegations of
child abuse and neglect, determine whether the charges are substantiated, and
take appropriate action to protect the safety of children. A CPS worker assigned to a case will go to the child's home (and often the child's school) to
interview the child and any adults involved to determine whether there is
evidence for abuse or neglect. A CPS worker may call any therapists or physicians involved with the family as well, and can set up specialist evaluations
(e.g., a physical exam for alleged sexual abuse) if needed. CPS will then present findings in court, and a judge will determine whether the allegations
are founded (substantiated) or unfounded (not supported by evidence). The
job of a CPS worker is difficult, because often there is no overt evidence of
abuse (even physical or sexual abuse often leaves no marks) and a child or
teen may be too scared or ashamed to tell the CPS worker what happened.
A CPS investigation may end in the child's being removed from the home
and placed in foster care, or other steps may be recommended. For example,

CPS may require one of the adults to leave the home (e.g., the stepfather who was physically abusive) while allowing the child to stay home with another adult (e.g., the mother or a grandparent). CPS may alternatively allow the child to stay at home but recommend additional services and supports or assist the family to connect to services that will reduce the risk for future maltreatment. CPS cannot charge or prosecute adults for acts connected to alleged maltreatment; this is done by law enforcement.

Foster Care

After CPS personnel determine that a child cannot safely remain with their family, they request the court to order (remand) an out-of-home placement (with family, called kinship foster care, or with a foster family, group home, or residential program). At that point, the child and family transition from protective services to foster care. Each state organizes foster care services differently. Services may be organized and regulated at the county or the state level. The state or regional government's department of health and human services, private agencies contracted by the government, or some integration of the two recruit, support, and monitor foster parents. Foster parents typically have the authority to make routine parenting decisions, including schedules, recreation, and basic health care, but some decisions (including accessing psychiatric treatment) remain with birth or legal parents as long as they retain parental rights. The laws and regulations parsing authority between the birth or legal parents and the foster parents vary. Still other decisions are made by the foster care worker or other service providers. For youth in foster care to do well, all the adults—the family of origin, foster family, foster care worker, and other services and supports such as school, health, and mental health providers—need to work as a team. The teen should be part of that team whenever possible.

When a youth enters foster care, all members of the team have much to do. The youth needs to adjust to the new environment and begin to grapple with his or her history and experiences. Birth or legal parents need to take stock and work on making life changes needed to be successful at reunifying with the child. Foster parents need to learn about, support, and parent the new young person in their home and support others in the household, including each other. The foster care worker needs to learn about the child and family, help identify goals and a plan to achieve them, support the foster parents, help the child adjust to the new family, ensure that health and mental health services occur, and document all these activities. Teachers and health care providers need to engage all the parties to learn about the child and family so they can develop effective educational and health plans.

Throughout the child's and family's journey in foster care, the full team needs to be in regular contact to identify and address challenges effectively. The reality of foster care is that placements change, foster care workers change, moves to new homes and communities occur, and new supports need to integrate into the team. Documenting the ongoing process of planning and monitoring successes and persistent challenges is critical to ensuring continuity in the child's and family's journey. All of this information is also important to determine permanency planning, such as whether reunification remains possible or whether the plan needs to shift to formal termination of parental rights adoption or an alternative permanency plan.

Being a foster parent is extremely demanding, emotionally and in terms of time, space, and other resources. Therefore, most states struggle to recruit and retain foster parents. The pool of foster parents who can provide more intensive, treatment-related services, such as treatment or therapeutic foster care, is typically even more limited. Given that essentially all children in foster care have experienced maltreatment or other forms of trauma and its subsequent emotional and behavioral complications, the health, mental health, and child welfare systems must engage effectively to develop robust services and supports that will be accessible to children in foster care.

> Two months pass. Joan follows the rules at home with Mary and Steve and doesn't get into trouble at school, but she's not doing well. She is sullen and isolative at home, sleeps poorly, and becomes unreasonably upset when Mary and Steve make suggestions or provide direction. At school, she is doing poorly in all her classes and hasn't connected with any other kids. Mary calls Joan's insurance carrier to find a therapist. They take her to a few appointments, but Joan refuses to talk and after a few sessions refuses to go to appointments altogether.

Mental health care services are an integral part of comprehensive medical care, but whether they are available and how they are integrated with the rest of medical care vary significantly depending on the state and region. The federal Mental Health Parity Act enacted in 1996 and updated as the Mental Health Parity and Addiction Equity Act of 2008 requires insurance carriers to cover mental health services as they cover other health care services. However, barriers to full parity still exist; for example, carriers may limit the number of outpatient visits allowed or designate all local providers as "out of network." In addition, commercial insurance providers and Medicaid health plans typically only cover services provided at the outpatient or inpatient levels of care rather than supporting intermediate levels of care such as home-based therapy services or partial hospitalization. Youth who need these intermediate levels of care must undergo a process to determine eligibility for care covered by public mental health systems. This complicated and time-consuming process requires that someone step up as the youth's advocate to submit the necessary paperwork and applications.

The organization of public mental health systems varies from state to state. In many states, children with "mild to moderate" mental health problems receive services provided by Medicaid managed care, whereas children meeting criteria for "serious emotional disturbance" receive services through the community mental health system. Children typically receive services within their legal county of residence, which bears the financial responsibility for providing these services. However, children in foster care may be relocated to another county; therefore, arranging services when a child is living in a county different from his or her legal county of residence can present a challenge.

There are many resources for those looking to find good mental health care for teens who have experienced trauma, and for mental health providers wanting to learn more about treating them.

- The Academy on Violence and Abuse (http://www.avahealth.org) has guides for best practices and competencies in caring for youth who have experienced trauma and other adverse childhood experiences.

- The Substance Abuse and Mental Health Services Administration (SAMHSA; https://www.samhsa.gov) provides information about mental health and substance abuse treatment services, including practical tools such as suicide screening tools as well as apps and information about where to find treatment.

- SAMHSA partners with other organizations, such as the Children's Bureau and Administration for Children and Families, to provide specific resources on topics related to foster care and trauma (e.g., "Making Healthy Choices: A Guide on Psychotropic Medications for Youth in Foster Care" [https://www.childwelfare.gov/pubPDFs/makinghealthychoices.pdf], which is a guide for youth, and the corresponding guide for caregivers and caseworkers, "Supporting Youth in Foster Care in Making Healthy Choices" [https://www.childwelfare.gov/pubPDFs/mhc_caregivers.pdf]).

As Mary and Steve are considering the next steps, the school guidance counselor calls. The school nurse told her that Joan is in the office frequently with minor physical complaints, and the nurse noticed cut marks on Joan's arms. Steve goes in to meet with the guidance counselor and figure out what to do. The counselor recommends that Joan should be in therapy or that maybe Steve should take her to an emergency room to "get evaluated." Steve is frustrated and goes to meet with the principal. In the waiting room, he starts talking to another parent, who tells him to ask the school to "have Joan tested." She had her son tested, she says, and now he gets counseling at school twice a week plus extra time for tests.

Schools are another critical source of support for traumatized teens. Schools provide the environment and resources that allow youth to gain knowledge and skills needed to reach their maximum potential. School systems are governed at the local, state, and federal levels. Public schools (district schools and charter schools) are funded by local, state, and federal taxes, and must follow all local, state, and federal regulations. Private and parochial schools get private funding and are thus freed from some regulations, including those that regulate special education for children with disabilities.

Because trauma has such profound impact on the brain, many teens who have experienced trauma struggle in the classroom and need either brief or long-term special education services. Federal law regulates special education services through the Individuals with Disabilities Education Act of 1990 (IDEA). IDEA requires state and public agencies to provide early intervention, special education, and related services to children from birth to young adulthood who meet eligibility criteria. The child needs to have a multidisciplinary evaluation to determine eligibility under cognitive impairment, autistic impairment, learning disability, emotional impairment, or other health impairment. This assessment should be done through the school (and any parent can request an evaluation for their child); however, families may need to go outside the school to get specialist evaluations such as for autism or specific learning disabilities. If the student is eligible for special education services, the team, including the child (especially as he or she gets older), family, educators, and sometimes a therapist or caseworker, develops an Individualized Education Plan (IEP). The IEP should give the student the support needed while keeping the student in the least restrictive placement, meaning inclusion in mainstream classroom settings wherever possible, and placement in specialized settings for the shortest time necessary. Foster parents and foster care workers can be important advocates during the IEP process, but if a biological parent is still involved, only he or she can make IEP decisions unless a court determines otherwise.

That evening after Joan is asleep, Steve and Mary sit down to brainstorm what to do. Mary looks over the pamphlets the pediatrician gave them. Steve starts looking online and finds the National Child Traumatic Stress Network (NCTSN) "Resources for Parents and Caregivers" page (https:// www.nctsn.org/audiences/families-and-caregivers). Reading through it, they realize that Joan needs not just any therapy, but evidence-based trauma therapy.

> The NCTSN Web site houses an amazing collection of resources and reading material (e.g., information sheets on complex trauma [https://www.nctsn.org/ what-is-child-trauma/trauma-types/complex-trauma] and other types of childhood trauma, and about treatments that work and where to find them), as well as trainings, webinars, and workshops for clinicians and parents. The Web site can be tough to navigate because so much information is available, but don't miss the NCTSN Learning Center (https://learn.nctsn.org) for free online trainings and toolkits to learn how to better help youth who have experienced trauma.

Mary and Steve ask Joan's foster care worker about setting up trauma-informed therapy, so he helps them get an intake appointment at their local community mental health clinic. Mary and Steve are frustrated that the therapist asks little about Joan's exposure to traumatic events. They call the foster care worker to share their concerns, but he says there aren't any other clinics that have openings and encourages them to "give this therapist a try." Mary and Steve feel frustrated that trauma-informed services are not available or are not being offered to Joan.

Sensing their frustration, the foster care worker mentions a support group for foster parents in their area. Mary and Steve decide to attend, hoping to find out more about systems and resources so they can be effective advocates for Joan.

Youth and families often need to be their own advocates. Advocacy can be small, such as requesting an IEP evaluation or a more intensive treatment for a child, or large, such as working on a local or national level to change the way systems (e.g., child welfare, mental health, schools, juvenile justice, or others) work. Youth and families should always be part of any systems change. Youth and families can teach the clinicians, workers, and providers they see about how trauma affects youth and families, what youth and families need to change and recover, and how to make systems and services work better for them. As advocates, families with lived experience as consumers of health and mental health services and recipients of child welfare systems can have a powerful role in system change. National organizations such as the National Alliance on Mental Illness (NAMI) and National Federation of Families for Children's Mental Health (NFFCMH) lead and join coalitions to improve the systems of care. State and local chapters often organize support groups for families and other caregivers. It is important for caregivers to connect with others in their community who are facing similar challenges; they can be a great resource for learning about mental illness, offering support, and finding avenues to create change.

There are many online resources for parents and caregivers.

- The American Academy of Child and Adolescent Psychiatry (AACAP) has easy-to-read handouts called Facts for Families on various mental health issues, including drugs, alcohol, and tobacco; eating disorders; mood disorders; psychiatric care and treatment; suicide; and trauma (https://www.aacap.org/AACAP/Families_and_Youth/Facts_for_Families/FFF-Guide/FFF-Guide-View-by-Topic.aspx). These handouts are available in Chinese, Spanish, and Vietnamese, as well as English.

- The American Academy of Pediatrics' Healthy Foster Care America provides a handout titled "Parenting After Trauma: Understanding Your Child's Needs" (https://www.healthychildren.org/English/family-life/family-dynamics/adoption-and-foster-care/Pages/Parenting-Foster-Adoptive-Children-After-Trauma.aspx).

- A fact sheet on supporting youth in finding treatment is available through the Child Welfare Information Gateway, under the U.S. Department of Health and Human Services (https://www.childwelfare.gov/pubPDFs/mhc_caregivers.pdf).

Creating Change

Anyone who identifies a gap in systems serving children who have experienced trauma can build a coalition to meet that gap. Change won't happen overnight, given the complexity of the systems involved. Partners involved in change efforts will need to establish intermediate objectives in the service of the long-term goal, and to understand and engage the different systems involved to effect change. Although every process is slightly different, change typically follows these seven steps: 1) identify the gap or challenge, 2) seek information from system partners to refine goals, 3) develop partnerships, 4) identify factors responsible for the gap or challenge, 5) develop a plan to address the gap or challenge, 6) monitor markers of progress, and 7) ensure sustainability.

> Mary and Steve attend the parent support group meeting. The group includes some foster parents working directly with counties and others working with private agencies that have state contracts. The group meets regularly for support and to share information. At this meeting, three other foster families also describe challenges with accessing trauma-informed mental health services for the children in their care. The other families had been struggling with this problem for over 2 years. One family had to tell the foster care agency that they couldn't take care of one young teen because his behavior was really scary and they couldn't get any services or treatment for him. A few other families speak up to share that they've had the same difficulty. The parent group decides to make this issue a priority for organized advocacy.

Identify the Gap or Challenge

The experiences of individual children and families or observations by system team members may cause team partners to explore gaps in the systems of care serving children and youth who have experienced trauma. First, formulate a clear statement of the concern, such as "The foster parents in my support group have said that they have a lot of trouble accessing mental health services for kids who come into their homes" or "The pediatricians in this practice never seem to get background health history or ask about trauma exposure when attempting to complete a comprehensive medical examination."

> The parent support group decides to reach out to local parent support groups across the state and send them surveys. The local parent support groups work with state child welfare, which shares the parent support groups' mailing lists. The survey asks about what kinds of mental health services and trauma-informed services are available in each county, and whether families feel this has impacted placement stability. Sixty percent of the members across the state respond. The survey shows that in the region where Steve and Mary live, 80% of families had similar problems finding trauma-informed care. Three other parts of the state had similar problems, whereas families in two regions said they had easy access to excellent child- and family-responsive trauma-informed services. The parents from the regions with a service shortage contact their state legislators, the religious and community organizations that recruited them, and the foster agencies that trained them

and matched them with kids. The legislators and leadership from the different organizations all pledge their support. Finally, the parent support group requests a meeting with state-level officials responsible for child welfare services and mental health services.

Seek Information From System Partners to Refine Goals

Sometimes when there appear to be gaps, they turn out to be rare issues or individual complications, rather than problems that require broad systems change. At other times the gaps or barriers found in one case are part of a bigger issue. Contacting individuals in other communities is often an effective way to determine if a problem is widespread. If the team uses support systems contacts to do this outreach, then those same contacts can be a good source of networking and advocacy to accomplish change. Checking in with others' experiences can also clarify what the problem or barrier is; for example, if accessing mental health services is difficult, is the problem due to a lack of providers, a referral system that isn't working, or an issue with insurance coverage or eligibility. After the preliminary investigation, the team can draft a specific problem statement and prepare to move to the next step. The statement might read, for example, "Foster care workers in these three counties ask foster parents to obtain community mental health services for the kids in their home, but when the parents call for services, the intake teams tell them the children are not eligible."

> At the meeting, state child welfare and mental health officials hear the concerns of Mary and Steve's parent support group and review the results of their survey. The officials seem to appreciate the importance of recognizing and treating trauma among kids in foster care. They say they have been trying to implement trauma screening tools statewide within the child welfare system to expedite referrals from child welfare to community mental health service providers. The state agencies also used materials from the California Evidence-Based Clearinghouse for Child Welfare (CEBC; http://www.cebc4cw.org). The CEBC is an organization that evaluates the evidence base for assessment and treatment practices and provides guidelines to organizations that want to engage in system change. The strategic planning process included reviewing the kinds of evidence-based treatments that were readily available and developing a strategic plan to ensure that all providers train and support case managers and therapists in evidence-based treatment approaches for children exposed to trauma. The officials acknowledged that progress had been slow and that two of the regions (including the county where Mary and Steve live) hadn't yet even begun the training process outlined by the state. Not surprisingly, those are some of the same regions where the parent support group's survey found that trauma-informed services weren't available. Two other re-

gions where the survey showed service gaps had done the training, so no one is sure why services aren't more accessible there.

Develop Partnerships

Depending on the problem that needs to be solved, the team may need to enlist a range of different partners, from youth and families to schools to religious or community groups to school officials. The team will of course want to invite partners from any systems directly connected to the problem, especially those responsible for making changes. However, even partners not directly connected to the problem, if the team can get them invested in solving it, might bring an important perspective and additional resources or incentives for system change. Recruiting all of the partners may take some time. The team can start with close contacts and allies and use those network contacts to expand the team. The team can consider establishing a primary team most closely connected to the problem and a resources team of allies and content experts who can apply strategic advocacy and support when needed. The agenda for early meetings of these teams should include agreeing on the core problem, developing a strategic plan and initial steps, making plans to share information efficiently (e.g., through in-person meetings, conference calls, or e-mail), and determining a preliminary timeline to complete the project.

> To address the gap in services in the four regions of the state with limited trauma-informed services, the group assembles a team consisting of foster parents from those regions and representatives from child welfare and children's mental health both locally from the four regions and from the state. Mary decides to join an effort to address trauma-informed services, while Steve continues to work on getting an IEP for Joan. The trauma-informed services team splits into two subgroups. Mary joins the subgroup for the region that is "pre-training" (since that is where she lives). The other subgroup is for the regions that are "post-training" but still have poor access. The "pre-training" subgroup, which Mary joined, does not have sufficient resources to lead and sustain the project, but they are able to obtain a limited grant from a private funder.
>
> The "post-training" subgroup discovers two main causes. The first is that referrals to the regional community mental health provider are too low to sustain hiring and training of any new therapists. The local pediatricians and primary care offices, which should be the main sources of referrals, are not well integrated with the mental health provider. The second is that the local child welfare system, including private and public foster care providers, and the local community mental health providers do not communicate directly about the needs of foster children in the community.
>
> Mary's "pre-training" subgroup finds that the local community mental health organization in her region plans to participate in the next wave of

training, which will start in 6 months. The team also discovers that a local private nonprofit mental health clinic just hired a therapist trained and certified in an evidence-based trauma treatment.

Identify What Factors Are Responsible for the Gap or Challenge

Starting with the problem statement, the core team breaks down the problem into the most concrete factors possible. There are several ways to accomplish this.

One approach is to use a root cause analysis (RCA) process. The RCA process is used to look at all the different factors that contribute to the problem, organized by category. The first step is to identify the categories of barriers (e.g., insurance issues or caseworkers not knowing about existing resources). The second step is to identify the specific, concrete-action barriers (e.g., that a document describing insurance access needs to be developed, and that an in-service training must be developed for caseworkers) within each category barrier. One way to organize the process visually is to use a "fishbone" graphic (Figure 15–1); each "rib" identifies the "category" barriers, and along the rib the team lists the concrete action barriers in each category. The team reviews each concrete action barrier in turn, determining whether it presents a major or minor barrier, how difficult it would be to change, and who would have to be involved to change it.

Another approach to the RCA is to conduct an "as is" (Figure 15–2) and "to be" (Figure 15–3) process (see "Process Mapping" at https://www.visual-paradigm.com). This approach lays out what currently happens (the "as-is" process—e.g., the existing steps for screening and referral for mental health services), then identifies what the process should look like once the problem is solved (e.g., an efficient and effective way of screening all youth entering foster care for mental health needs). This allows the team to identify what is working and what isn't to determine the priorities for change.

In this instance, after reviewing the "as-is" process for recognizing and addressing the impact of trauma, the "post-training" subgroup develops the "to be" process. In this process, they suggest moving trauma screening to occur at foster care entry so that a child's needs are recognized as early as possible.

The team working with the communities that have trained personnel but limited access develops the following action plan:

1. Set a series of meetings between the leadership of the primary care offices and the local community mental health organization to develop a referral process that works with the practice flow of the primary care offices.

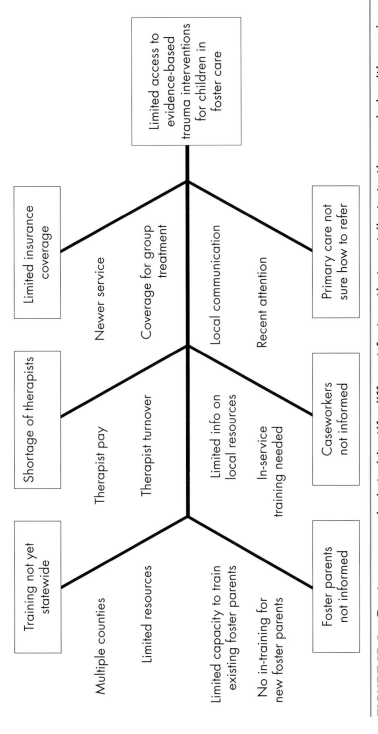

FIGURE 15–1. Root cause analysis to identify different factors that contribute to the gap in health services.

Source. Ishikawa K: *Guide to Quality Control.* Tokyo, JUSE, 1968.

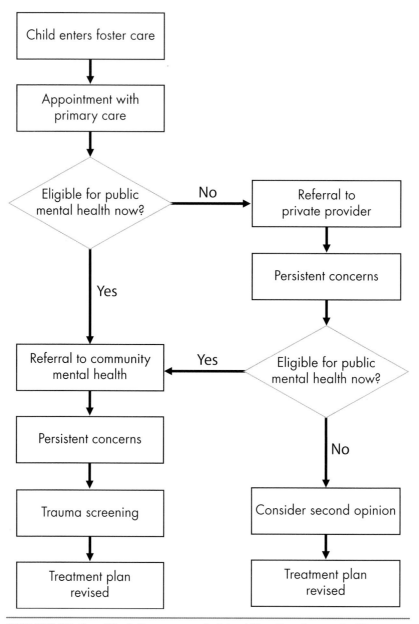

FIGURE 15–2. "As is" map—early identification impact of trauma.

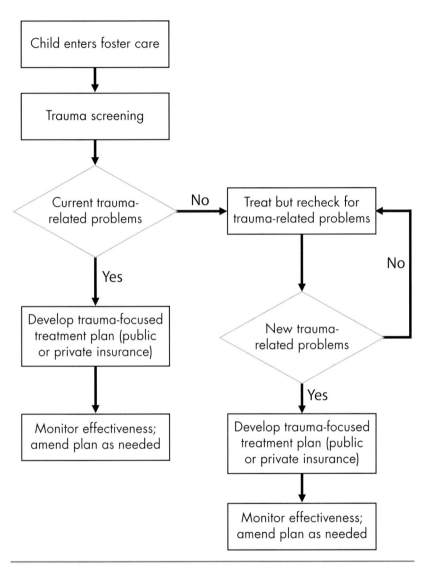

FIGURE 15-3. "To be" map—early identification impact of trauma.

Note. Assumes that all evidence-based trauma-informed services are available in public and private treatment provider systems.

2. Develop written materials for foster parents describing the process of trauma screening, assessment, and treatment so that they can advocate effectively for the children in their care.
3. Establish a formal connection between the child welfare leadership and the community mental health provider leadership to improve collaboration between the two organizations.

The team presents this plan to the leadership of the primary care organizations, community mental health, and child welfare. The leadership approves this plan and agrees to move forward with implementation.

> Education is an important part of any advocacy effort. The materials available online from the National Child Traumatic Stress Network, the American Academy of Pediatrics Healthy Foster Care America, and the Substance Abuse and Mental Health Services Administration can be useful for educating families, clinicians, politicians, or anyone who needs to understand why effective treatment for traumatized teens is so important. (See "Resources" at end of this chapter for brief descriptions of these organizations.)

Because the trainings won't start for another 6 months, Mary's team recommends some interim measures to the local leadership of child welfare and community mental health for her region: 1) Establish a temporary team consisting of child welfare and community mental health providers to review the youth in foster care in their community, determine those most in need of evidence-based trauma services, and explore an agreement with the surrounding counties that have completed trauma training to provide services for these children. 2) Contract with a local private nonprofit mental health clinic that has therapists with expertise in trauma to provide services for youth who cannot travel to the community mental health clinics in the surrounding counties. 3) Develop the formal relationships, including those between local child welfare, mental health, and primary care groups, that are needed to facilitate the better integration among local systems of care. The leadership members hear these recommendations. Although they are not sure of the feasibility of the first two recommendations, they agree to explore them, and agree to pursue the third recommendation.

Develop a Plan to Address the Gap or Challenge

After identifying the concrete barriers that keep the system from serving kids and families well, the team has to decide what needs to be changed to remove those barriers. The team identifies who is responsible for the change, who will be affected, what resources are needed, how long it will take, and what level of permission is needed (e.g., whether a change will require any revision of policy or law vs. revised practice). The team should draft a document of the proposed changes and present this plan to leaders responsible for endorsing and implementing the changes. Once leadership of the key system partners has reviewed and endorsed the change, it is time to plan how to implement the change. The team may need different partners or a different group structure for implementation than for planning.

> The parent support group meets again a few months later. Mary is excited to report back from her "pre-training" subgroup and hear what the other subgroup has accomplished. For implementation, they break into two teams, one focusing on access and the other focusing on interim resource development.
>
> The "post-training" subgroup reports the following successes:
>
> 1. Primary care and community mental health leadership met twice and established a referral process and a plan to monitor the progress from initial referral to treatment engagement and to posttreatment/discharge planning. The leadership also established a schedule for quarterly meetings to monitor the collaboration and amend as needed.
> 2. Child welfare developed a measure to track referrals to community mental health trauma treatment. Child welfare will join the quarterly meetings with primary care and community mental health providers to address any access issues specific to children in foster care.
> 3. Within 6 months the foster care agencies will start providing information sheets on trauma-informed care for parents.
>
> The interim resource development team marks the following successes:
>
> 1. Community mental health and child welfare has started identifying all the youth and families in need of trauma treatment.
> 2. One of the contiguous county community mental health organizations has the resources to treat a few of these youth, so they contracted to start treatment with those children living closest to the county border within 3 months.
> 3. Community mental health leadership has initiated outreach to primary care to develop collaboration.

Joan's foster care worker arranges for Joan to be one of the youth seen by the mental health clinic in the adjacent county. After some initial resistance, Joan starts working with a new therapist with experience and training in working with teens exposed to trauma. Within several weeks, Joan is starting to show some improvement. The therapist also works with Steve on the IEP process. Because Joan's biological parents have been unreachable since she was removed, the court identifies a "guardian ad litem" or "law guardian" and gives that person permission to sign off on Joan's IEP and let her start receiving services.

Monitor Markers of Progress

The primary implementation team, whether involved in implementation directly or acting in a steering capacity, should develop a strategy to document the change plan. This document contains the overall goal, each concrete change statement, and the interim steps needed to accomplish that change. It also defines "completion" for each task. Finally, it establishes the time line expected for each concrete change and for the overall change plan. This document serves as the record of the implementation process, notes items for discussion or decision, and ensures that all members stay on track. The leadership of the organization reviews the change plan documentation as well. The implementation team and organization leadership also determine how to mark important milestones in the change process. Publicizing successes during the change process and at project completion is part of the culture change that improves sustainability.

There may be times when the change process seems to stall or lose momentum. If so, the team can meet, review the process, and identify barriers to ongoing progress. Then the team can determine what steps are needed, such as shifting goals, engaging partners that did not participate in earlier stages of planning and implementation, or seeking guidance from leadership in the organizations involved in the change process.

> The parent support group maintains regular contact with the parents in the communities undergoing change through quarterly surveys and at regular in-person meetings. The parents in each community report that access to trauma-informed therapy services has improved, but there are occasional problems—waiting lists, lost referral forms, or therapists out on leave. The parent support group leadership reports the data to the other system partners at the quarterly meetings, but also engages directly when they hear of a situation that calls for more immediate attention. The data gathered by the parent support group generally match the data gathered by child welfare and community mental health.

Ensure Sustainability

Each implementation plan should include a measurable outcome and steps to complete the measurement process. The plan also needs to include steps to address challenges arising from turnover in the organization and in any of the stakeholder groups. Finally, the implementation plan should identify teams or individuals who will incorporate measuring key outcomes into standard operating procedure to identify future challenges requiring ongoing system change. This last step requires discussion with the leadership of organizations involved in system change. The implementation team can also discuss whether a subset of its membership remains connected in an "advisory" capacity to the organizations involved in the system change project.

Summary

It is possible to address gaps in the systems of care for children who have experienced trauma through identifying gaps, engaging all partners, and developing a plan based on consensus of the partners. Building on existing systems and supports, acknowledging real limitations, grounding change in best available evidence, and celebrating successes are essential to accomplish sustained systems change.

Resources

Academy on Violence and Abuse (AVA; http://www.avahealth.org) has created a document, "Adverse Childhood Experiences: Informing Best Practices," that helps professionals learn to integrate knowledge about the Adverse Childhood Experiences Study and subsequent related investigations into their care of patients. AVA also has the following guide for health systems, institutions, and individuals: "Competencies Needed by Health Professionals for Addressing Exposure to Violence and Abuse in Patient Care."

American Academy of Child and Adolescent Psychiatry (AACAP; https://www.aacap.org) has published Clinical Updates and Clinical Practice parameters to guide assessment and treatment of specific psychiatric disorders; brief handouts called Facts for Families to educate the public about mental health issues that commonly affect children and adolescents; and Resource Centers containing information in more detail on a variety of topics.

American Academy of Pediatrics (AAP; https://www.aap.org) maintains a Healthy Foster Care America site (a comprehensive resource for children and families who have been involved in foster care services, and for the professionals who are treating them).

California Evidence-Based Clearinghouse for Child Welfare (CEBC; http://www.cebc4cw.org) is a California Department of Social Services–supported partnership. The CEBC's mission is to advance the effective implementation of evidence-based practices for children and families involved with the child welfare system. The CEBC provides evidence-based measurement tools to assess child abuse and trauma. It also provides a centralized database for child welfare–related programs, along with descriptions and ratings for each program. It also provides guidance to child welfare agencies for evaluating, selecting, and implementing programs.

National Alliance on Mental Illness (NAMI; https://www.nami.org) is the nation's largest grassroots mental health organization dedicated to building better lives for the millions of Americans affected by mental disorders. NAMI Parents and Teachers as Allies is a free on-site presentation to help educate, support, and increase awareness to local communities. NAMI Family-to-Family is an evidence-based course to help family caregivers of individuals with mental illness. NAMI Basics provides similar education and support to parents and other caregivers of children with mental illness. In addition, NAMI's state and local chapters connect people to their local communities and supports.

National Child Traumatic Stress Network (NCTSN; http://www.nctsn.org) is a clearinghouse for a broad range of information and technical assistance related to traumatic stress. The NCTSN provides educational toolkits and an online Learning Center with resources for screening, assessment, and treatment.

National Federation of Families for Children's Mental Health (NFFCMH; https://www.ffcmh.org) is a national family-run organization to provide advocacy, leadership/technical assistance, and collaboration with other family-run and child-serving organizations to ensure the rights and treatment for children and youth with mental illness. NFFCMH has state chapters that extend this mission at the state and local levels.

National Health Collaborative on Violence and Abuse (NHCVA; http://www.nhcva.org) is a collaborative that comprises professional and advocacy organizations and that advocates for health policy and reform targeting violence and abuse. NHCVA organizes educational events and webinars to raise awareness, improve knowledge, and advance policy. NHCVA briefs the U.S. Congress annually on the public health implications of violence and abuse with the purpose of advancing public policy. The NHCVA Web site is a source of information on the health impact of violence and abuse with links to key content from its members' Web sites.

Substance Abuse and Mental Health Services Administration (SAMHSA; https://www.samhsa.gov) maintains a National Registry of Evidence-based Programs and Practices (NREPP; https://www.samhsa.gov/nrepp), which is a comprehensive database of treatments. The SAMHSA Web site also includes directories and helplines for those seeking help and treatment for mental illness or addiction. As discussed earlier in this chapter, SAMHSA has published a guide, "Making Healthy Choices," for teens in foster care to assist them with engaging effectively in their mental health care and a companion guide targeting adults who support youth in foster care.

Index

Page numbers printed in **boldface** type refer to tables or figures.